Syncope

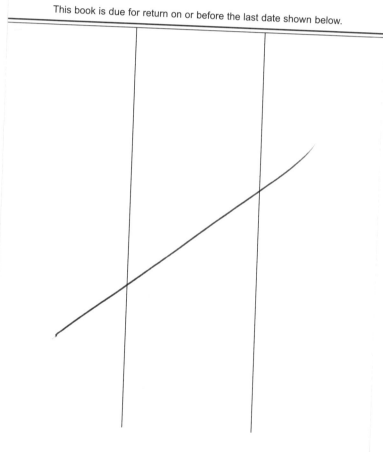

Michele Brignole · David G. Benditt

Syncope

An Evidence-Based Approach

Foreword by Richard Sutton

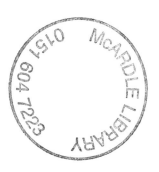
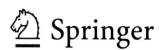 Springer

Dr. Michele Brignole
Dipartimento di Cardiologia
Centro Aritmologico
Ospedali del Tigullio
Via Bobbio 24
16033 Lavagna
Italy
mbrignole@ASL4.liguria.it

Dr. David G. Benditt
Cardiac Arrhythmia Center
Medical School
University of Minnesota
420 Delaware St. SE
55455 Minneapolis Minnesota
USA
bendi001@umn.edu

ISBN 978-0-85729-200-1   e-ISBN 978-0-85729-201-8
DOI 10.1007/978-0-85729-201-8
Springer London Dordrecht Heidelberg New York

British Library Cataloguing in Publication Data
A catalogue record for this book is available from the British Library

Library of Congress Control Number: 2011921118

Printed on acid-free paper

Springer is part of Springer Science+Business Media (www.springer.com)

Foreword

Syncope has, in recent years, drawn considerable scientific and health economic attention. Scientific study of syncope began, perhaps with Morgagni describing heart block followed by Adams and Stokes adding their views of this condition. Fainting has been a human phenomenon probably as long as the species has existed. It was well recorded by such authors as Jane Austen, who named it a swoon. Gower in the early twentieth century termed the common faint as vasovagal syncope, a term reiterated by Sir Thomas Lewis in the 1930s. He was also well aware of carotid sinus syndrome, although credit for its description is usually given to Roskamm. Wayne added his detailed experience in the 1950s. The start of the present rush of scientific effort can be attributed to reports from the laboratories of Rosen, Kapoor, Klein, and Silverstein in the early 1980s. These articles highlighted the lack of knowledge then existing about syncope and provided the inspiration for the introduction of tilt testing. Tilt studies offered a means of reproducing vasovagal syncope in a laboratory permitting heart rhythm and hemodynamic studies. At the outset it was thought that the event precipitated by tilt mimicked spontaneous occurrences and the hemodynamics observed were those also of naturally occurring attacks. Unfortunately, this has not proved to be the case now that we can record spontaneously occurring events with implanted ECG loop recorders.

Growth of scientific efforts in the field of syncope prompted the American College of Cardiology, led by one of the authors of this text, Dr. David Benditt, to produce a consensus report on tilt testing for syncope in 1996. The European Society of Cardiology (ESC) then took the lead in attempting to define the nature of syncope and how to manage it inspired by Dr. Michele Brignole, the other author of this text. The ESC reports were presented in 2001, 2004, and 2009. The most recent of these drew together a very large number of scientific bodies to approve it. This was an important step in gaining recognition of the work of cardiologists and their close associates by other disciplines, which are clinically involved in the care of patients with syncope including neurology, geriatrics, pediatrics, emergency medicine, autonomic neurology, primary care, and internal medicine. Thus, there could be no two better scientists than Drs. Brignole and Benditt to undertake a textbook on syncope.

The scope of *Syncope: An Evidence-Based Approach* is very complete comprising as it does an up-to-date review of all aspects of the study of syncope including related health economic issues. This is very timely and important as syncope is often managed in an uneconomic manner with hospital admission implying numerous costly but not necessarily clinically valuable tests. A recent estimate of the annual cost of syncope in the USA is US $2.4 billion in 2006, which is comparable with the annual budget for the treatment of HIV disease. In these times of economic restraint there is a huge potential to save large amounts of health-care expenditure. The authors indicate, how savings can be achieved by improving effectiveness of the syncope evaluation, by risk stratification and by greater utilization of Syncope Management Units. The authors are at pains to place syncope in the context of transient loss of consciousness (T-LOC), which is precisely what is needed for the physician in the front line seeing a patient, who may have syncope.

This text is very warmly commended to a broad range of physicians, paramedical disciplines, and health economists.

London, UK   Richard Sutton

Preface

Rationale for a New Book

Syncope, better known to most people as "fainting" or "blacking out," represents a complete albeit temporary loss of consciousness leading to interruption of awareness of ones surroundings and falls with risk of injury. Syncope has been estimated to occur at least once in about a half of all individuals during their life; many people suffer multiple faints. In terms of medical burden, syncope accounts for approximately 1% of emergency room visits. In 2006, syncope/collapse resulted in >1.1 million emergency department visits in the USA.

Syncope has many possible causes, but in each case the underlying mechanism is a transient insufficiency of blood flow to the brain. The result is a temporary disturbance of brain function causing loss of consciousness and collapse. By virtue of it being due to a self-limited hemodynamic problem (resulting, for example, from a heart rhythm disturbance or a drop in blood pressure of other cause), syncope differs from other conditions that cause loss of consciousness such as seizures, concussions, intoxications, or metabolic disorders. For example, seizures cause loss of consciousness due to a primary electrical problem in the brain, while concussion causes loss of consciousness secondary to brain trauma. It is crucial that the physician be able to differentiate syncope from these other forms of transient loss of consciousness.

Since syncope can be the result of any condition that results in a temporary loss of brain blood flow, it is best considered to be a syndrome (i.e., a set of symptoms that may be due to many possible causes) rather than a disease itself. Most often, when the fainter seeks medical attention, he/she has fully recovered from the event. Consequently, determining what happened is often very challenging.

Aims and Scope

Inasmuch as syncope and other causes of transient loss of consciousness (T-LOC) share many features, the diverse expertise of cardiologists, neurologists, emergency medicine specialists, general practitioners, geriatricians, and other clinicians is often needed in order to establish an accurate diagnosis and optimize treatment. Unfortunately, however, each of these subspecialities have tended to develop and use different terminology, methodology, and management guidelines; the result, rather than facilitating management of affected patients, has complicated effective inter-action among these various caregivers and has made evaluation and treatment more complex than it needs to be.

The authors of this book provide a thorough multidisciplinary review of the topic. As much as possible they offer recommendations consistent with the most recent European Society of Cardiology (ESC) guidelines which were developed in con-junction with multiple European subspeciality societies, as well as the Heart Rhythm Society and the American Autonomic Society.

The initial sections of the book discuss the scientific basis behind the diagnosis and management of T-LOC/syncope (both terms are often used together in this book since in the literature it is often unclear whether a specific "syncope" diagnosis was established). They detail the clinical pathways leading to syncope and the pathology behind them. The last section of the book then takes a more practical approach, defining recommendations for the practice of syncope management (i.e., evaluation and treatment). The most common procedures and tests are discussed along with their indications, methodology (when appropriate), interpretation, and limitations.

This book has been designed to fulfill the needs of the wide range of medical practitioners involved in the care of patients who present with transient loss of consciousness and in particular those who are thought to have had syncope. All specialties will benefit from the concentration on the importance of medical his-tory taking. Emergency room physicians and internists will be aided by the focus on risk stratification. Cardiologists and cardiac electrophysiologists will find up-to-date recommendations regarding the indications for and appropriate interpretation of noninvasive and invasive cardiac testing. Neurologists and psychiatrists may find particular utility in the sections exploring the often difficult topic of distinguishing true syncope from other important conditions that may present as transient loss of consciousness or seeming loss of consciousness (e.g., seizures, sleep disorders, and psychiatric disturbances). A degree of redundancy has been inserted on purpose into the book, so that in large measure each chapter is able to "stand on its own", and readers can then focus on the chapters that are most pertinent to their practice.

In closing, the authors wish to thank their many friends and colleagues (and especially those who served on the ESC Syncope Task Force) for their crucial input through invaluable discussions and debates over many years. These individuals have educated us and influenced our thinking; inevitably their ideas and contributions have made their way into and substantially improved this volume.

Lavagna, Italy   Michele Brignole
Minneapolis, MN   David G. Benditt

Contents

Section IA
Current Evidence-Based Knowledge: Classification, Pathophysiology, and Social/Economic Impact

Chapter 1
Syncope: Definition, Terminology, and Classification

Contents

Key points: Definition, Terminology, and Classification

- Syncope is a symptom in which transient loss of consciousness (T-LOC) occurs as a consequence of a self-limited, relatively brief, and spontaneously self-terminating period of inadequate cerebral nutrient delivery (most often due to transient hypotension).
- The following four points highlight the key diagnostic features of syncope:
  - loss of consciousness (incorporating loss of postural tone),
  - relatively rapid onset,
  - spontaneous, complete, and usually prompt recovery (although in some conditions causing syncope, recovery may be accompanied by a variable period of fatigue and diminished energy),
  - underlying mechanism is transient global cerebral hypoperfusion.

- A transient fall of systemic arterial pressure to a level below the minimum needed to sustain cerebral blood flow (i.e., the lower end of the

M. Brignole, D.G. Benditt, *Syncope*, DOI 10.1007/978-0-85729-201-8_1,
© Springer-Verlag London Limited 2011

> cerebrovascular "autoregulatory" range) is the most common cause of syncope. Other causes, such as acute hypoxemia, are rare.
>
> • The European Society of Cardiology (ESC) syncope guidelines classify syncope into three primary etiologic subsets: reflex (or neurally mediated), orthostatic, and cardiac (cardiovascular).
>
> • Delineating the underlying etiology (or etiologies) in a given patient is often challenging, but it is important, since syncope, while most often relatively benign from a mortality perspective, tends to recur and leave the affected individual subject to risk of physical injury and diminished quality of life.

Syncope is a symptom in which transient loss of consciousness (T-LOC) occurs as a consequence of a self-limited, relatively brief, and spontaneously self-terminating period of inadequate cerebral nutrient delivery.[1] The possible causes of syncope are numerous, but a transient fall of systemic arterial pressure to a level below the minimum needed to sustain cerebral blood flow (i.e., the lower end of the cerebrovascular "autoregulatory" range) is by far the most common. Other causes, such as acute hypoxemia, are possible, but rare. In any case, whether the underlying problem is "innocent" or potentially life-threatening, syncope may lead to physical injury, accidents that put others at risk, and economic loss (e.g., reduced employment options). Consequently, the management goals are to identify the specific causes(s) of the symptoms and thereafter develop a treatment plan designed to prevent recurrences.[1]

"Syncope" is not, for the most part, a term used by individuals when they present for evaluation of an abrupt apparent loss of consciousness event (Table 1.1).

Table 1.1 Some common terms used by patients to describe T-LOC events (some of which may be syncope)

1. *English (USA)*
   – Blackout
   – Collapse
   – Faint
   – Fit
   – Spell

2. *English (UK)*
   – Funny turns
   – Giddiness

3. *Dutch*
   – Flauw (weak /feeble/faint)
   – Vallen (to fall) or "vallen flauw" (falling weak or becoming feeble)
   – Aanval or (attack)
   – Wegraking' (becoming away)

4. *French*
   – Evanouissement
   – Perte de connaissance (loss of consciousness)
   – Tomber dans les pommes (fall in the apples!)

Table 1.1 (continued)

5. *German*
   – Bewußtlosigkeit (unconsciousness)
   – Ich hatte einen "blackout" (I suffered from a "blackout")
   – Ich bin umgefallen (I had a collapse)
   – Kollaps (collapse)
   – Ohnmacht (without power, without control)

6. *Italian*
   – Perdita dei sensi (colloquial, means loss of sensorial functions)
   – Perdita di conoscenza (colloquial and medical, loss of consciousness)
   – Sincope (medical term, but sometimes colloquial)
   – Svenimento (colloquial, means fainting)

7. *Japanese*
   – Kiwo-ushinau (colloquial, loss of consciousness)
   – Shisshin (medical term, syncope)
   – Kizetsu (colloquial, loss of consciousness)
   – Ishikisyougai (medical term, loss of consciousness)

8. *Spanish*
   – Desmayo (syncope, mostly used for the most common vasovagal situations)
   – Lipotimia (used probably for "common faint"; it really describes the typical vasovagal reaction with prodrome)
   – Mareo (literally is closer to "dizziness," and sometimes it means just "nausea," but it can be also used to describe syncope)

Affected individuals or witnesses (in English-speaking countries) will more often use lay terms such as "faint," "blackout," "spell," "collapse," "fit," or "seizure." In such circumstances, the physician must attempt to determine whether the event was indeed true syncope. In many instances it may even be difficult to be certain that transient loss of consciousness (T-LOC) actually occurred or whether an accidental "fall" or some other event (e.g., "drop attack" without T-LOC or "pseudosyncope") mimicked loss of consciousness. In essence, not every loss of consciousness spell is "syncope" (a neurologist might have written this as "not all loss of consciousness spells are epilepsy"). T-LOC may have been due to "syncope," but may also have been due to other relatively common conditions that are not syncope, such as concussion (i.e., trauma induced), epilepsy (a primary electrical abnormality in the brain), or intoxications (due to extrinsic "chemicals" or drugs). Furthermore, it is not unusual in current clinical practice for conditions that do not even result in true loss of consciousness to be mistaken for syncope; examples include psychogenic pseudosyncope, simple falls, sleep disorders, and drop attacks without T-LOC.

1.1 Definition

As noted already, "syncope" is defined by its pathophysiology: "a self-limited, relatively brief, period of inadequate cerebral nutrient delivery."[1–3] However, from the clinician's problem-solving perspective when confronted by a patient with complaints suspected of being true syncope, additional considerations are needed. To this end, the following four points highlight key diagnostic features of syncope.

1.1.1 Loss of Consciousness

True transient loss of consciousness (T-LOC) is an essential requirement to make a diagnosis of "syncope." Occurrence of T-LOC can only be derived from a detailed history of the symptomatic events taken from the patient and/or from witnesses to the episodes (i.e., "eyewitnesses"). In this context, loss of consciousness implies not only loss of awareness and appropriate responsiveness to external stimuli but also loss of postural tone. Consequently, if standing, the fainter falls down; if seated he/she slumps over. Syncope may occur with the patient supine or prone, but this is relatively rare and its occurrence suggests a hemodynamically serious arrhythmia as the cause.

Occasionally, symptoms may suggest that "syncope" is imminent, but the full T-LOC picture does not evolve at that time. This circumstance, which physicians may consider as being a "near-syncope," is often described by patients as a "near faint," but less specific terms such as "dizziness," "light-headedness," "brain fog" may also be used. However, these latter complaints (especially in the elderly) are nonspecific, and one should not assume that all complaints of "light-headedness" are indeed "near-syncope." Distinguishing transient cerebral functional disturbances due to modest hypoperfusion from "light-headedness" of nonspecific origin or drug effects is difficult and, if possible at all, requires meticulous attention to the history taking.

If the history indicates that there has not been loss of consciousness associated with the "spell," then "true" syncope is excluded. On the other hand, one can be misled. Due to lack of recall, cognitive impairment (especially in elderly "fallers"), or embarrassment, the patient may deny having lost consciousness. Reports from eyewitnesses may be crucial to clarify the story. Often, however, despite best efforts, it is not possible to distinguish true loss of consciousness of a faint from other conditions (e.g., an accidental fall).

1.1.2 Onset Is Relatively Rapid

The timing of events surrounding an apparent syncope is unreliable, as many fainters either do not experience or have no recall of premonitory symptoms. Most patients, and even eyewitnesses, are incapable of assessing the passage of time accurately. Nonetheless, a best estimate is that true syncope tends to be characterized by a relatively abrupt onset, perhaps within 10–20 s of warning symptoms.[1]

1.1.3 Recovery Is Spontaneous, Complete, and Usually Prompt

A spontaneous, complete, and prompt recovery from the faint excludes a number of non-syncope conditions that may cause T-LOC, but which do not reverse promptly on their own, or alternatively, require medical intervention. Examples of such non-syncope T-LOC conditions include coma, intoxicated states, and strokes (which may cause loss of consciousness in some instances). On the other hand, in certain forms of syncope, particularly the vasovagal faint, recovery of consciousness is rapid but may be accompanied by fatigue and a general sense of diminished energy for a lengthy period of time (often hours in duration). The latter must be distinguished from post-ictal symptoms after a true epileptic seizure.

1.1.4 Underlying Mechanism Is Transient Global Cerebral Hypoperfusion

Cerebral hypoperfusion differentiates "true syncope" from T-LOC due to trauma (e.g., concussion), seizures (epilepsy), intoxications, or metabolic disturbances. Both trauma and epilepsy may lead to loss of consciousness with complete and spontaneous recovery, but their origins are not inadequacy of cerebral perfusion.

1.2 Terminology

The importance of distinguishing "syncope" from the many other conditions that can be responsible for T-LOC or "T-LOC-mimics" has been alluded to already, and the principal considerations are summarized in Fig. 1.1. Unfortunately, there remains a persistent lack of clarity among many physicians faced with patients who are experiencing "spells" or "blackouts" regarding the importance of and how to go about differentiating true "syncope" from other forms of T-LOC.[2] The often imprecise writing found in medical literature addressing "syncope" has not been helpful in this regard.[4-6] Ultimately, imprecision in the literature muddies the water and is detrimental to advancing care.[7]

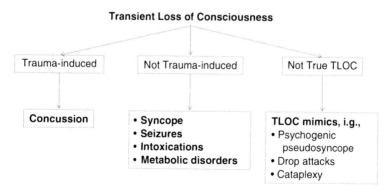

Fig. 1.1 Classification of the causes of transient loss of consciousness (T-LOC). Note that "syncope" is only one of many possible etiologies of T-LOC

The European Society of Cardiology (ESC) Syncope Task Force has, through its comprehensive syncope guidelines initiatives, attempted to bring a degree of consistency to the terminology.[1,8] Certain of the key definitions are summarized here:

1. Transient loss of consciousness (T-LOC): A term meant to encompass an abnormal state of unawareness with lack of normal responsiveness to external stimuli (i.e., looking asleep but unable to be awoken) in which there is absence of voluntary motor control (i.e., extends beyond "loss of postural tone" to include lack of voluntary muscle control even while supine and occasionally smooth muscle control resulting in incontinence).
2. Faint is a nonspecific lay term frequently used at the initial presentation of the patient; a "faint" encompasses all disorders characterized by transient, self-limited, nontraumatic loss of consciousness. When the cause of a faint is transient cerebral hypoperfusion, the term "syncope" is appropriate with the addition of terms indicating specific etiologies (e.g., neurally mediated syncope). Other nonspecific lay terms that are used in various English-speaking geographies include "blackout," "giddiness," and "collapse."
3. Syncope (see above): A self-limited, relatively brief, and self-terminating period of inadequate cerebral nutrient delivery resulting in transient loss of consciousness (including loss of postural tone).
4. Presyncope refers to symptoms and signs that may occur in advance of a true syncope event. Thus its use is a literal descriptor of events associated with a temporally closely associated subsequent syncope event.
5. Near-syncope is a term used to describe a clinical state that resembles "presyncope" but is not immediately followed by a true syncope event.
6. Seizure (epileptic seizure): A condition that may cause T-LOC due to a primary electrical disturbance of the brain, without need for diminution of cerebral perfusion.
7. Stroke (cerebrovascular accident): A condition in which a usually regional abnormality of cerebral perfusion (such as that may be induced by a thrombotic vascular obstruction) results in persistent and often irreversible neurological deficits. T-LOC may occur in rare cases, but the absence of prompt self-termination of the neurological deficit excludes "syncope."

1.3 Classification

Table 1.2 provides the ESC classification of the principal causes of syncope.[1,9] There are three primary etiologic subsets for syncope: reflex (neurally mediated), orthostatic, and cardiac (cardiovascular). In the recent past, cardiovascular causes of syncope were separately considered as "primary arrhythmias" and "structural cardiovascular disease." The recent update to the European Society of Cardiology has combined these two groups, and consequently they are presented below as subsets of "cardiac (cardiovascular) causes" of syncope. Furthermore, previous classifications of syncope included a section on "cerebrovascular and neurologic

Table 1.2 ESC classification of the principal causes of syncope[1]

Reflex (neurally mediated) syncope

Vasovagal:
– *Mediated by emotional distress: fear, pain, instrumentation, blood phobia*
– *Mediated by orthostatic stress*

Situational:
– *Cough, sneeze*
– *Gastrointestinal stimulation (swallow, defecation, visceral pain)*
– *Micturition (post-micturition)*
– *Postexercise*
– *Postprandial*
– *Others (e.g., laughing, brass instrument playing, weightlifting)*

Carotid sinus syncope
Atypical forms (without apparent triggers and/or atypical presentation)

Syncope due to orthostatic hypotension

Primary autonomic failure:
– *Pure autonomic failure, multiple system atrophy, Parkinson's disease with autonomic failure, Lewy body dementia*

Secondary autonomic failure:
– *Diabetes, amyloidosis, uremia, spinal cord injuries*

Drug-induced orthostatic hypotension:
– *Alcohol, vasodilators, diuretics, phenothiazine, anti-depressants*

Volume depletion:
– *Hemorrhage, diarrhea, vomiting, etc.*

Cardiac syncope (cardiovascular)

Arrhythmia as primary cause:
Bradycardia:
– *Sinus node dysfunction (including bradycardia/tachycardia syndrome)*
– *Atrioventricular conduction system disease*
– *Implanted device malfunction,*

Tachycardia:
– *Supraventricular*
– *Ventricular (idiopathic, secondary to structural heart disease or to channelopathies)*

Drug-induced bradycardia and tachyarrhythmias

Structural disease:
Cardiac: *cardiac valvular disease, acute myocardial infarction/ischemia*
Hypertrophic cardiomyopathy, cardiac masses (atrial myxoma, tumors, etc.)
Pericardial disease/tamponade, congenital anomalies of coronary arteries, prosthetic valves dysfunction

Others: *pulmonary embolus, acute aortic dissection, pulmonary hypertension*

---

causes," although it is widely agreed that such conditions are rarely the cause of true syncope. Consequently, despite the fact that certain of these conditions may result in a clinical picture that can be readily mistaken for syncope by even experienced practitioners (e.g., temporal lobe epilepsy may closely mimic [or induce] neurally mediated reflex bradycardia and hypotension), they have been removed from the classification and are considered separately as "syncope mimics."

The manner in which each of the conditions listed in the classification (Table 1.1) may cause syncope is discussed in more detail elsewhere in this volume. However, it should always be kept in mind that a single diagnosis may not be sufficient; more than one cause may contribute to the clinical picture (especially in the older patient).[10]

1.3.1 Reflex (Neurally Mediated) Syncope

The commonly used terms "reflex," "neurally mediated," and "neurally mediated reflex" mean the same thing. For consistency we used the ESC preferred term, namely reflex (neurally mediated) syncope. The vasovagal (or "common") and situational faints occur in virtually all age groups (although young and middle-aged adults predominate) and may be triggered by any of a variety of factors, including prolonged standing (particularly in "close," warm, emotionally charged environments [e.g., religious services]), unpleasant sights, and pain. The diagnosis is most often suspected from the medical history; however, the history is not always definitive, especially in the elderly.[11] In such cases, the accounts of eyewitnesses become crucial.

Carotid sinus syndrome (CSS) tends to occur in older patients with a male predominance probably related to both higher predilection to atherosclerotic cardiovascular disease and neurological disturbances in that population. For many years, CSS was thought to be relatively uncommon, but recent published experience suggests that it may be an important cause of non-accidental "falls" in older individuals.[12] Consequently, this often overlooked diagnosis warrants careful consideration in all older patients who faint or present with falls and/or injuries that are not readily explained.

The so-called situational faints are generally considered to be the same as vasovagal syncope, but with a clear-cut trigger being identifiable. Thus, by way of examples, post-micturition syncope, defecation syncope, and cough syncope are clearly associated with known triggers. In many cases, modification of or avoidance of triggers is the treatment strategy of choice.

1.3.2 Orthostatic (Postural) Syncope

Frank syncope induced by moving from the supine or seated to the upright posture is uncommon in healthy persons (although brief "near-syncope" or "gray-out" immediately after postural change is common), but is a relatively important problem in elderly or less physically fit individuals, or patients who are volume depleted. Iatrogenic factors such as excessive diuresis or aggressive prescription of antihypertensive drugs are the most important contributors to development of orthostatic syncope. Inadequate fluid intake, especially by older persons who have diminished thirst drive, is another important contributor. Secondary forms of autonomic dysfunction such as that occurs in diabetics or individuals who have abused alcohol over many years are also important considerations. Less often, primary disease of the autonomic nervous system dysfunction is the underlying cause. Some of the more important of these conditions include pure autonomic failure, multiple system atrophy, and Parkinson's disease with autonomic failure.[13–15]

1.3.3 Cardiac (Cardiovascular)

1.3.3.1 Primary Cardiac Arrhythmias

Primary cardiac arrhythmias (i.e., those rhythm disturbances arising as a result of cardiac conduction system disturbances, anomalous electrical connections, myocardial disease, or "channelopathies") are less frequent causes of syncope than either the neurally mediated or the orthostatic syncopes, but they are of importance due to their more worrying prognostic implications (see later chapters for more complete discussion). In general terms, the arrhythmias most often associated with syncope or near-syncope are the bradyarrhythmias accompanying sinus node dysfunction (SND) or AV block and the tachyarrhythmias of ventricular origin. In particular, the so-called channelopathies (i.e., long QT syndrome [LQTS], Brugada syndrome, short QT syndrome, catecholaminergic polymorphic VT) present special risks of both syncope and sudden death.[16–20]

1.3.3.2 Structural Cardiovascular or Cardiopulmonary Disease

Structural cardiac or cardiopulmonary disease is often present in syncope patients, particularly those in older age groups. However, in these cases it is more often arrhythmias or reflex effects that are responsible, rather than the structural disease itself.

In terms of syncope associated with structural disease, the most common is syncope occurring in conjunction with acute myocardial ischemia or infarction. Other acute medical conditions associated with syncope include pulmonary embolism and pericardial tamponade. However, as alluded to already, the basis of syncope in these conditions is most often multifactorial, including not only the hemodynamic impact of the specific lesion but also neurally mediated effects.

Syncope may also be a prominent feature of conditions in which there is fixed or dynamic obstruction to left ventricular outflow (e.g., aortic stenosis, hypertrophic cardiomyopathy [HCM]). In such cases symptoms are often provoked by physical exertion, but may also develop if an otherwise benign arrhythmia should occur (e.g., atrial fibrillation). The basis for the faint is in part inadequate blood flow due to the mechanical obstruction. However, especially in the case of valvular aortic stenosis, ventricular mechanoreceptor-mediated bradycardia and vasodilatation is thought to be an important contributor. Additionally, tachyarrhythmias (particularly atrial fibrillation) or ventricular tachycardia (even at relatively modest rates) may trigger syncopal events in these settings.[21–23]

1.4 Conclusion

Syncope is a symptom characterized by a period of transient loss of consciousness (T-LOC) that is brief in duration, self-limited, and due to a spontaneously reversible inadequacy of cerebral nutrient flow. The most common responsible factor is cerebral hypoperfusion due to transient hypotension. Syncope has many possible precipitating causes. However, the principal etiologies may be classified into three categories: (1) reflex (neurally mediated) faints, (2) orthostatic faints, and (3) cardiac (cardiovascular) faints. Delineating the underlying etiology (or etiologies) in a given patient is often challenging but is important, since syncope, while often relatively benign from a mortality perspective in most cases, tends to recur and may leave the affected individual subject to risk of physical injury and diminished quality of life.

References

1. Moya A, et al. Guidelines for the diagnosis and management of syncope (version 2009). The task force for the diagnosis and management of syncope of the European Society of Cardiology (ESC). *Eur Heart J.* 2009;30:2631–2671.
2. Thijs RD, et al. Unconscious confusion – a literature search for definitions of syncope and related disorders. *Clin Auton Res.* 2004;15:35–39.
3. van Dijk JG, et al. A guide to disorders causing transient loss of consciousness: focus on syncope. *Nat Rev Neurosci.* 2009;5:438–448.
4. Strickberger SA, et al. AHA/ACCF Scientific statement on the evaluation of syncope. *J Am Coll Cardiol.* 2006;47:473–484, and *Circulation.* 2006;113;316–327.
5. Soteriades ES, et al. Incidence and prognosis of syncope. *N Engl J Med.* 2002;347:878–885.
6. Chen-Scarabelli C, Scarabelli TM. Neurocardiogenic syncope. *Brit Med J.* 2004;329:336–341.
7. Benditt DG, et al. on behalf of the Ad Hoc Syncope Consortium. The ACCF/AHA Scientific Statement on Syncope: a document in need of thoughtful revision. *Europace.*2006;8: 1017–1021 and *Clin Auton Res.* 2006;18:363–368.
8. Brignole M, et al. Guidelines on management (diagnosis and treatment) of syncope-update 2004. *Europace.* 2004;6:467–537.
9. Benditt DG, Nguyen JT. Syncope: Therapeutic approaches. *J Am Coll Cardiol.* 2009;53: 1741–1751.
10. Benditt DG, Brignole M. Syncope: is a diagnosis a diagnosis? *J Am Coll Cardiol.* 2003;41:791–794.
11. Alboni P, et al. The diagnostic value of history in patients with syncope with or without heart disease. *J Am Coll Cardiol.* 2001;37:1921–1928.
12. Kenny RAM, et al. Carotid sinus syndrome: A modifiable risk factor for nonaccidental falls in older adults (SAFE PACE). *J Am Coll Cardiol.* 2001;38:1491–1496.
13. Mathias CJ. Autonomic diseases – clinical features and laboratory evaluation. *J Neurol Neurosurg Psychiatr.* 2003;74:31–41.
14. Mathias CJ. Autonomic diseases – Management. *J. Neurol Neurosurg Psychiatr.* 2003;74: 42–47.
15. Mathias CJ. Role of autonomic evaluation in the diagnosis and management of syncope. *Clin Auton Research.* 2004;14(S1):45–54.
16. Goldenberg I, et al. The long QT syndrome. *Curr Prob Cardiol.* 2008;33:629–694.
17. Sauer A, et al. Long QT Syndrome in Adults. *J Am Coll Cardiol.* 2007;49:329–337.

18. Brugada P, Brugada J. Right bundle branch block, persistent ST-segment elevation and sudden cardiac death: a distinct clinical and electrocardiographic syndrome. A multicenter report. *J Am Coll Cardiol.* 1992;20:1391–1396.
19. Antzelevitch C, et al. Brugada syndrome: report of the second consensus conference. *Circulation.* 2005;111:659–670.
20. Cerrone M, et al. Catecholaminergic polymorphic ventricular tachycardia: A paradigm to understand mechanisms of arrhythmias associated to impaired Ca^{2+} regulation. *Heart Rhythm.* 2009;11:1652–1659.
21. Thaman R, et al. Reversal of inappropriate peripheral vascular responses in hypertrophic cardiomyopathy. *J Am Coll Cardiol.* 2005;46:883–892.
22. Barletta G, et al. Hypertrophic cardiomyopathy: electrical abnormalities detected by the extended-length ECG and their relation to syncope. *Int J Cardiol.* 2004;97:43–48.
23. Fox WC, Lockette W. Unexpected syncope and death during intense physical training: evolving role of molecular genetics. *Aviat Space Environ Med.* 2003;74:1223–1230.

Chapter 2
Pathophysiology of Syncope

Contents

Key points: Pathophysiology

- Syncope is caused by a relatively brief period of inadequate delivery of oxygen, glucose, and other nutrients to brain tissues.
- In health, cerebral blood flow ranges from 50 to 60 mL/100 g of brain tissue/min (i.e., about 12–15% of resting cardiac output), and as such easily meets the minimum oxygen (O_2) requirement needed to sustain consciousness (approximately 3.0–3.5 mL O_2/100 g tissue/min).
- Blood flow to the brain is determined by multiple factors, including

  o heart rate,
  o stroke volume (determined by left ventricular volume and ejection fraction),
  o systemic vascular resistance,
  o systemic venous return to the heart,
  o cerebral vascular resistance, and
  o oxygen-carrying capacity of blood.

- Under most conditions, the brain's vascular system has the capability of stabilizing cerebral blood flow over a relatively wide range of systemic arterial pressures.

M. Brignole, D.G. Benditt, *Syncope*, DOI 10.1007/978-0-85729-201-8_2,
© Springer-Verlag London Limited 2011

- In older persons and in disease states, however, the safety factor for O_2 delivery may be markedly impaired. Additionally, in these settings, the autonomic nervous system is often encumbered by multiple drugs used to treat concomitant conditions (e.g., hypertension, ischemic heart disease, psychiatric problems). These agents (e.g., adrenergic blockers, vasodilators, anti-depressants) may further undermine cerebrovascular responsiveness to postural change and other stresses.
- A reduction in cerebral perfusion pressure below autoregulatory level for >10–15 s may cause sufficient cerebral dysfunction to result in syncope. Blood flow disturbances of this kind may be either neurally mediated (particularly neurally mediated hypotension such as in vasovagal syncope) or of primary cardiovascular origin such as those triggered by brady- or tachyarrhythmias.

As has been already introduced in Chapter 1, syncope is caused by a relatively brief period of inadequate delivery of oxygen, glucose, and other nutrients to brain tissues.[1,2] Since neuronal tissue has very limited energy storage capability, a well-maintained flow of oxygenated blood to the brain is crucial.

In healthy young persons cerebral blood flow ranges from 50 to 60 mL/100 g of brain tissue per minute, representing about 12–15% of resting cardiac output. A flow of this magnitude easily meets minimum oxygen (O_2) requirement to sustain consciousness (approximately 3.0–3.5 mL O_2/100 g tissue/min).[3] However, the safety factor for oxygen delivery may be markedly impaired in older individuals, in individuals with diseases such as hypertension, diabetes mellitus, or heart failure, and in hypoxemic states (e.g., chronic pulmonary disease).

Given the appropriate circumstance, any human may faint. However, some individuals seem to be more susceptible than others. The reasons for such differences (apart from enhanced susceptibility due to concomitant disease, frailty, or drug effects) are not adequately understood. However, differences in responsiveness of cardiac output and vascular tone to postural and other daily physiologic stresses may contribute. In some cases, a family history indicating an apparent predilection to syncope can be obtained and suggests a genetic predisposition (although environmental factors usually cannot be entirely excluded).

In this chapter, factors that control cerebrovascular perfusion and consequent cerebral nutrient delivery are reviewed. The goal is to provide an overview of the principal elements that, if sufficiently disturbed, may result in syncope.

2.1 Maintenance of Adequate Cerebral Blood Flow

As noted earlier, the brain, to a much greater extent than most organs, is dependent on stable blood flow; local nutrient storage capacity is limited. Consequently, maintenance of an adequate cerebrovascular perfusion gradient (determined in most cases by the systemic arterial pressure at the level of the carotid arteries, but

Table 2.1 Principal factors determining brain blood flow

(1) Heart rate

(2) Stroke volume (together with heart rate determines cardiac output)

(3) Systemic vascular resistance

(4) Systemic venous capacitance (determines venous return to the heart)

(5) Systemic venous pressure (along with systemic pressure determines pressure gradient across cerebral vascular system)

(6) Cerebral vascular steady-state and dynamic "autoregulation" capability (determines cerebral vascular resistance)

(7) Oxygen-carrying capacity of blood

influenced by central venous pressure as well) is essential to ensure normal cerebral function.

Blood flow to the brain is determined by a number of factors (Table 2.1), including, (1) heart rate, (2) stroke volume (determined by left ventricular volume and ejection fraction), (3) systemic vascular resistance, (4) systemic venous return to the heart, (5) systemic venous pressure, (6) cerebral vascular resistance, and (7) oxygen-carrying capacity of blood.[3] Together, the first four of these determine systemic arterial pressure; it is inadequacy of systemic arterial pressure that is responsible for the vast majority of syncope episodes. Systemic arterial pressure, cerebral vascular resistance, and systemic venous pressure establish the arterial–venous perfusion gradient across the brain; very high systemic venous pressure may adversely affect cerebral blood flow and may contribute to susceptibility to syncope in patients with severe heart failure. Item 7, the oxygen-carrying capacity of the blood, may be degraded by hypoxemic states (particularly acute hypoxemia) and chronic pulmonary disease, as well as in individuals with anemia or abnormal hemoglobin function, but is only rarely the sole explanation for syncope. Table 2.2 provides a pathophysiologic classification of causes of syncope.

Adequacy of cardiac output (the product of heart rate and stroke volume) is a crucial determinant of cerebral blood flow. Excessively rapid or slow heart rates or abrupt alteration of stroke volume (e.g., severe blood loss, acute myocardial infarction) may undermine the ability of the heart to pump sufficient blood. Similarly, appropriate prompt reactivity of arterial and venous vessel caliber (i.e., arterial vascular resistance, both systemic and splanchnic venous capacitance) necessitated by conditions such as postural change or other physical stress is crucial for maintaining systemic pressure.[3] With regard to cerebral perfusion, since gravitational force acts to diminish systemic arterial pressure at the level of the carotid vessels, arterial constriction elsewhere in the periphery (including the splanchnic bed) and maintenance of sufficient venous return to the heart are essential for salvaging an adequate cerebrovascular arterial pressure, especially as one moves from supine to upright posture (Fig. 2.1).

Apart from adjustments needed to accommodate for postural changes, systemic arterial pressure at the level of the brain must be adequately maintained during activities, ranging from food ingestion to exercise. These and other daily activities (e.g., mental stress) impose various unique demands on the vascular system by virtue of the need for rapid changes in blood flow to various organ systems.

Table 2.2 Mechanisms associated with cerebral hypoperfusion leading to syncope

---

Diminished venous return and systemic vascular resistance
Neurally mediated faints (particularly vasovagal syncope)
Prolonged exposure to warm environments (so-called thermal stress)
Vasodilator drugs
Autonomic neuropathies

Reduced oxygen supply
Rapid decompression at high altitude
Hematologic abnormalities

Primary reduced cardiac output states
Inadequate venous return
  – Excess systemic or splanchnic venous pooling
  – Dehydration
  – Hemorrhage
Cardiac arrhythmias
Valvular heart disease
Diminished cardiac output
  – Left ventricular function
  – Pericardial disease

Increased resistance to cerebral blood flow
Abrupt hypocapnia (e.g., extreme hyperventilation)

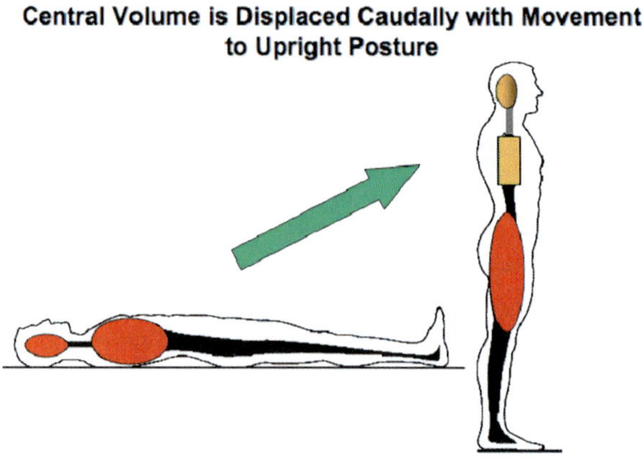

**Central Volume is Displaced Caudally with Movement
to Upright Posture**

Fig. 2.1 Movement to upright posture reduces intravascular volume in the thorax and diminishes venous return to the heart. Systemic pressure at the level of the brain is placed at risk in the absence of appropriate cardiovascular compensatory responses

2.1.1 Autonomic Neural Control

In health, prompt modification of systemic vascular caliber in response to physiologic stresses is dependent upon the flexibility and responsiveness of the autonomic nervous system. Afferents from mechanoreceptors in the carotid sinus, heart, and major cardiopulmonary vessels relay information to the brain through the vagus and glossopharyngeal nerves. Subsequently, hemodynamic changes are effected by sympathetic neural outflow to both the blood vessels and the heart and by parasympathetic (vagus) nerves to the heart. Circulating hormones (e.g., angiotensin II, epinephrine, and norepinephrine) and locally active hormones (e.g., endothelin and nitric oxide) also play a role but operate more slowly. Finally, intravascular fluid volume shifts, determined by multiple factors including hormones such as the renin–angiotensin–aldosterone system, atrial natriuretic peptide, and gastrointestinal hormones, modify arterial pressure, but only over a longer time course.

While neural control networks are generally highly efficient in healthy individuals, they may become less effective under a variety of conditions. For example, individuals returning from a weightless environment (e.g., astronauts) or others who experience prolonged bed rest may succumb to postural hypotension induced by presumed "deconditioning" of autonomic nervous system responsiveness. Similarly, disease states may act to diminish nervous system response either directly (e.g., Parkinsonism, pure autonomic failure) or indirectly (e.g., diabetes, chronic alcohol abuse). Additionally, in many patients, particularly the elderly, the autonomic nervous system is often encumbered by multiple drugs used to treat concomitant conditions (e.g., hypertension, ischemic heart disease, psychiatric problems). These agents (e.g., adrenergic blockers, vasodilators, anti-depressants) may through their pharmacologic actions further undermine cerebrovascular responsiveness to postural changes and other stresses.

2.1.2 Cerebrovascular Autoregulation

Under most conditions, the brain's vascular system has the capability of stabilizing cerebral blood flow over a relatively wide range of systemic arterial pressures (so-called autoregulation, Fig. 2.2). However, the physiology of this self-regulation

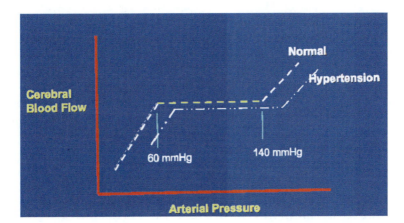

Fig. 2.2 Graph illustrating cerebrovascular autoregulation. In health, cerebral blood flow remains relatively constant over a wide range of systemic arterial blood pressures. Disease states may affect the autoregulatory zone. In this figure the impact of hypertension is depicted to shift the curve to the *right*

of blood flow delivery is inadequately understood and remains a subject of ongoing study.[3,4] In particular, recent interest has focused on the better understanding of dynamic changes in cerebral blood flow, such as might be associated with rapid changes of systemic blood pressure triggered by postural change, neurally mediated alterations of vascular tone, or cardiac arrhythmias. In terms of steady-state autoregulation, proposed mechanisms include myogenic responsiveness to increased vascular distending pressure, modulation of wall tension by adjustment of vessel radius, and metabolically induced changes in vessel diameter. Neural control is deemed to be of lesser importance than in other vascular beds,[3–7] but may become relevant for dynamic cerebrovascular autoregulatory adjustments. In any event, while the "autoregulatory" capacity of the cerebral vessels seems to be able to compensate well under most physiologic conditions (and even during atypical conditions such as space flight[4,5]), it has limitations. Dynamic autoregulation may not be able to compensate adequately for severe abrupt falls in systemic arterial pressure,[4–7] may be dysfunctional in certain disease states,[8] and may change with aging.[9]

At arterial pressures below the steady-state minimum value needed to maintain cerebral blood flow (a value which is not fixed but is, as has been noted already, affected by age and disease states), O_2 delivery may be compromised, and if sufficiently diminished may trigger syncope. It is also likely, but more difficult to establish, that lesser degrees of hypotension may cause "near syncope" or even less well-defined transient functional cerebral disturbances.

In summary, multiple factors contribute to maintenance of systemic blood pressure at a level adequate to provide carotid arterial pressures that lie safely within the cerebrovascular autoregulatory range. At any one time, this process encompasses contributions from the heart and vasculature, endocrine and paracrine systems, intravascular volume, the autonomic nervous system, and the status of gravitational forces (e.g., individual patient's posture). In essence, arterial vascular tone is appropriately adjusted for various moment-to-moment circumstances by autonomic nervous system control; the shunting of excessive amounts of oxygenated blood from the cerebrum to less critical but more "gravitationally advantaged" regions (e.g., the lower limbs) is prevented. Similarly, appropriate venous capacitance adjustments are equally important, as they determine the volume of venous return to the heart. The ability of systemic and splanchnic veins to maintain cardiac filling (preload) is especially important when subjects move abruptly to the upright posture. The heart cannot pump blood that it does not receive.

2.2 Failure to Maintain Cerebrovascular Perfusion

A reduction in cerebral perfusion pressure below autoregulatory level for >10–15 s may result in syncope.[1] In terms of possible causes, blood flow disturbances of this kind may be either neurally mediated or of primary cardiovascular origin.

2.2.1 Neurally Mediated Cerebral Hypoperfusion

Neurally mediated faints (discussed in more detail elsewhere in this volume) are the most common causes of syncope. In these conditions, systemic hypotension with consequent cerebral hypoperfusion is caused by a combination of vaso/venodilatation and bradycardia. The former results in some degree of diminished arterial resistance, but an even greater component of increased venous capacitance (with consequent diminished venous return to the heart). Neurally mediated causes are usually transient and functional (carotid sinus hypersensitivity may be an exception) in nature (e.g., vasovagal and situational faints and most orthostatic faints) and usually are not indicative of autonomic nervous system disease.

Primary autonomic nervous system disturbances causing syncope have in the past been thought to be relatively rare, but are becoming increasingly recognized.[10–14] On occasion these occur in the absence of other neurological disturbances, and subtle forms may be easily overlooked. Autonomic nervous system dysfunction may also occur in association with multiple system involvement (formerly termed Shy – Drager syndrome). However, far more common clinically than any of these primary autonomic nervous system disturbances are those which are of a secondary nature.[14] Examples of the latter include neuropathies of alcoholic or diabetic origin, dysautonomias occurring in conjunction with certain inflammatory and immunological conditions (e.g., Guillan – Barre, myasthenia gravis) or paraneoplastic syndromes.[14–18] Many patients who manifest postural orthostatic tachycardia syndrome (POTS) may also fall into this latter group.

Nervous system diseases that undermine vascular responsiveness to physiological stresses of daily life are less frequent than "functional" nervous system problems (i.e., neurally mediated reflex disturbances) but are important and often difficult to treat effectively.[13,14] Examples include Parkinsonism and pure autonomic failure, both of which are associated with increased susceptibility to orthostatic hypotension.

Movement from the supine or seated to upright posture with induction of a posture-induced fall in systemic pressure (i.e., orthostatic hypotension) is one of the most important triggers leading to abrupt fall of cerebral blood flow. On moving from the supine to the erect posture there is a large gravitational shift of blood away from the chest to the lower body systemic and splanchnic venous capacitance system. This shift of approximately 500–1,000 mL of blood occurs relatively rapidly (usually within the first 10 s of standing) and might induce an immediate sensation of "graying out" or "blacking out" if not adequately compensated (so-called immediate orthostatic hypotension). Somewhat later, with prolonged upright posture (and especially if muscle pump activity is relatively inactive), the high capillary transmural pressure in dependent parts of the body causes loss of fluid from the vascular space into the interstitial spaces. These vascular losses may cause a further decrease of about 15–20% (700 mL) in plasma volume over 10 min in healthy humans and possibly a greater percentage more quickly in older or diseased individuals. The net effect of posture-induced fluid shifts is to reduce venous return to the heart and decrease stroke volume.[19–21] On the other hand, in healthy individuals vasoconstriction of systemic and splanchnic vessels and an increased heart rate compensate for fluid shifts in order to maintain systemic pressure and cerebral blood flow in the upright posture.

As alluded to earlier, in healthy individuals, immediate compensation for orthostatic stress is mediated by the autonomic nervous system, with the principal sensory receptors being the aortic arch and carotid sinuses arterial mechanoreceptors (baroreceptors). Mechanoreceptors located in the heart and the lungs (cardiopulmonary receptors) are thought to play a lesser role. Autonomic influences are aided by local mechanisms such as the veno-arteriolar reflex and a myogenic response of the smooth blood vessels of resistance vessels in the dependent parts of the body. During longer periods of upright posture, additional hemodynamic compensation is provided by the neuro-endocrine system (i.e., renin–angiotensin–aldosterone and vasopressin), the skeletal muscle pump, and the "respiratory pump" (i.e., negative intra-thoracic pressure during inspiration facilitates venous return to the heart).

In terms of diagnostic criteria, orthostatic hypotension is customarily defined as a postural fall of systolic pressure >20 mmHg with upright posture. This value appears to be accepted in normotensive individuals, but for patients with higher baseline blood pressures, a systolic drop of >30 mmHg with postural change is probably a more appropriate criterion.[21] In any case, before a clinical diagnosis of orthostatic syncope is established, the blood pressure findings must be consistent with the medical history (i.e., postural change inducing near-syncope or syncope).

Neurally triggered cerebrovascular spasm causing syncope seems to be very rare. Spasm is common with intra-cranial bleeding and on occasion may occur spontaneously.[22,23] However, headache is the primary presenting feature rather than syncope. On the other hand, cerebrovascular spasm has been considered to be a contributory pathophysiologic factor in at least certain cases of vasovagal syncope.[24,25]

2.2.2 Non-neurally Mediated Causes of Hypotension

Cardiovascular causes of cerebral hypoperfusion, such as hypotensive primary cardiac arrhythmias, and structural cardiovascular disease are less frequent than neurally mediated syncope or orthostatic hypotension. The basis for cerebral hypoperfusion is most often systemic arterial hypotension induced by a diminished cardiac output due to tachy- or bradyarrhythmias. However, in the case of structural heart diseases (e.g., aortic stenosis, pulmonary hypertension), as well as during certain primary tachyarrhythmias, a neurally mediated reflex component may contribute to hypotensive episodes.[26–28]

Other situations commonly encountered in daily life may transiently degrade the ability to maintain systemic pressure and thereby lead to periods of cerebral hypoperfusion. For instance, food ingestion, warm environments, and physical exertion can lower blood pressure, especially when autonomic compensatory mechanisms are inadequate. Specifically, splanchnic vasodilatation during food ingestion (with both reduction of systemic venous return and shunting of blood from systemic arterial circulation) and increased skeletal muscle blood flow during exercise can reduce systemic arterial pressure and contribute to inadequate cerebral perfusion. On the other hand, strategically timed meals may ameliorate supine hypertension in the many autonomic dysfunction patients whose upright hypotension is complicated by supine hypertension (i.e., during sleeping hours).

Transient failure of compensatory mechanisms or interference by other factors such as vasodilator drugs, diuretics, dehydration, or hemorrhage (any of which may reduce systemic blood pressure below the cerebrovascular autoregulatory range) may induce a syncope episode. Risk of failure of normal protective compensatory mechanisms is greatest in older or ill patients, especially those with other markers of autonomic dysfunction, or in whom coexisting heart failure requires systemic pressure to be kept low by medications yet central venous pressure remains relatively high.[29,30] In the latter instance the pressure gradient for maintenance of cerebral perfusion is diminished.

2.3 Clinical Perspectives

Transient abrupt falls in systemic arterial pressure with cerebral hypoperfusion are the most frequent cause of syncope. Neural reflex vasodilatation (e.g., vasovagal and situational faints) or orthostatic fluid shifts (e.g., orthostatic faints) with consequent inadequate venous return leading to diminished cardiac output is the pathophysiologic disturbance underlying the most common causes of cerebral hypoperfusion and syncope. These faints tend to occur with the patient in the upright position, since the risk to stability of arterial pressure at the level of the brain is greatest in that circumstance. However, while less frequent, other causes of low cardiac output remain important clinically. Marked bradycardia or abrupt onset of tachyarrhythmias can also cause syncope. In these cases, a primary fall in cardiac output plays a key role; the duration of the episode and the ability (or inability) of the periphery to compensate (especially in the case of tachycardia) are the principal determinants of whether syncope occurs. In the latter cases, so-called cardiac syncope, symptoms may even occur with the patient in a supine position. Finally, it should be noted (as has already been pointed out earlier) that cerebral perfusion depends on the integrity of the cerebrovascular autoregulatory mechanism and on central venous pressure. Disease states such as hypertension and diabetes are known to compromise the former, while heart failure with elevated venous pressure and low arterial pressure might be expected to diminish trans-cranial pressure gradient and thereby reduce the safety factor for cerebral perfusion.

References

1. Moya A, et al. Guidelines for the diagnosis and management of syncope (version 2009). The task force for the diagnosis and management of syncope of the European Society of Cardiology (ESC). *Eur Heart J.* 2009;30:2631–2671.

2. Brignole M, et al. Guidelines on management (diagnosis and treatment) of syncope – update 2004. *Europace*. 2004;6:467–537.
3. Rowell LB. *Human circulation. Regulation during physical stress*. New York, NY: Oxford University Press; 1986.
4. Folino FA. Cerebral autoregulation and syncope. *Prog Cardiovasc Dis*. 2007;50:49–80.
5. Schondorf R, et al. Cerebral autoregulation in orthostatic intolerance. *Ann N Y Acad Sci*. 2001;940:514–526.
6. Iwasaki K, et al. Human cerebral autoregulation before, during and after spaceflight. *J Physiol*. 2007;579:799–810.
7. Ogoh S. Autonomic control of cerebral circulation: exercise. *Med Sci Sports Exerc*. 2008;40:2046–2054.
8. Xu W-H, et al. Disparate cardio-cerebral vascular modulation during standing in multiple system atrophy and Parkinson disease. *J Neurologic Sci*. 2009;276:84–87.
9. Brodie FG, et al. Long-term changes in dynamic cerebral autoregulation: a 10 years follow up study. *Clin Physiol Funct Imaging*. 2009;29:366–371.
10. Low PA. Autonomic nervous system function. *J Clin Neurophys*. 1993;10:14–27.
11. Low PA, et al. Prospective evaluation of clinical characteristics of orthostatic hypotension. *Mayo Clin Proc*. 1995;70:617–622.
12. Mathias CJ. Autonomic diseases – clinical features and laboratory evaluation. *J Neurol Neurosurg Psychiatr*. 2003;74:31–41.
13. Mathias CJ. Role of autonomic evaluation in the diagnosis and management of syncope. *Clin Auton Res*. 2004;14(S1):45–54.
14. Freeman R. Autonomic peripheral neuropathy. *Neurol Clinics*. 2007;25:277–301.
15. Edmonds ME, Sturrock RD. Autonomic neuropathy in the Guillian-Barre syndrome. *Brit Med J*. 1979;2:668–670.
16. Vernino S, Lennon VA. Neuronal ganglionic acetylcholine receptor autoimmunity. *Ann N Y Acad Sci*. 2003;998:211–214.
17. Vernino S, et al. Autoantibodies to ganglionic acetylcholine receptors in autoimmune autonomic neuropathies. *New Engl J Med*. 200;343:847–855.
18. Camdessanche JP, et al. Paraneoplastic peripheral neuropathy associated with anti-Hu antibodies. A clinical and electrophysiological study of 20 patients. *Brain*. 2002;125:166–175.
19. van Dijk JG, et al. A guide to disorders causing transient loss of consciousness: focus on syncope. *Nature Rev Neurosci*. 2009;5:438–448.
20. Verheyden B, et al. Steep fall in cardiac output is main determinant of hypotension during drug-free and nitroglycerine-induced orthostatic vasovagal syncope. *Heart Rhythm*. 2008;5:1695–1701.
21. Wieling W, Schatz IJ. The consensus statement on the definition of orthostatic hypotension: a revisit after 13 years. *J Hyperten*. 2009;27:935–938.
22. Garcin B, et al. Reversible cerebral vasoconstriction syndrome. *J Clin Neurosci*. 2009;16:147–150.
23. Ducros A, et al. The clinical and radiological spectrum of reversible cerebral vasoconstriction syndrome. A prospective series of 67 patients. *Brain*. 2007;130:3091–3101.
24. Silvani S, et al. Cerebral vasoconstriction in neurally mediated syncope: relationship with type of head-up tilt test response. *Ital Heart J*. 2003;4:768–775.
25. Grubb BP, et al. Cerebral syncope: loss of consciousness associated with cerebral vasoconstriction in the absence of systemic hypotension. *Pacing Clin Electrophysiol*. 1998;21:652–658.
26. Atwood JE, et al. Exercise testing in patients with aortic stenosis. *Chest*. 1988;93:1083–1087.
27. Johnson AM. Aortic stenosis, sudden death and the left ventricular baroreceptors. *Br Heart J*. 1971;33:1–5.
28. Leitch JW. Syncope associated with supraventricular tachycardia: An expression of tachycardia or vasomotor response. *Circulation*. 1992;85:1064–1071.

29. Giese AE, et al. Impact of age and blood pressure on the lower arterial pressure limit for maintenance of consciousness during passive upright posture in healthy vasovagal fainters: preliminary observations. *Europace*. 2004;6:457–462.
30. Gisolf J, et al. Human cerebral venous outflow pathway depends on posture and central venous pressure. *J Physiol*. 2004;560:317–327.

Chapter 3
Epidemiology of Syncope (Fainting)

Contents

Key points: Epidemiology

- Transient loss of consciousness (T-LOC) is a common clinical presentation. However, since syncope is only one of several explanations for T-LOC, and it is often unclear whether other causes have been adequately excluded, available estimates of the frequency of syncope based on T-LOC occurrences can only be considered an approximation.
- Inasmuch as T-LOC/syncope events are so brief, conventional epidemiological measures such as "prevalence" (proportion of people with the disease) and "incidence" (proportion of people acquiring the disease in a sampling interval) are not useful (e.g., the true prevalence approaches 0 at any time). As recommended by Sheldon et al., measures such as cumulative proportion, cumulative event rate, or cumulative incidence are more meaningful.
- Most epidemiological reports indicate an apparent bimodal distribution of syncope incidence over a broad age range. Peaks occur in adolescence and in older years.
- Data derived from several studies reveal a cumulative incidence of approximately 10% by age 80 years.

- Certain subpopulations have a higher frequency of syncope. Thus, older individuals and patients with structural heart disease appear to be at highest risk.
- In certain conditions such as valvular aortic stenosis and dilated cardiomyopathy syncope is associated with increased mortality risk. However, while of concern in many other conditions, such as hypertrophic cardiomyopathy and the channelopathies, the relation of syncope to increased mortality is more controversial. Neurally mediated syncope and syncope in the absence of structural heart disease is associated with much lower sudden death risk.
- Even though syncope may not be associated with high mortality in all patients, it does have a tendency to recur and can have important negative quality-of-life impact.

Transient loss of consciousness (T-LOC) is a common clinical presentation, with numerous such patients being evaluated annually in emergency departments, hospitals, and physicians' offices. In many of these cases, especially those in whom T-LOC was not due to trauma, the patient may well have suffered a syncope spell (i.e., T-LOC due to a brief self-terminating period of inadequate cerebral perfusion). However, since in many reports it is unclear whether other causes of T-LOC have been adequately excluded, current estimates of frequency of syncope in the population can only be considered an approximation.

3.1 Prevalence and Incidence

"Prevalence" (the proportion of people with the disease) and "incidence" (the proportion of people acquiring the disease in a sampling interval) are measures commonly used to provide a quantitative description of the occurrence of medical conditions in a population. However, as has been pointed out by Chen et al.[1] and by Sheldon and Serletis,[2] these measures are difficult to apply in characterizing T-LOC/syncope. Inasmuch as T-LOC/syncope events are so brief, the true prevalence approaches zero at any time. Terms such as cumulative proportion of the population affected by the condition, cumulative event rate, or cumulative incidence are more meaningful. Furthermore, as emphasized by Sheldon and Serletis,[2] the epidemiological outcome is very different when community-based measures are used compared to statistics derived from medical institutions.

3.1.1 Community-Based Estimates

Early community studies, based on recollection of syncope events, provide insight into the cumulative incidence of presumed syncope by assessment of the percentage of individuals who have experienced at least one T-LOC/syncope episode. However,

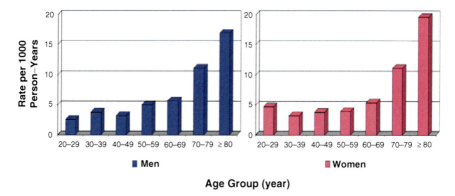

Fig. 3.1 Approximate percent of the population of men (*blue*) and women (*red*) with a history of syncope at each age group. Findings are based on report by Soteriades et al.[4]

the estimates are at times quite varied. Thus, Savage et al.[3] found that only 3.2% of adults (women 3.5%, men 3%) followed in the Framingham study admitted to one or more syncope spells. By contrast, in a subsequent Framingham report,[4] Soteriades et al. provided a substantially greater cumulative incidence for syncope. Among 7,814 Framingham participants (3,563 men, 4,251 women), there were 822 who reported having experienced "syncope." Thus, omitting for the moment the possibility that not all events were in fact true "syncope" (i.e., there is some uncertainty regarding precision of diagnosis), 10.5% of subjects admitted to at least one syncope spell over a 17-year sampling time. Furthermore, there appeared to be a greater incidence with advancing subject age (Fig. 3.1). Thus the estimated cumulative incidence was 3.5/1,000 patient-years in young individuals and approached 20/1,000 patient-years in subjects >80 years. In another, large but retrospective community-based study of more than 1,900 adults aged ≥45 years from Olmsted county, Minnesota (47% male, mean age 62 years), Chen et al.[1] noted that 364 subjects reported having experienced syncope; this finding results in an estimated cumulative incidence of 19%. Again, females reported a higher incidence than did males (22 versus 15%), but there were no age-related differences detected. When the Olmsted county data were reevaluated excluding individuals less than 20 years of age (in order to compare to the Framingham data set), the cumulative incidence of syncope was about 11%. The latter number is remarkably similar to the second Framingham report.[4] Finally, among fainters, Chen et al.[1] also noted that 47% reported recurrent events, 10% had suffered injury, and 21% (mainly younger fainters) indicated that syncope was in fact triggered by an injury. Figure 3.2 illustrates an apparent bimodal distribution of syncope incidence over a broad age range. Peaks occur in adolescence and in older years. These data derived from several studies reveal a cumulative incidence of approximately 10% by age 80. Figure 3.3 provides insight into the incidence of faints versus age in the State of Utah in 2009. Again, a bimodal distribution is evident, and females tend to report more events than do males.

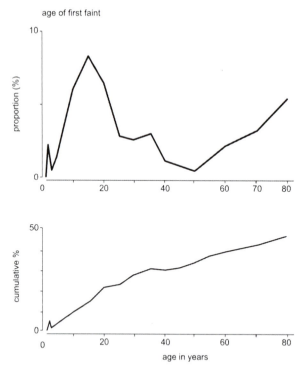

Fig. 3.2 Proportion of the population reporting a syncope versus age. *Upper panel* reveals a bimodal distribution with peaks in adolescence and at older age. The *lower panel* indicates a cumulative incidence of approximately 50% of the population by the age of 80 years. See text for discussion

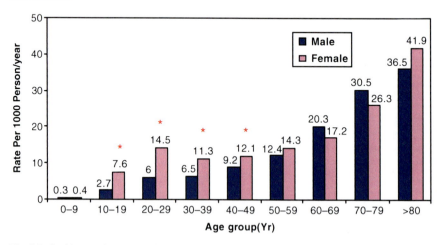

Fig. 3.3 Incidence of reported "faints" in the State of Utah versus age, * indicates $p < 0.01$. See text for discussion

3.1.2 Selected Population Estimates

Apart from the community-based epidemiological studies summarized above, a number of other reports have examined the cumulative incidence of syncope in more highly selected populations. In all cases, the estimates of syncope frequency are biased depending on the "site" at which the measurement is made (Fig. 3.4).

3.1.2.1 Medical Students

Ganzeboom et al.[5] in a survey by questionnaire of almost 400 Dutch medical students found that 47% of women reported having experienced syncope, while only 24% of men did. The overall average for syncope events having occurred in these medical students was 39%. Subsequently, a report from Calgary, Alberta, Canada, also assessing medical students, provided very similar estimates of lifetime cumulative incidence of syncope.[6] However, the Calgary group not only assessed the medical students, but in addition evaluated first-degree relatives. In that report, the likelihood of at least one faint was 37% by age 60, with almost all first spells having occurred by age 40. Furthermore, the Calgary study indicated that by age 60, 31% of males and 42% of females had fainted; findings were very similar to those reported from the Netherlands.[5,6] In addition, females were more likely to faint than males. Taken together, the two "medical student" studies suggest a higher cumulative syncope incidence (approximately 40%) than do the community-based studies (approximately 15–20%). All studies suggest that females are perhaps somewhat more susceptible to syncope or are perhaps less reticent to report events.

Syncope frequency

(depending on the 'site' at which the measurement is made)

Site	Incidence (per 1000 patient-year)	Ratio
General population	18 – 40	1
Seeking for medical visit	9.3 – 9.5	1:2 – 1:4
Referred to hospital for investigations	3.6	1:5 – 1:10
Referred to Emergency Department	0.7 – 1.8	1:10 – 1:50

Fig. 3.4 Schematic illustrating the frequency with which syncope is estimated to occur in the general population, versus the frequency observed by general practitioners, in-hospital referral for further investigations and referral to the emergency department[30,31]

3.1.2.2 Athletes

Syncope in athletes is a frequent clinical problem and one that raises considerable concern among medical practitioners, and both affected individuals and their families. In this regard, Colivicchi et al.[7] examined findings in over 7,500 young athletes (5,132 males and 2,436 females, average age 16 ± 2 years) who were undergoing pre-participation physical assessments as required in Italy. Among these individuals, 6.2% (474 individuals) reported an apparent syncope within the previous 5 years. Most events (whether associated with exertion, post-exertion, or unassociated with exertion) were deemed to be neurally mediated reflex syncope. In only two cases of exertion-associated syncope was a structural cardiac basis for syncope uncovered (one hypertrophic cardiomyopathy, one right ventricular outflow tachycardia). Overall, the incidence of first syncope episodes was low in this population, being 2.2 per 1,000 subject-years for syncope unassociated with exertion and 0.26 per 1,000 subject years for post-exertion syncope. During 6 years of follow-up, syncope recurrences in this population were approximately 20 per 1,000 subject-years, with no other adverse outcomes noted. In essence, syncope in athletes is usually of neurally mediated reflex origin. Individuals who faint during "full flight" or while in the supine or prone position are the subgroups in need of most intensive evaluation, along with those in whom structural cardiac disease is uncovered during evaluation.

3.1.2.3 Infirm and Older Persons

The patient groups that appear to be at highest risk of syncope are those with cardiovascular disease and/or older patients in institutional care settings.[3,8] Among older (>70 years) institutionalized individuals living in a nursing home, Lipsitz et al. estimated that 23% had experienced syncope.[8]

Comparable estimates of syncope frequency in free-living older subjects are, however, harder to obtain and are likely suspect given that many of these individuals (perhaps 20%) have amnesia for loss of consciousness. Furthermore, in many of these older patients, amnesia may also mask any premonitory warning symptoms that could suggest a faint; the result is that the presentation may be suspected of simply having been an accidental "fall" (i.e., a "fall" that may have been due to a faint would be missed) rather than syncope.[9,10] In any case, in infirm and older persons and/or have concomitant cardiovascular disease, essential drug treatment often plays an important role in increasing syncope risk. Typically, antihypertensives, diuretics, and antianginal agents have been implicated. However, one report also emphasizes the importance of psychoactive agents. Specifically, Cherin et al.[11] undertook a case-controlled study of presumed drug-induced syncope in 588 older patients (mean age 80 years, 66% female) and 1,807 controls (mean age 76 years, 60% female). Multivariable analysis revealed that three drug classes proved to be associated with high risk of syncope: non-tricyclic antidepressants, neuroleptics, and antiparkinsonian agents. Aspirin and antiplatelet drugs were associated with diminished syncope risk.[11]

3.1.2.4 Other Populations

- 15% of children <18 years of age,[12]
- 25% of a military population aged 17–26,[13]
- 27% of an air force population (mean age 29),[14]
- 16 and 19% in men and women aged 40–59.[15]

3.2 Syncope Recurrences

About 30% of persons who have had a syncope spell will experience a recurrence by 3 years of follow-up, with most recurrences occurring within the first 2 years.[3,5,6]
Key predictors of greater tendency to syncope recurrences include

- age <45 years at initial presentation,
- a psychiatric diagnosis, and
- a history (generally over many years) of prior syncope recurrences; in particular, patients with multiple syncope events in the preceding year and/or >6 life-time syncope spells and a positive tilt-table test (i.e., suggestive that syncope is of neurally mediated reflex origin) have a high risk of syncope recurrence (>50% over 2 years).[16]

3.3 Mortality Concerns

Patients with syncope of cardiac or cardiovascular origin are at greatest mortality risk. Thus, in cardiac syncope (i.e., primary cardiac arrhythmia, acute ischemic episode, or severe valvular heart disease), the reported 1-year mortality ranges from 18 to 33% compared to 0–12% for patients with either non-cardiac causes of syncope or unexplained syncope. The differences are even more striking when considering "sudden cardiac death" events; the 1-year incidence of sudden death is approximately 24% in patients with a cardiac cause versus about 3% in the other two groups.[6,19] The presence and severity of coexisting structural heart disease are the most important predictors of mortality risk in syncope patients.[17–19] However, in most cases, syncope does not increase sudden death risk above that associated with the structural heart disease itself (exceptions may include dilated cardiomyopathy).

One-year mortality in patients with syncope due to cardiac arrhythmias increases exponentially from 4% (no other risk factor) to 80% in patients with three or more risk factors.[18] Conversely, some cardiac causes of syncope, such as sick sinus syndrome and most types of supraventricular tachycardias, are not typically associated with increased mortality.

Although patients with cardiac syncope have higher mortality rates compared with those of non-cardiac or unknown causes, it has long been thought that cardiac syncope patients do not exhibit a higher mortality when compared with matched controls having similar degrees of heart disease.[20-23] There are, however, some important exceptions. For example, Olshansky et al.[24] reported a greater mortality in SCD-HeFT (Sudden Cardiac Death in Heart Failure) trial patients who had experienced syncope. Specifically, syncope post-randomization was associated with a relative risk increase of 1.41 (1.13–1.76) for all-cause mortality, 1.55 (1.19–2.02) for cardiovascular mortality, and 1.41 (0.90–2.21) for sudden death.

Other reported exceptions include syncope due to:

- severe aortic stenosis,
- hypertrophic cardiomyopathy (HCM),[24,25]
- the channelopathies (e.g., Brugada syndrome, long QT syndrome), and arrhythmogenic right ventricular dysplasia (ARVD).

A number of subgroups of syncope patients appear to have a more benign prognosis. These include:

- young healthy individuals without heart disease and normal electrocardiogram (ECG),
- individuals with the most common forms of neurally mediated reflex syndromes (i.e., vasovagal faint, most situational faints) and syncope of unknown cause (5% first-year mortality).

3.4 Unresolved Prognostic Issues

The impact of syncope has been a particular concern in "channelopathy" patients, specifically in LQTS or Brugada pattern. In regard to LQTS, in one large prospective observational study encompassing >800 patients, cardiovascular end-points including apparent syncope, cardiac arrest, and sudden death occurred in 23% of patients. Syncope was associated with a fivefold increased risk of cardiac arrest or sudden death, but it was not a sensitive predictor of death risk.[26] Similarly, in patients with the so-called Brugada pattern on ECG who have a history of syncope, the observation has been made that syncope is not a sensitive predictor of or risk factor for sudden death. In a multicenter study[27-29] 40% of 220 Brugada patients implanted with an ICD had a history of syncope, but the patients with syncope were not at a higher risk of appropriate ICD discharge than those who had been asymptomatic. Similarly, in a preliminary report of a large meta-analysis encompassing 1,140 patients (262 [23%] having a history of syncope),[28] the patients with syncope had the same risk of ventricular tachyarrhythmias as those who had been without syncope, and significantly lower than those presenting with documented cardiac arrest. See also Chapter 15.

3.5 Clinical Perspectives

Syncope is widely known to be a common clinical problem, but one for which it is difficult to obtain reliable epidemiological data.[30] The frequency of syncope is obscured by the fact that it is only one of many causes of T-LOC, and it is often difficult for frontline medical practitioners to discern precisely whether it was syncope or some other cause (e.g., seizure, accident) that resulted in a patient to collapse. Consequently, precise epidemiological assessment of syncope frequency is difficult. Furthermore, conventional epidemiological terms do not readily apply to such transient phenomena as syncope. Thus, the frequency in the population is perhaps best described as "cumulative incidence" rather than conventional "incidence." With these limitations in mind, it is evident that certain subpopulations have a higher frequency of syncope than do others. In particular, older and frail institutionalized individuals are at greatest risk. In regard to mortality, most forms of syncope are not associated with increased risk. In addition, even in the setting of structural heart disease, syncope does not appear to increase mortality risk above that of disease-matched controls. Nevertheless, even though syncope may not be associated with high mortality in all patients, it does have a tendency to recur and can have an important negative impact on quality of life.

References

1. Chen LY, et al. Prevalence of syncope in a population aged more than 5 years. *Am J Med.* 2006;119(1088):e2.
2. Sheldon RS, Serletis A. Epidemiological aspects of transient loss of consciousness/syncope. In: Benditt DG, et al (eds). *Syncope and Transient Loss of Consciousness.* A multidisciplinary approach. Oxford: Blackwell Publishing;2007:pp 8–14.
3. Savage DD, et al. Epidemiologic features of isolated syncope: the Framingham Study. *Stroke.* 1985;16:626–629.
4. Soteriades ES, et al. Incidence and prognosis of syncope. *N Engl J Med.* 2002;347:878–885.
5. Ganzeboom KS, et al. Prevalence and triggers of syncope in medical students. *Am J Cardiol.* 2003;91:1006–1008.
6. Serletis A, et al. Vasovagal syncope in medical students and their first-degree relatives. *Eur Heart J.* 2006;27:1965–1970.
7. Colivicchi F, et al. Epidemiology and prognostic implications of syncope in young competing athletes. *Eur Heart J.* 2004;25:1749–1753.
8. Lipsitz LA, et al. Syncope in an elderly, institutionalised population: prevalence, incidence, and associated risk. *Q J Med.* 1985;55:45–54.
9. Kenny RA, et al. Impact of a dedicated syncope and falls facility for older adults on emergency beds. *Age Ageing.* 2002;31:272–275.
10. Kenny RAM, et al. Carotid sinus syndrome: a modifiable risk factor for nonaccidental falls in older adults (SAFE PACE). *J Am Coll Cardiol.* 2001;38:1491–1496.
11. Cherin P, et al. Risk of syncope in the elderly and consumption of drugs: A case control study. *J Clin Epidemiol.* 1997;50:313–320.
12. Lewis DA, Dhala A. Syncope in the pediatric patient. The cardiologist's perspective. *Pediatr Clin North Am.* 1999;46:205–219.
13. Murdoch BD. Loss of consciousness in healthy South African men: incidence, causes, and relationship to EEG abnormality. *S Afr Med J.* 1980;57:771–774.

14. Dermkasian G, Lamb I. Syncope in a population of healthy young adults: incidence, mechanisms, and significance. *JAMA*. 1958;168:1200–1207.

15. Feruglio GA, Perraro F. Rilievi epidemiologici sulla sincope nella popolazione generale e come causa di ricovero. *G Ital Cardiol*. 1987;17(suppl I):11–13.

16. Sheldon R, et al. Risk factors for syncope recurrence after a positive tilt-table test in patients with syncope. *Circulation*. 1996;93:973–981.

17. Middlekauff H, et al. Syncope in advanced heart failure: high risk of sudden death regardless of origin of syncope. *J Am Coll Cardiol*. 1993;21:110–116.

18. Martin TP, et al. Risk stratification of patients with syncope. *Ann Emerg Med*. 1997;29: 459–466.

19. Kapoor WN, et al. Diagnostic and prognostic implications of recurrences in patients with syncope. *Am J Med*. 1987;83:700–708.

20. Pires LA, et al. Comparison of event rates and survival in patients with unexplained syncope without documented ventricular tachyarrhythmias versus patients with documented sustained ventricular tachyarrhythmias both treated with implantable cardioverter-defibrillators. *Am J Cardiol*. 2000;85:725–728.

21. Olshansky B, et al. Clinical significance of syncope in the electrophysiologic study versus electrocardiographic monitoring (ESVEM) trial. *Am Heart J*. 1999;137:878–886.

22. Steinberg JS, et al. Follow-up of patients with unexplained syncope and inducible ventricular tachyarrhythmias: analysis of the AVID registry and an AVID substudy. Antiarrhythmics Versus Implantable Defibrillators. *J Cardiovasc Electrophysiol*. 2001;12:996–1001.

23. Knight BP, et al. Outcome of patients with nonischemic dilated cardiomyopathy and unexplained syncope treated with an implantable defibrillator. *J Am Coll Cardiol*. 1999;33: 1964–1970.

24. Olshansky B, et al. Syncope predicts the outcome of cardiomyopathy patients: Analysis of the SCD-HeFT study. *J Am Coll Cardiol*. 2008;51:1277–1282.

25. Spirito P, et al. Syncope and risk of sudden death in hypertrophic cardiomyopathy. *Circulation*. 2009;119:1703–1710.

26. Sauer AJ, et al. Long QT syndrome in adults. *J Am Coll Cardiol*. 2007;49:329–337.

27. Sacher F, et al Outcome after implantation of a cardioverter-defibrillator in patients with Brugada syndrome. A Multicenter Study. *Circulation*. 2006;114:2317–2324.

28. Sarkozy A, et al Long-term follow-up of primary prophylactic implantable cardioverter-defibrillator therapy in Brugada syndrome. *Eur Heart J*. 2007;28:334–344.

29. Paul M, et al. Role of programmed ventricular stimulation in patients with Brugada syndrome: a meta-analysis of worldwide published data. *Eur Heart J*. 2006;28:2126–2133.

30. Olde Nordkamp LRA, et al. Syncope prevalence in the ED compared to general practice and population: a strong selection process. *Am J Emerg Med*. 2009;27:271–278.

31. Malasana G, Brignole M, Daccaret M, Sherwood R, Hamdan M. The magnitude of the Faint and Fall Problem in the general population of Utah: a first step towards the creation of a cost-effective diagnostic approach. *Pacing Clin Electrophysiol*. 2010, Oct 4. doi: 10.1111/j.1540-8159.2010.02930.x. [Epub ahead if print].

Chapter 4
Syncope Burden: Economic Impact of Syncope on Health-Care Resources and Personal Well-Being

Contents

Key Points: Economic Impact of Syncope

- Transient loss of consciousness (T-LOC) accounts for approximately 1% of emergency department (ED) visits based on data from Italy, France, and the USA.
- The majority of T-LOC events are believed to be syncope and conditions that mimic syncope, with other important contributors including unexplained falls, seizures, and head injuries (concussions).
- Calculating the total cost of diagnosing and treating T-LOC/syncope is complex since indirect costs (e.g., loss of earning by patients and/or family members) are difficult to assess. Nevertheless, direct costs alone are substantial, with 75% driven by the relatively high "hospitalization rate."
- It is estimated that of the one-third of patients seen in emergency departments who are admitted to hospital, many could be safely evaluated as outpatients at considerable cost saving.
- The social impact of T-LOC/syncope is substantial (e.g., injury to the patient or to others, lost productivity, disability). Major morbidity such as fractures and motor vehicle accidents is reported in 6% of patients, and minor injury is reported (e.g., laceration, bruises) in 29% of patients.
- A structured guideline-based care model improves diagnostic efficiency and should reduce both direct and indirect costs while improving quality of life. However, to achieve this end, thorough training of clinic and hospital staff on optimal syncope/T-LOC evaluation is essential.

M. Brignole, D.G. Benditt, *Syncope*, DOI 10.1007/978-0-85729-201-8_4,
© Springer-Verlag London Limited 2011

Transient loss of consciousness (T-LOC) accounts for approximately 1% of emergency department (ED) visits based on data derived from various studies in Italy, France, and the USA.[1,2] In the USA, this percentage translated into >1,127 million ED visits in 2006 based on "primary diagnoses" of "syncope and collapse" recorded in the 2006 National Hospital Ambulatory Care survey, and >411,000 hospital admissions when these diagnoses were listed among discharge diagnoses. Furthermore, recent US estimates indicate that T-LOC accounts annually for >16 million physician office visits, ED visits, and outpatient clinic visits. This number appears to be growing (Figs. 4.1 and 4.2), with approximately one-third of these patients being admitted to hospital for additional assessment.

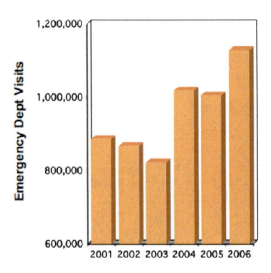

Fig. 4.1 Annual trend of US emergency department visits based on DRG-9 for syncope and collapse

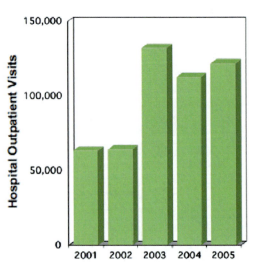

Fig. 4.2 Annual trend of US hospital outpatient clinic visits based on DRG-9 for syncope and collapse

The majority of T-LOC events are believed to be syncope and conditions that mimic syncope (see Chapter 14). Other important contributors include unexplained falls (some of which are likely to be due to unrecognized syncope while others are accidental), seizures, and head injuries. For unexplained falls, it may be difficult to determine if loss of consciousness was the trigger. This chapter reviews current estimates of the economic and social costs of syncope and summarizes its impact on quality of life.

4.1   Cost of T-LOC/Syncope Care

4.1.1   Current Status

Calculating the total cost of diagnosing and treating T-LOC/syncope is complex since the indirect costs related to loss of earning by patients and/or family members are difficult to assess. Nevertheless, direct costs alone are substantial and in large measure (about 75% of the cost) are driven by the relatively high "hospitalization rate" after initial visit to the emergency department (ED) or clinic.[3,4]

Patients with T-LOC/syncope, when admitted to hospital, often undergo expensive and often repeated investigations, many of which are unnecessary and most often do not provide a definite diagnosis. It is estimated that of the one-third of patients seen in emergency departments who are admitted to hospital, many of these could be safely evaluated as outpatients at considerable cost saving. Recent efforts from various organizations (mainly ED based) have focused on devising "risk stratification" techniques with the objective of reducing the number of hospital admissions for evaluation of T-LOC/syncope. Development of a consensus regarding "risk stratification" rules for determining which patients should be admitted and which could be evaluated in an outpatient environment may help control this otherwise substantial cost of care.

In the early 1980s, Kapoor et al.[5] reported that the length of hospital stay for patients being evaluated for syncope ranged from 5 to 10 days, with only about 50% of cases actually being diagnosed. A more recent report from Israel examining syncope evaluations in 1999 revealed similar hospitalization durations; patients admitted to internal medicine services remained in hospital for 4.6 ± 3.5 days, while those admitted initially to an intensive care unit were hospitalized for 7.2 ± 5.6 days.[6] On the other hand, in the SEEDS (Syncope Evaluation in the Emergency Department Study), hospital durations were only 2.9 ± 2.3 days suggesting that substantial shortening of in-hospital stay can be achieved by an experienced team.[7]

Although published information is limited, the magnitude of T-LOC/syncope care cost has been reported for the USA and the UK, and regional data are available from Italy and Spain:

4.1.1.1   The USA

An estimate of direct syncope/T-LOC costs in the USA may be obtained from the US Medicare database. In the year 2000 the total cost of treatment for patients with

Table 4.1 Utah study: Payments received for evaluation of faints and falls per patient

	Faint	Fall
Inpatient admission payment ($)	12, 640	19, 194
Outpatient visit payment ($)	499	366
Emergency department visit ($)	1, 105	711
Mean payment ($)	2, 517	3, 200
Payment per 1,000,000 inhabitants/year ($)	34, 825, 129	95, 357, 712
Payment for the State of Utah per year ($) (2,736,000 inhabitants)	95, 281, 552	260, 898, 701

syncope was $2.4 billion, and estimated total annual charges for syncope-related admissions were $5.4 billion. The mean charge was $12,000 per hospitalization. By way of comparison, in the same time frame, asthma and COPD accounted for $2.8 billion and $1.9 billion, respectively.[3,4]

More recently, payments for T-LOC/syncope care were examined in the State of Utah.[8] These payments reflect reimbursement for care, and for many conditions is less than the actual cost of care delivery. The average payment received per faint and fall evaluation was $2,517 and $3,200, respectively; the resultant estimated yearly payments were $4,825,129 and $ 95,357,712 per 1,000,000 inhabitants/year (Table 4.1).

4.1.1.2 The UK

In the UK, syncope and collapse are among the six commonest causes of emergency admission and most of the cost was incurred by those diagnostic categories deemed "emergency" activity (i.e., urgent admission and tests, rather than referral for outpatient assessment). Data in 2005–2006 from the UK[9] provide estimates of £70 million (approximately $105 million) annually for T-LOC/syncope care. There were approximately 83,000 hospital admissions, of which about 95% were considered to be emergent, with an average cost of £836 (approximately $1,250) per patient.

4.1.1.3 Italy

A detailed assessment of the direct cost of caring for T-LOC/syncope in Italy is found in a study comparing syncope management provided by a guideline-based "standardized" care strategy with that associated with "usual" care [10] (see also Chapter 10). The study evaluated outcomes in 745 patients undergoing a web-based standardized care protocol in 11 Italian hospitals. The control group comprised 929 patients cared for in an unregulated "usual" manner in similar hospitals. The overall cost per patient was $1,394 \pm 1,850$ € for "usual" care versus $1,127 \pm 1,383$ € for standardized care ($p = 0.0001$). The difference was even more striking when considered on a "cost per diagnosis" basis ("usual" care $1,753 \pm 2,326$ € versus standardized care, $1,240 \pm 1,521$ €, $p = 0.0001$). Hospital costs accounted for 75%

of the overall cost of care. If patients were diagnosed and discharged from the ED, the costs for "usual" and standardized care were only 226±79 € versus 198±83 €, respectively.

4.1.1.4 Spain

In Spain, Baron-Esquivias et al.[11] assessed direct costs of syncope care in a large tertiary care facility in Seville. Findings were assessed in 203 patients having a range of syncope diagnoses, with approximately 70% having a prior cardiac diagnosis (thereby increasing the likelihood of a cardiac etiology for syncope). In fact, 90% of cases were ultimately determined to have a cardiac etiology, thereby raising the overall cost of care compared to many other studies in which neurally mediated reflex syncope and orthostatic hypotension comprise the majority of diagnoses. In any event, with these caveats noted, the cost of care was 11,200 € per patient. However, the average cost per diagnosis was only 1,160 €. The majority of the cost (average 6,300 €) was that associated with the treatment due to the high penetration of cardiac diagnoses in this population. Hospital stay cost comprised the remainder.

4.1.2 Opportunity for Reducing Cost

Kenny et al.[9] lead the way in recognizing that a more organized approach to evaluation of "syncope and collapse" could result in effective diagnostic outcomes at lesser cost. These authors compared the outcomes in older adults (>65 years of age) of a dedicated syncope and falls unit at Royal Victoria Hospital, Newcastle, UK, with conventional care provided at 13 nearby peer inner-city teaching hospitals. The comparison focused on four diagnostic categories based on ICD-10 codes: orthostatic hypotension, syncope and collapse, unspecified abnormality of gait and mobility, and dizziness and giddiness. Findings revealed that the syncope/falls unit resulted in markedly shorter hospital stays (average 2.4 days versus 8.6 days in peer hospitals), and fewer over all hospital days despite greater volume in these diagnostic categories than most of the peer facilities. Furthermore, the percentage of admissions deemed to be "emergent" was substantially reduced (35 vs. 97%) in the presence of a syncope/falls unit. Thus, given the option of a rapid workup without hospital admission, many more emergency physicians and general physicians were able to opt for handling most cases as outpatients (day cases). Overall, the authors were able to compute a substantial healthcare savings despite the cost of staffing and equipping the "syncope/falls" unit.[9]

The potential for guideline-driven care to reduce hospitalization frequency and cost of care is also apparent from the report by Brignole et al.[10] summarized above and is further supported by the SEEDS experience from the Mayo Clinic.[7] In SEEDS, syncope patients coming to the ED were randomized to one of two treatment arms: evaluation in an ED-based "syncope unit" or "usual" care. For "syncope unit" patients, only 43% required in-hospital care, whereas 98% of "usual" care patients were hospitalized. Overall, availability of an ED-based syncope unit reduced total in-hospital time from 140 to 64 days with an improvement of diagnostic yield. Inasmuch as in-hospital time accounts for approximately 75% of evaluation cost, the difference observed in SEEDS could translate into important savings in care of T-LOC/syncope patients.

Despite the intuitive benefit of a structured approach to syncope/T-LOC assessment, the cost savings may not occur automatically. Farwell et al.[12] noted in their initial approach to structured evaluation that many physicians still ordered unnecessary tests. Thus, despite a greater overall diagnostic yield (structured evaluation: 78% vs. historical control: 71%), the cost/diagnosis actually rose. The ECSIT study (Epidemiology and Costs of Syncope in Trento) also observed the diagnostic benefit of a structured methodology but at greater cost.[13] In both reports, it appears that failure to follow protocol was likely at fault. In essence, then, aggressive teaching and use of on-site computer-based systems should be considered as essential components of structured care strategies in order to achieve a demonstrable cost-effective benefit.[14,15]

4.2 Quality of Life

The social impact of T-LOC/syncope is substantial. Syncope may result in injury to the patient or to others; this may occur for example when a patient is working in an environment where injury might result from loss of postural control. Major morbidity such as fractures and motor vehicle accidents is reported in 6% of patients, and minor injury such as laceration and bruises is reported in 29% of patients. There is no readily accessible data on the risk of injury to others; however, syncope while driving is thought to be a rare cause of motor vehicle accidents and consequent injury. Sleep deprivation and intoxication are much more important concerns. On the other hand, falls as a result of syncope are important, particularly in the elderly and infirm. Recurrent syncope is associated with fractures and soft tissue injury in >10% of fainters.[5]

Apart from physical injury, patients with recurrent syncope are reported to develop moderate to severe functional incapacity – similar to chronic disease states such as rheumatoid arthritis, low back pain, epilepsy, and psychiatric disorders. In general, impairment is evident in domains such as mobility, usual activities, self-care, pain and discomfort, and anxiety and depression. For example, Santhouse et al.[16] compared psychiatric assessment and quality-of-life (QoL) measures in 52 syncope patients, 96 patients with epilepsy, and 100 healthy controls. The syncope and epilepsy groups did not differ substantially in terms of psychiatric and QoL findings, and both manifested greater anxiety and depression and reduced QoL versus controls.

There is a marked negative relationship between the frequency of spells and overall perception of health.[17] Functional disturbance may also make these individuals more prone to injury. Measuring such impairment is not often done in clinics, but instruments for this purpose have been developed;[18,19] the scale developed by

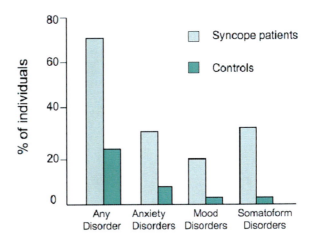

Fig. 4.3 Prevalence of psychiatric disorders in recurrent syncope (after Giada et al.[20])

Linzer et al.[19] is relatively straightforward to apply and while further validation remains needed, it has the benefit of simplicity with 11 yes/no queries and three graded queries.

As noted above,[18] recurrent syncope appears to be associated with both psychiatric disorders and impairment of QoL. For example, Giada et al.[20] compared findings in 61 patients with tilt-positive recurrent syncope to 61 gender and age-matched healthy controls. Psychiatric disorders were more prevalent in the syncope patients (71 versus 23%). Anxiety was present in 28% of fainters (versus 5% in controls), mood disorders in 18% (versus 3%) and somatization disorders in 29% (versus 3%) (Fig. 4.3). QoL scores were also lower in fainters, with an inverse relation to reported syncope burden. van Dijk et al.[21] also observed QoL disturbances in syncope patients compared to healthy Dutch population controls. The SFSQ scale (disease-specific functional status questionnaire) was used to assess QoL. Impairment was recorded in one-third of listed activities, particularly daily life routines, driving, and walking. Female gender, multiple syncope events, and the presence of presyncope symptoms were associated with worse QoL. On the other hand, the same group and others have found that QoL improves over time suggesting that appropriate treatment with symptom control is beneficial in these patients; benefit was less apparent in older patients and those with recurrent events.[22-24]

4.3 Clinical Perspectives

The direct and indirect economic burden of managing T-LOC/syncope is substantial. Direct costs reflect emergency room/clinic visits, hospital costs, testing, and physician/nursing expenses. Indirect costs are more difficult to calculate but include lost productivity. Beyond these, however, findings indicate that affected patients exhibit diminished QoL and a variety of psychiatric disturbances.

It appears that structured guideline-based care improves diagnostic efficiency and should reduce both direct and indirect costs while offering patients the potential for improved QoL. However, to achieve this end, thorough training of clinic and hospital staff on optimal syncope/T-LOC evaluation is essential; in the absence of effective education and careful monitoring to minimize T-LOC/syncope evaluation protocol violations, there remains a tendency to maintain the status quo (e.g., the ordering of low-yield tests) that undermines the potential for reducing cost per diagnosis.

References

1. Moya A, et al. Guidelines for the diagnosis and management of syncope (version 2009). The task force for the diagnosis and management of syncope of the European Society of Cardiology (ESC). *Eur Heart J*. 2009;30:2631–2671.
2. Brignole M, et al. Guidelines on management (diagnosis and treatment) of syncope – update 2004. *Europace*. 2004;6:467–537.
3. Sun BC, et al. Characteristics and admission patterns of patients presenting with syncope to US emergency departments, 1992–2000. *Acad Emerg Med*. 2004;11:1029–1034.
4. Sun BC, et al. Direct medical costs of syncope=related hospitalizations in the United States. *Am J Cardiol*. 2005;95:668–671.
5. Kapoor WN, et al. Diagnostic and prognostic implications of recurrences in patients with syncope. *Am J Med*. 1987;83:700–708.
6. Shiyovich A, et al. Admission for syncope: Evaluation, cost and prognosis according to etiology. *Israel Med Assoc J*. 2008;10:104–108.
7. Shen WK, et al. Syncope Evaluation in the Emergency Department Study (SEEDS): a multidisciplinary approach to syncope management. *Circulation*. 2004;110: 3636–3645.
8. Malasana G, Brignole M, Daccaret M, Sherwood R, Hamdan M. The magnitude of the Faint and Fall Problem in the general population of Utah: A first step towards the creation of a cost-effective diagnostic approach. *Pacing Clin Electrophysiol*. 2010. Nov 22. doi: 10.1111/j.1540-8159.2010.02968.x. [Epub ahead of print].
9. Kenny RA, et al. Impact of a dedicated syncope and falls facility for older adults on emergency beds. *Age Ageing*. 2002;31:272–275.
10. Brignole M, et al. Evaluation of Guidelines in Syncope Study 2 (EGSYS-2) GROUP. Standardized-care pathway vs. usual management of syncope patients presenting as emergencies at general hospitals. *Europace*. 2006;8:644–650.
11. Baron-Esquivas G, et al. Cost of diagnosis and treatment of syncope in patients admitted to a cardiology unit. *Europace*. 2006;8:122–127.
12. Farwell DJ, Sulke AN. Does the use of a syncope diagnostic protocol improve the investigation and management of syncope? *Heart*. 2004;90:52–58.
13. Del Greco M, et al. Diagnostic pathway of syncope and analysis of the impact of guidelines in a district general hospital. The ECSIT study (epidemiology and costs of syncope in Trento). *Ital Heart J*. 2003;4:99–106.
14. Brignole M, et al. Management of syncope referred urgently to general hospitals with and without syncope units. *Europace*. 2003;5:293–298.
15. Ammirati F, et al. Management of syncope: clinical and economic impact of a syncope unit. *Europace*. 2008;10:471–476.
16. Santhouse J, et al. A comparison of self-reported quality of life between patients with epilepsy and neurocardiogenic syncope. *Epilepsia*. 2007;48:1019–1022.
17. Rose MS, et al. The relationship between health-related quality of life and frequency of spells in patients with syncope. *J Clin Epidemiol*. 2000;53:1209–1216.

18. Linzer M, et al. Impairment of physical and psychological function in recurrent syncope. *J Clin Epidemiol.* 1991;44:1037–1043.
19. Linzer M, et al. Recurrent syncope as a chronic disease. *J Gen Intern Med.* 1994;9:181–186.
20. Giada F, et al. Psychiatric profile, quality of life and risk of syncopal recurrence in patients with tilt-induced vasovagal syncope. *Europace.* 2005;7:465–471.
21. van Dijk N, et al. Clinical factors associated with quality of life in patients with transient loss of consciousness. *J Cardiovasc Electrophysiol.* 2006;17:998–1003.
22. van Dijk N, et al. Quality of life within one year following presentation after transient loss of consciousness. *Am J Cardiol.* 2007;100:672–676.
23. Baron-Esquivas G, et al. Short-term evolution of vasovagal syncope: Influence on the quality of life. *Int J Cardiol.* 2005;102:315–319.
24. Mendu ML, et al. Yield of diagnostic tests in evaluating syncopal episodes in older patients. *Arch Intern Med.* 2009;169:1299–1305.

Section IB
Current Evidence-Based Knowledge: Structured Diagnostic Strategy

Chapter 5
The Initial Evaluation of T-LOC: Diagnostic Strategy Based on the Initial Findings

Contents

Key points: Identifying the mechanism of T-LOC based on the initial evaluation
- The starting point for evaluation of syncope is an "Initial evaluation" that consists of history, physical examination including orthostatic blood pressure measurements, and standard electrocardiogram. In selected cases, the initial evaluation includes also echocardiography in patients with suspected heart disease, immediate in-hospital monitoring when a potentially severe arrhythmia is suspected, and neurological evaluation or blood tests when there is suspicion of non-syncopal causes of transient loss of consciousness (T-LOC).
- The initial evaluation of T-LOC has two aims: to identify the specific cause of the loss of consciousness so as to be able to provide effective treatment and to assess the risk (immediate and long term) specific for each patient (this latter issue will be addressed in Chapter 6).

M. Brignole, D.G. Benditt, *Syncope*, DOI 10.1007/978-0-85729-201-8_5,
© Springer-Verlag London Limited 2011

- The initial evaluation may lead to a certain diagnosis or highly likely suspected diagnosis, that need to be confirmed by appropriate diagnostic tests, or to "no diagnosis" in which case more extensive history review and testing are required.
- The subsequent strategy of evaluation varies according to the severity and frequency of the episodes and the presence or the absence of heart disease.
- In general, the absence of suspected or certain heart disease excludes a cardiac cause of syncope. Conversely, the presence of heart disease is a strong predictor of cardiac cause of syncope and virtually includes all cardiac syncopes, but its specificity is low as about half of patients with heart disease have a non-cardiac cause of syncope.
- Determining the mechanism of syncope is a prerequisite for advising patients with regard to prognosis and to developing an effective mechanism-specific treatment.

5.1 The Initial Evaluation

The initial evaluation of a patient presenting with transient loss of consciousness (T-LOC) consists of careful history, physical examination including orthostatic blood pressure measurements (i.e., active standing test), and standard ECG.[1,2] In selected cases, the initial evaluation may include also echocardiography, in-hospital (telemetry) ECG monitoring (in the USA out-of-hospital telemetry ECG monitoring [e.g., Cardionet®] is available), and neurological evaluation or blood tests (Table 5.1).[3] The importance of the initial evaluation goes well beyond its capability to make a diagnosis as it determines the most appropriate subsequent diagnostic pathways and risk evaluation (this latter issue will be treated in Chapter 6).

Table 5.1 Initial evaluation recommended in the guidelines on syncope of the European Society of Cardiology[3]

To all:
– History
– Physical examination
– Standard 12-lead ECG
In selected cases (when appropriate):
– Echocardiogram
– In-hospital (telemetric) monitoring (out-of-hospital telemetry may be applicable where available)
– Neurological evaluation or blood tests

5.1.1 History and Physical Examination

A carefully obtained comprehensive history (incorporating eyewitness accounts) alone may be diagnostic of the cause of T-LOC/syncope or may suggest the strategy of evaluation.[1-3] The clinical features of the presentation are most important, especially the factors that might have predisposed to T-LOC/syncope.

The important parts of the *history* are listed in Table 5.2. They are the key features in the diagnostic workup. When taking the history, all items listed in Table 5.2 should be carefully sought.

Physical findings that are useful in diagnosing the cause of T-LOC/syncope include cardiovascular and neurological signs and orthostatic hypotension. For example, the presence of a murmur or severe dyspnea is indicative of structural heart disease and suggestive of a cardiac cause of syncope. Active standing is used to diagnose the classical form of orthostatic hypotension. In this regard, the sphygmomanometer is adequate for routine clinical testing because of its ubiquity and simplicity. Automatic arm-cuff devices, as they are programmed to repeat and confirm measurements when discrepant values are recorded, may be a disadvantage due to the rapidly falling blood pressure during orthostatic hypotension. With a

Table 5.2   Important historical features for T-LOC

Questions about circumstances just prior to attack:

- Position (supine, sitting, or standing)
- Activity (rest, change in posture, during or after exercise, during or immediately after urination, defecation, cough, or swallowing)
- Predisposing factors (e.g., crowded or warm places, prolonged standing, post-prandial period) and of precipitating events (e.g., fear, intense pain, neck movements)

Questions about onset of attack:

- Nausea, vomiting, abdominal discomfort, feeling of cold, sweating, aura, pain in neck or shoulders, blurred vision, dizziness

Questions about attack (eyewitness):

- Way of falling (slumping or kneeling over), skin color (pallor, cyanosis, flushing), duration of loss of consciousness, breathing pattern (snoring), movements (tonic, clonic, tonic–clonic or minimal myoclonus, automatism) and their duration, onset of movement in relation to fall, tongue biting
- Was T-LOC associated with an accident?

Questions about end of attack:

- Nausea, vomiting, sweating, feeling of cold, confusion, muscle aches, skin color, injury, chest pain, palpitations, urinary or fecal incontinence

Questions about background:

- Family history of sudden death, congenital arrhythmogenic heart disease or fainting
- Previous cardiac disease
- Neurological history (Parkinsonism, epilepsy, narcolepsy)
- Metabolic disorders (diabetes, etc.)
- Medication (antihypertensive, antianginal, antidepressant agent, antiarrhythmic, diuretics, and QT prolonging agents)
- (In case of recurrent syncope) Information on recurrences such as the time from the first syncopal episode and on the number of spells

sphygmomanometer more than four measurements per minute cannot be obtained without venous obstruction in the arm. When more frequent values are required continuous beat-to-beat non-invasive blood pressure measurement can be used.

5.1.2 Baseline Electrocardiogram

An initial ECG is most commonly non-diagnostic in patients with T-LOC/syncope. When abnormal, the ECG may disclose an arrhythmia associated with a high likelihood of syncope, or an abnormality (e.g., conduction system disease, long QT, preexcitation) which may predispose to arrhythmia development and syncope. Moreover, any abnormality of the baseline ECG is an independent predictor of cardiac syncope or increased mortality, suggesting the need for pursuing evaluation for cardiac causes in these patients. Equally important, a normal ECG is associated with a low risk of cardiac syncope as the cause, with a few possible exceptions, for example, in case of syncope due to a paroxysmal supraventricular tachyarrhythmia or certain poorly characterized channelopathies.[1-3]

5.1.3 Additional Tests

Echocardiography is indicated as part of the initial evaluation in patients in order to confirm the suspicion of structural heart disease; moreover it provides information about the type and severity of underlying heart disease, and therefore it plays an important role in risk stratification of the patients. In-hospital monitoring (usually telemetry) is warranted when a potentially severe arrhythmia is suspected. A few days of ECG monitoring may be of value, especially if the monitoring is applied immediately after syncope. However, the yield (up to 17%) is low and the cost is substantial. If an immediate life-threatening problem does not appear to be likely, out-patient telemetry monitoring (currently available in the USA) or long-term event monitoring (worldwide) may be preferable. Neurological evaluation or blood tests are indicated when there is suspicion of non-syncopal causes of transient loss of consciousness (T-LOC). Basic blood tests and metabolic assessment are indicated if syncope has occurred during an episode of myocardial ischemia, or may be due to loss of circulating volume (i.e., anemia), or if a syncope-like disorder with a metabolic cause is suspected.

5.2 The Three Main Questions to Be Addressed at Initial Evaluation

Three key questions should be addressed during the initial evaluation[1,2]:

– Is loss of consciousness attributable to syncope or not?
– Are there features in the history that suggest the causal diagnosis?
– Is heart disease present or absent?

5.2.1 Is Loss of Consciousness Attributable to Syncope or Not?

Differentiating true syncope from "non-syncopal" conditions associated with real or apparent transient loss of consciousness is generally the first diagnostic challenge and influences the subsequent diagnostic strategy. In most cases making this distinction can be accomplished during the initial evaluation.

Figure 5.1 shows a history-based flowchart for differential diagnosis between syncopal and non-syncopal causes of T-LOC. Note that it is based on the presence or the absence of the clinical features reported in the definition of syncope (see Section 1.1). While a complete loss of consciousness is consistent with a syncopal attack, in several other disorders consciousness only seems to have been lost but in reality it has not; this is the case in "psychogenic pseudosyncope" (known to neurologists as "pseudoseizures"), transient ischemic attack, falls, dizziness, cataplexy, and classic drop attacks.

In psychogenic pseudosyncope patients may seem to be unconscious when they are not. This condition may be a voluntary attempt to obtain secondary gain in the context of factitious disorders and malingering, but is involuntary in conversion disorders. Finally, some patients may voluntarily trigger true syncope in themselves to attract attention, as a game, or to obtain some other advantage. Transient ischemic

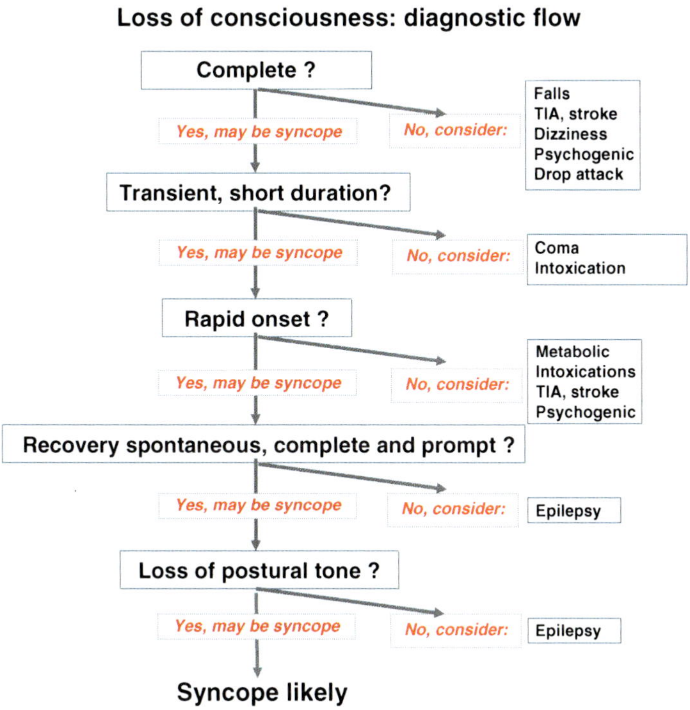

Fig. 5.1 Loss of consciousness: diagnostic flow

attacks (TIAs) in the territory of one carotid artery do not cause loss of consciousness. Only TIAs in the vertebrobasilar circulation may theoretically do so, but other signs such as ataxia, eye movement disorders, and vertigo then predominate.

Typically, falls, dizziness (vertigo), cataplexy, and drop attacks do not cause any impairment of consciousness. These disorders are described in Chapter 14. In general, the differential diagnosis between syncope and these latter disorders is sometimes difficult to establish due to lack of a reliable description of the attack. Obtaining further details from eyewitnesses becomes crucial.

Typical syncopal episodes are brief, lasting only a few seconds; rarely syncope duration may be longer, even lasting for few minutes. Longer duration of loss of consciousness argues against a syncopal nature and those lasting "many minutes" tend to suggest psychogenic disorders. The condition of "coma" is distinct from syncope and is usually reserved for long-lasting loss of consciousness such as those triggered by metabolic derangements such as hypoglycemia, various intoxications, or trauma.

Often, syncope occurs without apparent warning. In other cases syncope is preceded by prodromes (e.g., light-headedness, nausea, sweating, weakness, and visual disturbances), but also in these cases the onset of loss of consciousness is rapid; progressive deterioration of consciousness is in favor of non-syncopal attacks. Prolonged confusion following the attack typically suggests epilepsy; this feature should be differentiated from other symptoms which sometimes follow a syncopal episode such as tiredness, easy fatigue, and nausea. Syncope causes loss of postural tone; if standing patients will tend to fall. In "absence" (petit mal) epilepsy in children and partial complex epilepsy in adults patients remain upright during attacks in contrast to T-LOC. Complete flaccidity during unconsciousness argues against epilepsy.

If the features of the clinical presentation summarized above favor a non-syncopal cause of T-LOC, then the subsequent evaluation should be primarily directed to confirm such diagnoses and in general the patient should be referred to a neurologist, psychiatrist, or internist as appropriate. If a syncopal cause is likely, then the subsequent evaluation consists in defining its nature.

5.2.2 Is Heart Disease Present or Absent?

The absence of signs (including echocardiographic assessment) of suspected or overt heart disease virtually excludes a cardiac cause of syncope, with the exception of syncope accompanied by palpitations, which could be due to paroxysmal tachycardia (especially paroxysmal supraventricular tachycardia). Conversely, the presence of heart disease at the initial evaluation is a strong predictor of a cardiac cause of syncope, but its specificity is low; about half of patients with heart disease have a non-cardiac cause of syncope. In the study by Alboni et al.,[4] heart disease was an independent predictor of cardiac cause of syncope, with a sensitivity of 95% and a specificity of 45%; by contrast, the absence of heart disease allowed exclusion of a cardiac cause of syncope in 97% of the patients. In any case, the presence of structural heart disease has prognostic significance, independently of the mechanism of syncope and influences the subsequent investigations.

If structural heart disease is suspected, echocardiography is a necessary part of the initial evaluation. If confirmed, the subsequent evaluation is primarily aimed to ascertain a cardiac cause of syncope. If severe (potentially life-threatening) arrhythmias are suspected, immediate in-hospital ECG monitoring is warranted.

5.2.3 Are There Features in the History That Suggest the Diagnosis?

Table 5.3 lists how to use the history and physical findings in suggesting various etiologies of T-LOC/syncope. Apart from being diagnostic per se, the history may guide the subsequent evaluation strategy.

Reflex syncope is easily suspected when clear triggers and typical prodromes are present. This very often occurs in young subjects. Conversely, premonitory symptoms are reported less frequently in older people. Moreover, structural heart disease

Table 5.3 Clinical features suggestive of specific causes of syncope

Reflex syncope:
- Absence of structural heart disease
- Long history of syncope (>3 years)
- In relationship with emotional distress: fear, pain, instrumentation, blood phobia (triggers of vasovagal syncope)[i]
- Prolonged standing or crowded, warm places (triggers of vasovagal syncope)[1]
- Nausea, vomiting, abdominal pain, feeling of cold, or sweating associated with syncope (autonomic activation)[ii]
- During the meal or within 1 h from the meal (absorptive state)
- With head rotation, pressure on carotid sinus (as in tumors, shaving, tight collars)
- After exertion
- EGSYS score <3

Note:
(i) Uncertain in the absence of features of autonomic activations, otherwise vasovagal
(ii) Uncertain in the absence of features of typical vasovagal triggers, otherwise vasovagal

Syncope due to orthostatic hypotension:
- Asymptomatic orthostatic hypotension
- After standing up
- Temporal relationship with start of medication leading to hypotension or changes of dosage
- Presence of autonomic neuropathy or parkinsonism
- After exertion

Cardiac syncope:
- Presence of definite structural heart disease or ECG abnormalities
- During exertion or supine
- Absence of prodromes
- Preceded by palpitation
- Family history of sudden death

and comorbidities suggesting competing diagnoses are more often present in the elderly. As consequence, compared with younger patients, the medical history has a limited value in the diagnosis of the cause of syncope in older patients. For example, in the study of Del Rosso et al.,[5] the diagnosis of the cause of syncope was possible on the basis of the history alone in 26% younger and 5% older patients ($p < 0.0001$). In patients >65 years, the clinical features of cardiac and reflex syncope were very similar, thus making an initial clinical diagnosis less secure and additional testing more essential.

Distinguishing between benign reflex syncope and potentially life-threatening cardiac syncope is probably the most frequent and important diagnostic issue. In patients affected by syncopal T-LOC, the EGSYS score [6] has been shown to be able to predict cardiac cause of syncope and to differentiate these patients from those affected by reflex syncope. To each variable listed in Table 5.4 a point score was assigned on the basis of the regression coefficient. The probability of cardiac syncope is reported in Table 5.5. A point score ≥ 3 was considered the best discriminator for a diagnosis of cardiac syncope. The sensitivity for diagnosis of cardiac syncope was 95% and specificity was 61%; this means that a score of three points or more is virtually able to select all patients affected by cardiac syncope but many false positives are to be expected. The predictive negative value was 99%; this means that a score <3 is virtually able to exclude a cardiac syncope. Conversely, the predictive positive value and the predictive negative value of a score >4 were 88% and 88%, respectively, which virtually establishes a diagnosis of cardiac syncope.

Table 5.4 Predictors of cardiac cause of syncope and point scores for the diagnosis of cardiac syncope: the EGSYS score [6]

Variable	Score
Sudden-onset palpitations immediately followed by syncope	4
Heart disease and/or abnormal ECG	3
Syncope during effort	3
Syncope while supine	2
Precipitating and/or predisposing factors: – Warm-crowded place and/or prolonged orthostasis – In relationship with emotional distress (fear, pain, instrumentation)	−1
Autonomic activation: syncope preceded or followed by nausea/vomiting, abdominal pain, feeling of cold, or sweating	−1

Table 5.5 Probability of cardiac syncope according to the EGSYS score [6]

EGSYS score value	Probability of cardiac syncope (%)
<3 points	2
3 points	13
4 points	33
>4 points	77

5.3 The Diagnostic Strategy Based on the Initial Evaluation

The initial evaluation may lead to "certain" or "uncertain" diagnosis or no diagnosis (here termed as unexplained syncope, Fig. 5.2).

5.3.1 Certain Diagnosis

Initial evaluation may lead to a "certain" diagnosis based on symptoms, physical signs, ECG findings, and additional tests listed in Table 5.1. Under such circumstances, no further evaluation may be needed and treatment, if any, can be initiated. There is general consensus coming from the Guidelines on Syncope of the European Society of Cardiology[1-3] that the results of the initial evaluation are most often diagnostic of the cause of syncope in the following situations:

- *Classical vasovagal syncope* is diagnosed if syncope is precipitated by emotional distress (such as fear, severe pain, instrumentation, blood phobia) or prolonged standing and is associated with typical prodromal symptoms.
- *Situational syncope* is diagnosed if syncope occurs during or immediately after specific triggers:
  - gastrointestinal stimulation (swallow, defecation, visceral pain)
  - micturition (post-micturition)
  - post-exercise
  - post-prandial
  - cough, sneeze
  - others (e.g., laughing, brass instrument playing, weightlifting)

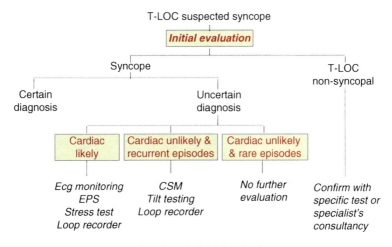

Fig. 5.2 The diagnostic evaluation based on the initial evaluation

- *Orthostatic syncope* is diagnosed when the history is consistent with the diagnosis and during an active standing test there is documentation of orthostatic hypotension (usually defined as a decrease in systolic blood pressure ≥ 20 mmHg or a decrease of systolic blood pressure to <90 mmHg) associated with syncope or presyncope (a fall >30 mmHg is needed in hypertensive subjects). Orthostatic hypotension due to acute severe anemia and bleeding may be diagnosed by clinical features and confirmed by a complete blood count. Most often prescribed drugs are the problem.
- *Arrhythmia-related syncope* is diagnosed by ECG (including ECG monitoring) when there is

  - sinus bradycardia <40 beats/min or repetitive sinoatrial blocks or sinus pauses >3 s in the absence of medications known to have negative chronotropic effect
  - second-degree Mobitz II or third-degree atrioventricular block
  - alternating left and right bundle branch block
  - paroxysmal supraventricular tachycardia or ventricular tachycardia
  - pacemaker (ICD) malfunction with cardiac pauses

- *Cardiac ischemia-related syncope* is diagnosed when symptoms are present with ECG evidence of acute ischemia with or without myocardial infarction and confirmed by the dosage of cardiac biomarkers for ischemia. However, in this case, the further determination of the specific ischemia-induced etiology may be necessary (e.g., neurally mediated hypotension, tachyarrhythmia, and ischemia-induced AV block).
- *Cardiovascular syncope* is diagnosed by echocardiography performed at initial evaluation when syncope presents in patients with prolapsing atrial myxoma or other intra-cardiac tumors, severe aortic stenosis, pulmonary hypertension, pulmonary embolus or other hypoxic states, acute aortic dissection, pericardial tamponade, obstructive hypertrophic cardiomyopathy, and prosthetic valve dysfunction. Syncope due to acute cardiopulmonary diseases and other hypoxic states may be diagnosed by clinical features and confirmed by a hemogasanalysis and other blood tests.

Despite the above lists, it is important to bear in mind that syncope is often multifactorial and multiple comorbidities often exist in syncope patients. The latter is especially true in older individuals. Thus, careful consideration should be given to multiple potentially interacting factors (e.g., diuretics in older patients already susceptible to orthostatic hypotension and myocardial ischemia in the setting of moderate aortic stenosis). The physician must always remember that an abnormality does not equate to a diagnosis in syncope patients.

5.3.2 Uncertain (or Suspected) Diagnosis

Commonly, the initial evaluation leads to a suspected diagnosis when one or more of the features listed in Table 5.3 are present.[1-3] A cardiac mechanism is suspected

Table 5.6 ECG abnormalities suggesting the possibility of an arrhythmic syncope

---

- Bifascicular block (defined as either left bundle branch block or right bundle branch block combined with left anterior or left posterior fascicular block)
- Other intraventricular conduction abnormalities (QRS duration ≥ 0.12 s)
- Mobitz I second-degree atrioventricular block
- Asymptomatic sinus bradycardia (<50 bpm) or sinoatrial block
- Preexcited QRS complexes
- Prolonged QT interval
- Right bundle branch block pattern with ST elevation in leads V1–V3 (Brugada syndrome)
- Negative T waves in right precordial leads, epsilon waves, and ventricular late potentials suggestive of arrhythmogenic right ventricular dysplasia
- Q waves suggesting myocardial infarction

---

when ECG abnormalities such as those listed in Table 5.6 are present;[1-3] the higher is the EGSYS score,[6] the higher is the likelihood of cardiac syncope.

When a cardiac syncope is likely, cardiac evaluation (comprising one or more of the following; electrophysiological study, stress testing, and prolonged ECG monitoring including implantable loop recorder) is recommended (Fig. 5.2).

Specific situations are as follows:

- In patients with palpitations associated with syncope, electrocardiographic monitoring is recommended as first evaluation steps.
- In patients with chest pain suggestive of ischemia before or after loss of consciousness, cardiac biomarkers for ischemia, stress testing, and eventually coronary angiography are recommended as first evaluation steps.
- In patients with syncope during or after effort, stress testing are recommended as first evaluation steps.

If cardiac evaluation does not show evidence of arrhythmia as a cause of syncope, re-evaluation for a neurally mediated syndrome is recommended only in those with recurrent or severe syncope. The latter evaluation includes tilt-table testing, carotid sinus massage, and ECG monitoring and often further necessitates implantation of an implantable loop recorder (ILR).

When cardiac syncope is unlikely and the patients have recurrent severe syncopal episodes, evaluation for reflex (neurally mediated) syndromes and delayed orthostatic hypotension are recommended only in those with recurrent or severe syncope. Recommended evaluation includes tilt testing, carotid sinus massage, ECG monitoring and often further necessitates of implantation of an implantable loop recorder. Carotid sinus massage is indicated in patients >40 years without suspicion of heart or neurological disease and recurrent syncope. Orthostatic challenge (i.e., head-up tilt test) is indicated when loss of consciousness is related to standing. Neurological evaluation or blood tests are indicated when there is suspicion of non-syncopal causes of T-LOC. Finally, the majority of patients with single or rare T-LOC episodes and findings suggesting that cardiac syncope is unlikely have a high probability of reflex syncope. Tests for confirmation are usually not effective, but are helpful if the symptoms are reproduced.

Neurologic disease may cause T-LOC (e.g., epileptic seizures), but is almost never the cause of true syncope (see Chapter 14). Nonetheless, neurological testing may be needed to distinguish epilepsy from syncope in some patients or to exclude intra-cranial injury after a T-LOC-induced fall, but such testing should be an exception and is not warranted in the evaluation of the basis of true syncope. The possible contribution of electroencephalography (EEG), computed tomography, and magnetic resonance imaging of the brain is to disclose abnormalities related to epilepsy or intra-cranial abnormalities (e.g., subdural hematoma); there are no specific EEG findings for any loss of consciousness other than epilepsy (and the inter-ictal EEG is often normal even in these cases). Accordingly, several studies conclusively show that EEG monitoring was of little use in unselected patients with presumed syncope. Thus, EEG is not recommended for patients in whom syncope is the most likely cause of T-LOC. Carotid transient ischemic attacks (TIAs) are not accompanied by loss of consciousness. Therefore, carotid Doppler ultrasonography is not required in patients with syncope. In patients with frequent recurrent syncope who have multiple other somatic complaints and initial evaluation raises concerns for stress, anxiety, and possible psychiatric disorders, psychiatric assessment is recommended (see Chapter 14).

If the cause of syncope is undetermined once the evaluation is completed, *reappraisal* of the workup is needed because subtle findings or new historical information may change the strategy. Reappraisal may consist of obtaining additional details of history and re-examining the patient, placement of an implantable loop recorder if not previously undertaken, as well as review of the entire evaluation to-date. If new clues to possible cardiac or neurological disease are found, further cardiac and neurological assessments are recommended. In these circumstances, consultation with appropriate specialists may be useful. Psychiatric assessment is recommended in patients with frequent recurrent "syncope" who have multiple other somatic complaints. The occurrence of many "syncopes" per day or week is highly suggestive of "pseudo-syncope". These patients may be experiencing psychogenic pseudosyncope and need specialized psychiatric care for their management. If no diagnosis can be established at the end of the complete workup as described above, the syncope is termed unexplained.

5.4 Diagnostic Yield of the Initial Evaluation

Pooled data from population-based studies show that the history and physical examination identified a potential cause of syncope in approximately 50% of the patients. Reflex syncope (vasovagal, situational) accounts for approximately 75% of diagnoses at initial evaluation. The diagnostic yield of standard ECG obtained in the emergency department is on average 6% and accounts for about half of total diagnoses of cardiac syncope. In-hospital (telemetry) monitoring is very helpful in a

Table 5.7 Diagnostic yield of the initial evaluation of syncope in two different clinical settings

	Emergency department (a) (541 pts)			Syncope unit (b) (891 pts)		
	Performed % patients	Positive % tests	NND	Performed % patients	Positive % tests	NND
History and physical examination	541 (100%)	224 (41%)	2.1	891 (100%)	191 (21%)	4.5
Electrocardiography	541 (100%)	34 (6%)	16	Excluded*		
Basic blood tests	166 (31%)	21 (13%)	7.9	298 (33%)	5 (2%)	60
Echocardiography	49 (9%)	5 (10%)	10	269 (30%)	8 (3%)	34
In-hospital ECG monitoring	21 (4%)	13 (62%)	1.6	80 (9%)	14 (17%)	5.7

Sources: (a) Evaluation of Guidelines in Syncope Study 2 (EGSYS-2) study.[8] (b) Syncope Unit Project (SUP) study.[9]

NND, number needed for diagnosis (number of patients tested every one patient diagnosed).

*Patients with arrhythmia-related syncope diagnosed by 12-lead standard ECG were not referred to syncope unit because the diagnosis was already established.

minority of selected high-risk patients.[7] Routine blood tests rarely yield diagnostically useful information. In selected cases, blood tests can confirm a clinical suspicion of acute anemia, acute myocardial infarction, pulmonary embolism, and other hypoxic states and more rarely hypoglycemia and intoxications. However, the diagnostic yield very much depends on the prevalence of these types of syncope, and the prevalence of the cause of T-LOC are different depending on the clinical settings in which the patient is evaluated and by the age of the patients. Tables 5.7 and 5.8 compare the diagnostic yield and case mix in the setting of the emergency department [8] with that observed in the syncope unit [9] in two large multicenter prospective

Table 5.8 Case mix of diagnoses obtained at the initial evaluation of syncope in two different clinical settings

	Emergency department (a) (297 pts)	Syncope unit (b) (218 pts)
Patients with a diagnosis established at initial evaluation:	297 (55%)	218 (24%)
– Reflex (vasovagal, situational)	202 (70%)	169 (77%)
– Orthostatic hypotension	36 (12%)	18 (8%)
– Cardiac (arrhythmic, structural)	34 (12%)	Excluded*
– Non-syncopal T-LOC (to be confirmed by specialist, if appropriate)	25 (8%)	42 (19%)

Source: (a) Evaluation of Guidelines in Syncope Study 2 (EGSYS-2) study.[8] (b) Syncope Unit Project (SUP) study.[9]

*Patients with arrhythmia-related syncope diagnosed by 12-lead standard ECG were not referred to syncope unit because the diagnosis was already established.

Table 5.9   More useful and less useful tests for syncope evaluation

	Test	Suspected diagnosis
More useful	Carotid sinus massage	Neurally mediated
	Tilt testing	Neurally mediated
	Echocardiogram	Cardiac
	Electrophysiological test	Cardiac
	Exercise stress testing	Cardiac
	Holter/external loop monitoring	Neurally mediated and cardiac
	Implantable loop recorder	Neurally mediated and cardiac
Less useful (indicated only in selected cases)	Electroencephalography	Epilepsy and TIA
	Brain computed tomography	Epilepsy and TIA
	Brain magnetic resonance imaging	Epilepsy and TIA
	Carotid Doppler sonography	Epilepsy and TIA
	Coronary angiography	Cardiac
	Pulmonary computed tomography/ scintigraphy	Cardiopulmonary diseases
	Chest X-ray	Cardiac
	Abdominal ultrasound examination	Comorbidities

TIA, transient cerebral ischemic attack.

studies. Due to the different clinical situations, while initial evaluation is diagnostic in 55% of patients referred to emergency department, it is diagnostic in only 24% of the patients referred to a syncope unit. Furthermore, other reported differences depend on diagnostic definitions, geographical factors, and local care pathways making a comparison between different studies difficult. Table 5.9 summarizes the clinical usefulness of most of the tests commonly used for the management of the patients with T-LOC.

5.5 Clinical Perspectives

Readers should be aware of the limitations and pitfalls of the current standard strategy for evaluation of the T-LOC/syncope patient. A major issue in the use of diagnostic evaluation is that T-LOC/syncope is a transient symptom and not a disease. Typically, patients are asymptomatic at the time of evaluation and the opportunity to capture a spontaneous event during diagnostic testing is rare. As a result, the diagnostic evaluation has focused on physiological states that could cause loss of consciousness. This type of reasoning leads, of necessity, to uncertainty in establishing a cause. In other words, the causal relationship between a diagnostic abnormality and T-LOC/syncope in a given patient is often presumptive. A further concern about tests used for evaluation of the etiology of syncope in particular is that measurements of test sensitivity are not possible because of a lack of reference or gold standard for most of the tests employed for this condition. Since syncope is an episodic symptom, a reference standard could be an abnormality observed during a spontaneous event. This is possible, for instance, if syncope occurred concurrently with an arrhythmia detected by an implantable loop recorder. However, most of the time decisions have to be made based on the patient's history or abnormal findings during asymptomatic periods. Uncertainty is further compounded by the fact that there is a great deal of variation in how physicians take a history and perform a physical examination, the types of tests requested, and how they are interpreted and the definitions they use. Uncertainty regarding diagnostic definitions hampers comparison between different studies and the evaluation of treatments. Finally, it seems that the most complex (i.e., with competing possible causes) and potentially severe cases – which therefore would require more specific treatment – remain undiagnosed by means of conventional investigations. This occurs more often in older patients who frequently have structural heart disease and multiple comorbidities. The paradox seems to be that the more we need a precise diagnosis the more difficult is to obtain one.

In summary, there is a need for specific criteria for diagnosis and clear-cut guidelines for choosing tests, determining test abnormalities, and interpreting test outcomes in establishing a cause of syncope. This chapter is largely based on consensus documents from a large multidisciplinary task force, designed by the European Society of Cardiology to write Guidelines on Syncope in the years 2001–2009.

References

1. Brignole M, et al. Guidelines on management (diagnosis and treatment) of syncope: Update 2004. *Europace*. 2004;6:467–537.
2. Brignole M, et al. Guidelines on management (diagnosis and treatment) of syncope: Update 2004. Executive summary and recommendations. *Eur Heart J*. 2004;25:2054–2072.
3. Moya A, et al. Guidelines for the diagnosis and management of syncope (Version 2009). *Eur Heart J*. 2009;30:2631–2671.
4. Alboni P, et al. The diagnostic value of history in patients with syncope with or without heart disease. *J Am Coll Cardiol*. 2001;37:1921–1928.
5. Del Rosso A, et al. Relation of clinical presentation of syncope to the age of patients. *Am J Cardiol*. 2005;96:1431–1435.
6. Del Rosso A, et al. Clinical predictors of cardiac syncope at initial evaluation in patients referred urgently to a general hospital: the EGSYS score. *Heart*. 2008;94:1620–1626.
7. Benezet-Mazuecos J, et al. Utility of in-hospital cardiac remote telemetry in patients with unexplained syncope. *Europace*. 2007;9:1196–1201.
8. Brignole M, et al. A new management of syncope: prospective systematic guideline-based evaluation of patients referred urgently to general hospitals. *Eur Heart J*. 2006;27:76–82.
9. Brignole M, et al. Prospective multicentre systematic guideline-based management of patients referred to the Syncope Units of general hospitals. *Europace*. 2010;12:109–118.

Chapter 6
Transient Loss of Consciousness (T-LOC) Risk Stratification

Contents

Key points: Stratifying the risk of T-LOC based on the initial evaluation.

- The process of risk stratification is an essential part of the initial evaluation and is especially important in the emergency department or urgent care settings when T-LOC patients first present.
- Risk stratification assesses the probability of serious clinical events (e.g., death, severe adverse event, or recurrence of syncope) occurring within a relatively short period of time (usually <1 month) for each patient. The risk assessment determines the need for immediate hospitalization and/or early intensive evaluations, and subsequent management.
- The prognosis (i.e., the risk of future adverse clinical events) may be either directly related to the faint or more generally (and usually more often) related to the underlying disease of which syncope is only one of the presenting symptoms.
- Patients at greatest risk of death or injury require immediate hospitalization or early intensive evaluation.
- Patients at low risk but who present with a severe event (e.g., injury, accident) or have recurrent unpredictable episodes require prompt assessment as outpatients or day cases preferably with referral to a specialized

M. Brignole, D.G. Benditt, *Syncope*, DOI 10.1007/978-0-85729-201-8_6,
© Springer-Verlag London Limited 2011

syncope facility or clinic (so-called syncope unit or syncope clinic) if available.
- In patients at low risk with less severe presentations (single or rare episodes), further investigation is usually unnecessary. Nonetheless, these patients should be educated so as to recognize early stages of syncope and reassured of the benign nature of their symptoms.
- The strategy of management of patients with syncope should be aimed at reduction of unnecessary hospitalizations and referral to specialized outpatient syncope diagnostic and treatment facilities.

6.1 Introduction

There are two main reasons for evaluating a patient with T-LOC:[1–3]

1. To identify the specific cause of the loss of consciousness in order to apply an effective mechanism-specific treatment strategy. In this regard, it is recognized that in the vast majority of the patients, T-LOC/syncope is a disturbing or disabling condition that while not immediately life-threatening may nonetheless substantially diminish quality of life and lead to physical injury. Defining the mechanism is the prerequisite for finding a specific therapy to prevent syncopal recurrences.
2. To assess the prognostic risk for the patient (death, severe adverse event, or recurrence of syncope). The prognosis (i.e., the risk of future adverse clinical events) may be either directly related to the T-LOC/syncope or more generally (and more often) related to the underlying disease of which T-LOC/syncope is only the presenting symptom. Physicians should be aware not to confound the prognostic significance of T-LOC/syncope with that of the underlying disease. The treatment of T-LOC/syncope frequently differs from the treatment of the underlying disease (e.g., an ICD may be an appropriate part of the management of the underlying disease in a syncope patient with severe left ventricular dysfunction, but the ICD is not usually effective for preventing syncope recurrences). Consequently, therapy must consider both targeting the cause of T-LOC/syncope and curing/ameliorating the underlying disease.

The process of risk stratification is an essential part of the initial evaluation because it defines as best as possible the probability of the occurrence of serious clinical events for each patient (e.g., death, severe adverse event, or recurrence of syncope). The risk assessment of necessity can only be predictive of a short-term horizon. Nonetheless, it is useful for determining the need for immediate hospitalization, early intensive evaluations, and subsequent management.

6.2 Assessing the Risk

With regard to risk stratification associated with syncope in particular, two important elements should be considered: (1) risk of death and life-threatening events and (2) risk of syncopal recurrence.

6.2.1 Risk of Death and Life-Threatening Events

Structural heart disease is a major risk factor for sudden death and overall mortality in patients with syncope.[1–3] Orthostatic hypotension which occurs in older patients is associated with a twofold higher risk of death owing to the severity of comorbidities compared with the general population. Conversely, young patients without structural heart disease and patients affected by neurally mediated syncope or isolated orthostatic hypotension have an excellent prognosis with respect to mortality (although injury and accidents remain a concern). Life-threatening diseases (e.g., acute coronary syndrome, pulmonary embolism, acute heart failure) are often suspected by findings obtained during the noninvasive initial assessment. The presence of additional signs and symptoms, such as chest pain or dyspnea, suggests the possible presence of concomitant conditions that require prompt and targeted confirmatory testing. Nonspecific markers such as brain natriuretic peptide (BNP) have been associated with increased risk.

Most of the deaths and many detrimental outcomes in syncope patients seem to be related to the severity of the underlying disease rather than to syncope per se. Life-threatening diseases may also include severe arrhythmias (e.g., third-degree AV block or ventricular tachyarrhythmias). In the EGSYS follow-up study,[4] among 398 patients referred for syncope to the emergency departments (EDs) of 11 general hospitals, death of any cause occurred in 9.2% patients during a mean follow-up of 614 days. Among the patients who died, 82% had an abnormal ECG and/or heart disease; conversely, only six (3%) deaths occurred in patients without abnormal ECG and/or heart disease, indicating a negative predictive value of 97%. Mortality was significantly worse in patients with structural cardiac or cardiopulmonary cause of syncope (37%) compared to patients with other syncope causes in whom mortality was 11% for orthostatic syncope, 10% for primary cardiac arrhythmia, 7% for unexplained syncope, and 7% for neurally mediated syncope (Fig. 6.1).

Several clinical factors helpful for predicting outcome have been identified in prospective population studies[5–12] involving a validation cohort (Table 6.1) and will be described in detail later in Chapter 16.

6.2.1.1 Short-Term Risk

The risk of life-threatening conditions in the few days or weeks after referral is the main reason for immediate hospital admission and exhaustive evaluation. Few studies have evaluated the short-term risk of death, injury, or syncope recurrence (i.e., within few days of initial presentation). In the San Francisco Syncope Rule,[5] an

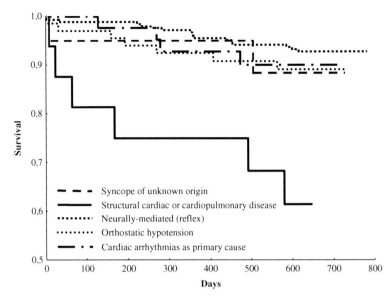

Fig. 6.1 Mortality according to the diagnosis of syncope among 398 patients referred for syncope to the emergency department in the EGSYS 2 study[4]

abnormal ECG (defined as new changes or non-sinus rhythm), shortness of breath, systolic blood pressure ≤90 mmHg, hematocrit ≤30%, and congestive heart failure (by history or examination) predicted the likelihood of a serious adverse event within 7 days of ED evaluation. Serious adverse events were defined as death, myocardial infarction, arrhythmia, pulmonary embolism, stroke, subarachnoid hemorrhage, significant hemorrhage, or any condition causing a return ED visit and hospitalization for a related event. The rule was determined to exhibit a sensitivity of 98% and a specificity of 56%. However, these results could be only partially confirmed by three validation studies that showed a high rate of both false-positive and false-negative results (Table 6.1).

In the ROSE rule,[9] brain natriuretic peptide (BNP) concentration ≥300 pg/mL, positive fecal occult blood, hemoglobin ≤90 g/L, oxygen saturation ≤94%, Q wave on the electrocardiogram, chest pain at the time of syncope, and bradycardia <50 bpm predicted the likelihood of serious adverse event within 1 month of ED evaluation. Serious adverse events were defined as death, acute myocardial infarction, life-threatening arrhythmia, decision to implant a pacemaker or cardiac defibrillator within 1 month of index collapse, pulmonary embolus, cerebrovascular accident, hemorrhage requiring a blood transfusion, acute surgical procedure, or endoscopic intervention.

In the STePS study,[13] abnormal ECG, concomitant trauma, absence of symptoms of impending syncope, and male gender were associated with higher risk of death or serious adverse events (defined as cardiopulmonary resuscitation, pace maker or defibrillator implant, intensive care unit admittance) at 10 days and early readmission to hospital. However, owing to the relative low rate of events, the clinical utility was hampered by a very low positive predictive value which ranged between 11 and 14%.

Table 6.1 Risk stratification at initial evaluation in some prospective population studies including a validation cohort

Study	Risk factors	Score	Outcome	Results (validation cohort)
S. Francisco rule[5]	– Abnormal ECG* – Congestive heart failure – Shortness of breath – Hematocrit <30% – Systolic blood pressure <90 mmHg	No risk = 0 item Risk = ≥1 item	Serious events* at 7 days	98% sensitive and 56% specific[5] 89% sensitive and 42% specific[6] 76% sensitive and 37% specific[7] 74% sensitive and 57% specific[8]
ROSE rule[9]	– BNP concentration ≥300 pg/mL – Positive fecal occult blood – Hemoglobin ≤90 g/L – Oxygen saturation ≤94% – Q wave on ECG – Syncope during chest pain – Bradycardia <50 bpm	No risk = 0 item Risk = ≥1 item	Serious events* at 1 month	Sensitivity 87% Specificity 65% Positive predictive value 16% Negative predictive value 98%
Martin et al.[10]	– Abnormal ECG* – History of ventricular arrhythmia – History of congestive heart failure – Age >45 years	0–4 (1 point each item)	1-year severe arrhythmias* or arrhythmic death	0% score 0 5% score 1 16% score 2 27% score 3 or 4
OESIL score[11]	– Abnormal ECG* – History of cardiovascular disease – Lack of prodrome – Age >65 years	0–4 (1 point each item)	1-year total mortality	0% score 0 0.6% score 1 14% score 2 29% score 3 53% score 4

Table 6.1 (continued)

Study	Risk factors	Score	Outcome	Results (validation cohort)
EGSYS score[12]	– Palpitations before syncope (+4) – Abnormal ECG and/or heart disease (+3) – Syncope during effort (+3) – Syncope while supine (+2) – Autonomic prodrome[a] (–1) – Predisposing and/or precipitating Factors[b] (–1)	Sum of + and – points	2-year total mortality Cardiac syncope probability	2% score <3 21% score $\geq$3 2% score <3 13% score 3 33% score 4 77% score >4

*See for definition
[a]Warm-crowded place/prolonged orthostasis/fear–pain–emotion
Nausea/vomiting
BNP = brain natriuretic peptide concentration

All studies have shown that the risk of death and of adverse outcome is high in the few days following the index syncopal episode among high-risk patients, thus justifying the effort for identification and immediate hospitalization with intensive management of these patients. Most of the deaths and many detrimental outcomes seemed to be related to the severity of the underlying disease rather than to syncope per se.[14]

6.2.1.2 Long-Term Risk

More studies have evaluated the long-term (1-year or more) risk of a T-LOC/syncope presentation (Table 6.1). In the study by Martin et al.,[10] four risk factors were identified: (1) abnormal ECG result (defined as rhythm abnormalities, conduction disorders, hypertrophy, old myocardial infarction, and atrioventricular [AV] block); (2) history of ventricular arrhythmia; (3) history of congestive heart failure; or (4) age >45 years; these were found to be predictors of severe arrhythmia (sustained ventricular tachycardia, symptomatic supraventricular tachycardia, pauses >3 s, AV block, pacemaker malfunction) or 1-year mortality. The event rate (clinically significant arrhythmia or arrhythmic death) at 1 year ranged from 0% for those with none of the four risk factors to 27% for those with three or four risk factors.

In the STePS study,[13] a long-term severe outcome was correlated with age >65 years, history of neoplasm, cerebrovascular disease, structural heart disease, and ventricular arrhythmia. In the OESIL study,[11] 1-year predictors of mortality were found to be age >65 years, history of cardiovascular disease, lack of prodromes, and abnormal ECG (defined as rhythm abnormalities, conduction disorders, hypertrophy, old myocardial infarction, possible acute ischemia, and AV block). In the OESIL risk assessment, mortality within 1 year increased progressively from 0% for no factor to 57.1% for four factors. In the EGSYS score,[12] six predictive factors were identified (Table 6.1). The patients were considered to have heart disease if they had a history of ischemic heart disease, valvular dysfunction, myocardiopathies, congenital heart disease, or clinical evidence of congestive heart failure. The ECG was considered abnormal if there was sinus bradycardia, AV block greater than first degree, bundle branch block, acute or old myocardial infarction, supraventricular or ventricular tachycardia, left or right ventricular hypertrophy, ventricular preexcitation, long QT, or Brugada pattern. Although specifically designed to identify cardiac syncope, the EGSYS score also proved able to predict a 2-year mortality of 21% in those with a score ≥3 compared with 2% in those with a score <3 (Fig. 6.2).

In summary, increasing age, abnormal ECG, a history of cardiovascular disease (especially ventricular arrhythmia or heart failure), syncope occurring without prodromes or during effort or supine were found to be predictors of increased susceptibility to worrisome sustained arrhythmia and/or 1-year mortality. Again, similar to the short-term events, most deaths and serious outcomes seemed to be correlated to the severity of underlying disease rather than to syncope per se.

High-risk patients need to be assessed carefully; optimal therapy and management must be provided. However, the presumption that an immediate in-hospital evaluation improves a patient's long-term clinical outcome has never been

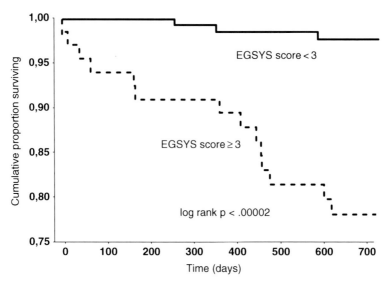

Fig. 6.2 Mortality according to the EGSYS risk score in the validation cohort of the EGSYS 2 study[11] among 256 patients referred for syncope to the emergency department

demonstrated, and alternative strategies could be considered. In particular, referral to a specialized outpatient "blackout" or syncope clinic is highly recommended.

6.2.2 Risk of Syncopal Recurrence

In population studies, approximately one-third of patients have recurrences of syncope by 3 years of follow-up. The number of episodes of syncope during life and their frequency especially in the immediate preceding year are the strongest predictors of recurrence. In "low-risk" patients with uncertain diagnosis and age >40 years (see Table 8.4), a history of less than three syncopes yields a probability of recurrence of syncope of 20% during the next 2 years whereas a history of three syncopes yields a probability of recurrence of syncope of 42% during the same period. A psychiatric diagnosis and age <45 years are also associated with higher rates of syncope recurrence. Conversely, gender, tilt test response, severity of presentation, and presence or absence of structural heart disease have minimal or no predictive value.

In population studies, syncope recurrence rates seem to remain high despite available treatments. Thus, in the EGSYS follow-up study[4] syncope recurred in 16.5% of patients during a mean of 614 days. The incidence of syncope recurrence was similar irrespective of the presumed mechanism (Fig. 6.3). Syncope rate was 12.5/100 patient-years in patients with syncope due to primary cardiac arrhythmia; among

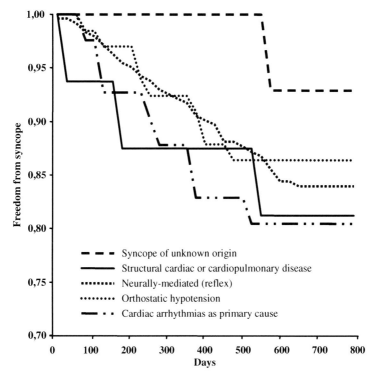

Fig. 6.3 Syncopal recurrence rate according to the final diagnosis among 398 patients referred to the emergency department in the EGSYS 2 study[4]

these, the rate was 9.1/100 patient-years in those who received some specific treatment (pacemaker, ablation, or ICD) and 20.0/100 patient-years in those who did not ($p = 0.28$). The recurrence rate was 14.9/100 patient-years in patients with structural cardiac (or cardiopulmonary) syncope, 9.8/100 patient-years in patients with neurally mediated syncope, 8.8/100 patient-years in patients with orthostatic syncope, and 4.1/100 patient-years in patients with unexplained syncope. Potentially, the persistence of recurrences may in part reflect inadequate diagnostic precision and/or the possibility that there may be more than one cause of syncope in individual patients.

Major morbidity such as fractures and motor vehicle accidents were reported in 6% of syncope patients and minor injury such as laceration and bruises in 29%. In patients presenting to an ED, minor trauma was reported in 29.1% and major trauma in 4.7% of cases; the highest prevalence of trauma (43%) was observed in older individuals with carotid sinus hypersensitivity.[15] Recurrent syncope is associated with fractures and soft tissue injury in 12% of patients. Morbidity is particularly high in the elderly and ranges from loss of confidence, depressive illness, and fear of falling to fractures and subsequent institutionalization. The risk of events (i.e., trauma) is higher if syncope recurrence is unpredictable and occurs in the absence of a prodrome.

In general, the risk related to recurrence of syncope is higher (emphasizing the importance of finding a specific diagnosis) in the following settings:

- syncope is very frequent, e.g., alters the quality of life;
- syncope is recurrent and unpredictable (absence of prodrome) and exposes patients to a "high risk" of trauma;
- syncope occurs during the prosecution of a "high-risk" activity (e.g., driving, machine operation, flying, competitive athletics).

6.3 Management According to Risk Stratification

According to the 2009 Guidelines on Syncope of the European Society of Cardiology,[3] physicians should be able, at the end of the initial evaluation, to stratify patients with syncope of uncertain cause into three categories: those at high risk, those at low risk with recurrent episodes, and those at low risk with single or rare episodes (Fig. 6.4). The subsequent management varies accordingly.

The patients at high risk of death or life-threatening arrhythmias are those listed in Table 6.2. In particular these patients are those:

- with a clear indication for an ICD according to guidelines who should undergo this therapy before more comprehensive evaluation of the mechanism of syncope;
- with previous myocardial infarction who should undergo an electrophysiological study which includes premature ventricular stimulation. An implantable loop recorder (ILR) should be considered only at the end of a negative complete workup;
- with clinical or ECG features suggesting an arrhythmic mechanism of syncope who should undergo in-hospital prolonged telemetric monitoring and eventually an electrophysiological evaluation; ILR should be considered if the initial workup is non-diagnostic.

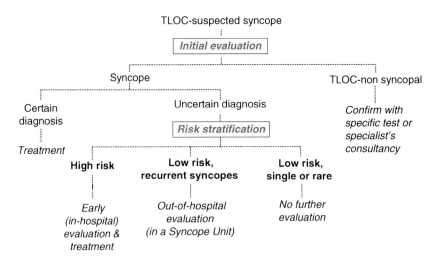

Fig. 6.4 Management according to risk stratification

Table 6.2   High-risk criteria which require early intensive evaluation (in-hospital or in specialized facilities)

- Situations in which there is a clear indication for implantable defibrillator (ICD) or pacemaker treatment independently of a definite diagnosis of the cause of syncope
- Severe structural cardiovascular or coronary artery disease (heart failure or low ejection fraction or previous myocardial infarction)
- Clinical or ECG features suggesting an arrhythmic syncope:
  - Syncope during exertion or supine
  - Palpitations at the time of syncope
  - Family history of sudden death
  - Non-sustained ventricular tachycardia
  - Bundle branch block (QRS duration ≥0.12 s)
  - Sinus bradycardia (<50 bpm) or sinoatrial block in the absence of negatively chronotropic medications and physical training
  - Pre-excited QRS complexes
  - Prolonged or short QT interval
  - Right bundle branch block pattern with ST elevation in leads V1–V3 (Brugada syndrome)
  - Negative T waves in right precordial leads, epsilon waves, and ventricular late potentials suggestive of arrhythmogenic right ventricular dysplasia

Patients at high risk should be evaluated immediately and intensively. Some of these will require prompt hospitalization, and others will be safely evaluated in a specialized facility, i.e., syncope unit.

When high-risk features are absent or, if present, the subsequent workup is negative, the risk of life-threatening events is low. Evaluation can then be aimed at prevention of syncope recurrence. Patients at low risk with severe presentation (because their episodes are recurrent and unpredictable or occur in settings that may result in injury) are reasonably assessed as outpatients or day cases preferably with referral to a specialized syncope facility (i.e., syncope unit). These patients require careful diagnostic assessment and, given their susceptibility to recurrent events, will benefit from a mechanism-specific therapy. ECG documentation of a spontaneous syncopal relapse is the preferred method for diagnosis in patients in whom an arrhythmia is likely (see Chapter 8).

Finally, in patients with the less severe forms of syncope, no further investigation is warranted because specific treatment is not necessary, and patients can be educated and reassured about the benign nature of their symptom (e.g., most instances of vasovagal syncope).

6.4   Clinical Perspectives: In-Hospital Versus Outpatient Evaluation in Specialized Facilities

Inasmuch as syncope may be a harbinger of sudden death among patients thought to be at risk of cardiac causes of syncope, physicians generally take a "safe" approach and tend to admit more patients to hospital than is really necessary. Approximately 35–50% of patients referred to emergency department are hospitalized. Although the rationale for this approach is understandable, the presumption that in-hospital evaluation improves a patient's clinical outcome has never been demonstrated; consequently, alternative strategies should be considered.

The hospital admission decision can be justified by: (1) high risk of short-term adverse events, (2) establishing the correct diagnosis, and (3) initiating optimal therapy (Table 6.3). The risk of life-threatening conditions in the few days after referral is the main reason for immediate hospital admission and exhaustive evaluation (see short-term risk section). Apart from the safety issues, hospitalization is still necessary when in-hospital monitoring or invasive tests (i.e., electrophysiological study, coronary angiography, etc.) are required. In the EGSYS 2[16] and SUP[17] population studies, 4% and 9% of patients, respectively, underwent in-hospital monitoring and 14% and 8%, respectively, underwent invasive tests (see Chapters 5 and 7). All other noninvasive investigations can safely be performed on an outpatient basis. Finally,

Table 6.3 Basis for hospital admission in patients with transient loss of consciousness

For high short-term risk:
- Cardiac
  - Documented potentially life-threatening arrhythmias/conduction disturbance (such as but not limited to)
    - √ Mobitz II or 2:1 second-degree or third-degree AV block
    - √ Long and short QT pattern
    - √ Brugada pattern
    - √ ARVD
    - √ WPW pattern
    - √ Non-sustained or sustained VT
    - √ SVT/atrial fibrillation with rapid ventricular response
    - √ Interruption of the cardiac rhythm >3 s by sinus pauses or AV block or heart rates <40/min
  - Moderate to severe systolic dysfunction (e.g., <40%)
  - Documented or suspected acute coronary syndromes
  - Heart failure
- Non-cardiac
  - Acute hemorrhage (hematocrit <30)
  - Stroke or focal neurologic disorders
  - Pulmonary embolism
  - End-stage diseases (cancer, etc.)
  - Major physical injuries secondary to T-LOC/syncope
  - New seizure

For diagnosis of T-LOC/syncope:
- Need of in-hospital monitoring because of suspected arrhythmias (brady- or tachy-)
- Need to perform electrophysiological study and other eventual invasive evaluations
- That occurred when patient was supine ("supine syncope")
- That occurred when patient was in the midst of exercise ("full flight")
- Strong family history of unexpected sudden death or channelopathy

For treatment of T-LOC/syncope:
- Cardiac arrhythmias as cause of syncope
- Syncope due to cardiac ischemia
- Syncope secondary to the structural cardiac or cardiopulmonary diseases
- Cardioinhibitory neurally mediated syncope when a pacemaker implantation is planned

hospitalization is required when therapeutic interventions are indicated (i.e., cardiac pacing, catheter ablation, automatic defibrillator, coronary revascularization, cardiac surgery, etc.). In population studies,[16,17] this accounted for 62/465 patients (13%) referred to the emergency department and for 53/891 (10%) referred to specialized syncope facilities.

Thus, the modern strategy of management of patients with syncope should be aimed at reduction of unnecessary hospitalizations. We estimate that fewer than 20% of patients require hospitalization for diagnosis and 10–13% for therapy. Lower risk patients may be satisfactorily managed by assessment as outpatients or day cases preferably with referral to a specialized syncope facility, i.e., syncope unit.

References

1. Brignole M, et al. Guidelines on management (diagnosis and treatment) of syncope: Update 2004. *Europace*. 2004;6:467–537.
2. Huff JS, et al. Clinical policy: critical issues in the evaluation and management of adult patients presenting to the emergency department with syncope. *Ann Emerg Med*. 2007;49:431–444.
3. Moya A, et al. Guidelines for the Diagnosis and Management of Syncope (Version 2009). *Eur Heart J*. 2009;30:2631–2671.
4. Ungar A, et al. Early and late outcome of treated patients referred for syncope to emergency department. The EGSYS 2 follow-up study. *Eur Heart J*. 2010;31:2021–2026.
5. Quinn J, et al. Prospective validation of the San Francisco Syncope Rule to predict patients with serious outcomes. *Ann Emerg Med*. 2006;47:448–454.
6. Sun BC, et al. External validation of the San Francisco Syncope Rule. *Ann Emerg Med*. 2007;49:420–427.
7. Schladenhaufen R, et al. Application of San Francisco Syncope Rule in elderly ED patients. *Am J Emerg Med*. 2008;26:773–778.
8. Birnbaum A, et al. Failure to validate the San Francisco Syncope Rule in an independent emergency department population. *Ann Emerg Med*. 2008;52:151–159.
9. Reed M, et al. Risk stratification of syncope in the emergency department: The ROSE study. *J Am Coll Cardiol*. 2010;55:713–721.
10. Martin TP, et al. Risk stratification of patients with syncope. *Ann Emerg Med*. 1997;29: 459–466.
11. Colivicchi F, et al. Development and prospective validation of a risk stratification system for patients with syncope in the emergency department: the OESIL risk score. *Eur Heart J*. 2003;24:811–819.
12. Del Rosso A, et al. Clinical predictors of cardiac syncope at initial evaluation in patients referred urgently to general hospital: the EGSYS score. *Heart*. 2008;94:1620–1626.
13. Costantino G, et al. Short and long-term prognosis of syncope, risk factors and role of hospital admission. Results from the STePS (Short-Term Prognosis of Syncope) Study. *J Am Coll Cardiol*. 2008;51:276–283.
14. Benditt DG, Can I. Initial evaluation of "syncope and collapse". the need for a risk stratification consensus. *J Am Coll Cardiol*. 2010;23(55):722–724.
15. Bartoletti A, et al. Physical injuries caused by a transient loss of consciousness: main clinical characteristics of patients and diagnostic contribution of carotid sinus massage. *Eur Heart J*. 2008;29:618–624.
16. Brignole M, et al. A new management of syncope: prospective systematic guideline-based evaluation of patients referred urgently to general hospitals. *Eur Heart J*. 2006;27:76–82.
17. Brignole M, et al. Prospective multicentre systematic guideline-based management of patients referred to the Syncope Units of general hospitals. *Europace*. 2010;12:109–118.

Chapter 7
Indications for and Interpretation of Laboratory Diagnostic Tests

Contents

M. Brignole, D.G. Benditt, *Syncope*, DOI 10.1007/978-0-85729-201-8_7,
© Springer-Verlag London Limited 2011

Key points: Identifying the mechanism of syncope by means of laboratory tests

- Selected diagnostic laboratory tests are performed soon after the initial evaluation when the cause of syncope remains uncertain. Test selection should be based on the initial assessment.
- Carotid sinus massage is recommended in patients over age 40 years with uncertain syncope. Carotid sinus syncope is generally accepted to be likely if syncope is reproduced by the carotid sinus massage in the presence of asystole longer than 3 s and/or a fall in systolic blood pressure >50 mmHg, in the absence of competing diagnoses.
- Active standing test is part of the initial evaluation. Due to the marked day-to-day variability of postural response, the active standing test should be repeated on different days when orthostatic hypotension is suspected. An active standing test resulting in symptomatic orthostatic hypotension is considered diagnostic of the cause of syncope if consistent with the medical history.
- Tilt testing is recommended in patients with uncertain syncope when syncope is suspected to be vasovagal in nature and/or mediated by orthostatic stress. The end-point is the induction of vasovagal syncope or delayed (progressive) orthostatic hypotension.
- ATP test cannot be used alone as a diagnostic test to select patients for cardiac pacing.
- Electrophysiological study is indicated when cardiac arrhythmic syncope is suspected at initial evaluation in patients with previous myocardial infarction, bundle branch block, sinus node dysfunction, or sudden and brief undocumented palpitations.
- Exercise testing is indicated in patients who experience syncope during or shortly after exertion and in patients with chest pain suggestive of coronary artery disease. The development of advanced AV block or hypotension during exertion and/or a hypotensive reflex immediately after the exercise are diagnostic.
- Other (non-provocative) tests investigate the underlying substrate. Their utility is in general limited to the evaluation of structural cardiac and cardiovascular diseases which may be the cause of syncope.
- Overall, diagnostic laboratory tests are able to establish an evidence-based diagnosis in about a half of the patients with uncertain syncope. Most of these have a reflex syncope diagnosed by tilt-table testing or carotid sinus massage; relatively few patients with cardiac syncope are diagnosed with such testing.

7.1 Introduction

The diagnostic evaluation strategy for patients with syncope of uncertain etiology (i.e., syncope that remains of uncertain nature after the initial evaluation) consists of either trying to formulate a diagnosis by employing selected laboratory tests or alternatively using a long-term monitoring approach until a syncope recurrence (or related event) can be documented (Table 7.1). In this chapter we describe the indication and the interpretation of the most commonly performed laboratory tests. In the next chapter (Chapter 8) we describe the indication and the interpretation of various systems for prolonged ECG monitoring.

7.2 Carotid Sinus Massage

Carotid sinus massage (CSM) is a test used to unmask the clinical condition carotid sinus syndrome (CSS) in patients with syncope. However, as discussed below, a "positive" CSM may be observed in the absence of CSS. Consequently, the test result must be carefully considered in the setting of both the patient's medical history and possible competitive syncope etiologies.

The carotid sinus reflex arc is composed of an afferent limb arising from the mechanoreceptors of the carotid artery and terminating in midbrain centers, mainly the vagus nucleus and the vasomotor center. The efferent limb is via the vagus nerve and the parasympathetic ganglia to the sinus and atrioventricular nodes and via the sympathetic nervous system to the heart and the blood vessels.[1] Whether the site of dysfunction resulting in a hypersensitive response to the massage is central or at the level of brainstem nuclei or peripheral at the level of carotid baroreceptors is still a matter of debate.

It has long been observed that pressure at the site where common carotid artery bifurcates produces a reflex slowing in heart rate and fall in blood pressure. In some patients with syncope, especially those >40 years of age, an abnormal response to carotid massage can be observed. A ventricular pause lasting 3 s or more and a fall

Table 7.1 Diagnosing syncope after the initial evaluation

Laboratory tests:
  Provocative tests:

  – Carotid sinus massage
  – Orthostatic challenge (active standing test and tilt testing)
  – ATP (adenosine) test
  – Electrophysiological study (EPS)
  – Exercise testing

  Other tests (coronary angiography, chest and abdominal computed tomography, pulmonary
    scintigraphy, chest X-ray, abdominal ultrasound examination)
Prolonged ECG monitoring (Holter, external loop recorders, remote at-home telemetry, and
  implantable loop recorders [ILRs])

---

in systolic blood pressure of 50 mmHg or more are considered abnormal and define *carotid sinus hypersensitivity (CSH)*[1–3] (Fig. 7.1). However, abnormal responses are frequently observed in up to 40% patients without syncope, especially if they are older and affected by cardiovascular diseases.[4] The specificity of the test increases if reproduction of spontaneous syncope during carotid massage is made a requisite for positivity of the test (this usually requires undertaking carotid massage [CSM] with the patient in an upright position). For this reason the laboratory diagnosis of *carotid sinus syndrome (CSS)* requires reproduction of spontaneous symptoms associated with documentation of CSH and exclusion of competing mechanisms.[2,3] CSS may be misdiagnosed in half of the cases if the massage is not performed in the upright position.[5] Furthermore, even if an asystolic response is evoked by CSM, the possibility still exists that the patient may also exhibit a marked vasodepressor response; in order to assess the contribution of the vasodepressor component (which

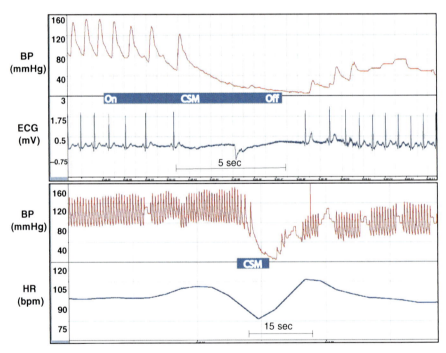

Fig. 7.1 Typical falling of blood pressure (BP) and heart rate (HR) during a positive response to 7 s of carotid sinus massage performed in upright position. *Upper panel.* The BP and electrocardiographic tracing shows, after the start of the massage, sinus slowing for three beats followed by 6 s sinus pause. According to the "method of symptoms" the massage was stopped as soon as syncope occurred. Heart beats resumed quickly after the end of the massage. *Lower panel.* The compressed BP pressure and electrocardiographic tracing shows that the vasodepressor component of the massage is prolonged for several seconds after the end of the massage and complete recovery to baseline values is not yet reached after 45 s. Recorded by Nexfin device (BMEYE, the Netherlands)

may otherwise be hidden) CSM is usually repeated after intravenous administration of atropine. Atropine usually eliminates the vagally induced cardioinhibitory response and permits the unmasking of the vasodepressor phenomenon.[5]

An appropriate methodology is necessary for correct classification of CSM responses; these are generally classified as cardioinhibitory (i.e., asystole), vasodepressive (fall in systolic blood pressure without substantial bradycardia), or mixed (Table 7.2). This classification has a practical importance for treatment; not surprisingly, cardiac pacing is more likely to be effective for pure cardioinhibitory forms than for vasodepressor or mixed forms. The methodology of the test is described in more detail in Chapter 17.

There is a relationship between CSH and spontaneous, otherwise unexplained, syncope. This relationship is important and has been studied by two different methods. The first was a comparison of the recurrence rate of syncope between patients with and without pacemaker treatment. Some nonrandomized as well as two randomized studies demonstrated fewer recurrences at follow-up in patients implanted with pacemakers than in patients without pacing.[6,7] The second method was to analyze the occurrence of asystolic episodes registered in patients with cardioinhibitory response to carotid sinus massage by an implanted device. In the two trials that employed this latter methodology, recordings of long spontaneous pauses were very common.[8,9] These results suggest that a positive response to CSM in patients with syncope is highly predictive of the occurrence of spontaneous asystolic episodes.

Carotid sinus syndrome (CSS) is a frequent cause of syncope, especially in elderly men; the prevalence of CSS as a cause of syncope ranges from 4% in patients <40 years of age to 41% in patients >80 years old in a selected population of patients evaluated in a tertiary center (Fig. 7.2). Puggioni et al.[5] performed CSM in a large population of 1,719 consecutive patients with syncope of uncertain cause after the initial evaluation (mean age 66 ± 17 years); CSH was found in 56% and syncope was reproduced in 26% of cases. The response was cardioinhibitory in 46% of patients, mixed in 40%, and vasodepressor in 14%.

Table 7.2 Carotid sinus massage: classification of the positive responses

---

Dominant cardioinhibitory form
- Carotid sinus massage, baseline: asystole ≥3 s with reproduction of spontaneous symptoms
- Carotid sinus massage after atropine (1 mg or 0.02 mg/kg body weight): no further symptoms[a]

Mixed form
- Carotid sinus massage, baseline: asystole ≥3 s and fall in systolic blood pressure ≥50 mmHg with reproduction of spontaneous symptoms
- Carotid sinus massage after atropine (1 mg or 0.02 mg/kg body weight): milder symptoms due to systolic blood pressure fall ≥50 mmHg

Dominant vasodepressor form
- Carotid sinus massage, baseline: reproduction of the spontaneous symptoms due to systolic blood pressure fall ≥50 mmHg without asystole
- Carotid sinus massage after atropine (1 mg or 0.02 mg/kg body weight): unchanged

---

[a] In this case vasodepressor reflex is absent or, if present, asymptomatic

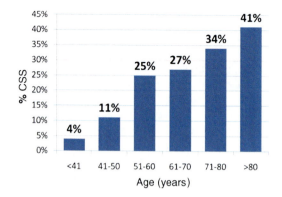

Fig. 7.2 Prevalence of carotid sinus syndrome (*CSS, ordinate*) per decade of age (*abscissa*) in a population of patients referred to a tertiary center for evaluation of syncope of uncertain cause

The main potential complication of CSM is neurological, i.e., transient ischemic attack (TIA) and stroke; the incidence of such complications ranges between 0.17 and 0.45%.[5,10] The risk of stroke is increased in the setting of carotid artery disease; in such cases CSM is best avoided.

7.2.1 Indications

CSM is recommended in patients >40 years of age with uncertain syncope after the initial evaluation. Massage is best avoided if there is evidence of carotid vascular disease (i.e., prior ipsilateral stroke, carotid bruits).[2,3]

7.2.2 Interpretation of Results

Carotid sinus syncope is diagnosed if syncope is reproduced by CSM in the presence of asystole longer than 3 s and/or a fall in systolic blood pressure >50 mmHg, in the absence of competing diagnoses.[2,3]

7.3 Orthostatic Challenge (Active Standing Test and Tilt-Table Testing)

Changing from supine to upright posture causes a large gravitational shift of blood from the chest to the venous capacitance system below the diaphragm. Failure of compensatory reflexes to counteract this orthostatic stress is the basic cause of clinical features of orthostatic intolerance (see Chapters 1 and 2). Two orthostatic challenge tests are widely applied in practice to diagnose forms of orthostatic hypotension and vasovagal syncope triggered by prolonged standing: the active standing test and head-up tilt-table test. Tests involving simulated orthostatic stress such as applying lower body negative pressure, or undertaking the "squat-stand" maneuver, are mainly used in research.[3]

Beat-to-beat noninvasive blood pressure measurement is widely used in research and tilt-table testing laboratories and is recommended when tilt testing is performed. The preferred devices are those which employ the photoplethysmographic volume clamp method of Penaz to record the arterial waveform indirectly from a finger. Studies on its accuracy have suggested little systematic bias versus intra-arterial pressure but substantial variability. In combined data from 20 published studies the average systolic bias was 2.2 ± 12.4 mmHg.[11] While the sphygmomanometer is used for routine clinical testing because of its reliability and simplicity, it is less desirable when testing clinical conditions such as vasovagal syncope that involve evaluation of the autonomic nervous system. Furthermore, both standard sphygmomanometers and automatic arm-cuff devices that are programmed to repeat and confirm measurements are at a disadvantage in following rapidly falling blood pressure during orthostatic hypotension and are discouraged. Heart rate recording is integral to orthostatic challenge and is indispensable to the separation of the various clinical syndromes.

Day-to-day variability of postural blood pressure response is well documented with both lying-to-standing test and tilt-table testing. In a study of patients with clinical orthostatic hypotension by Ward and Kenny,[12] reproducibility of classic orthostatic hypotension in the elderly was observed in about 67% of the tested subjects. Reproducibility was greater in patients with evidence of autonomic dysfunction and less evident in individuals with normal autonomic function. Moreover, postural responses show diurnal (worse in the morning) and seasonal (worse during summer) variability. In addition, in patients with post-prandial hypotension, the effect is almost immediately apparent after a meal and peaks within 30–60 min. Consequently, given the variability of test responses, a single orthostatic test is insufficient for diagnosis. As orthostatic intolerance is poorly reproducible, it has been shown that several measurements may be required to establish the diagnosis.[11]

The reproducibility of tilt testing for evaluation of vasovagal syncope has been widely studied. The overall reproducibility of an initial negative response (85–94%) is higher than the reproducibility of an initial positive response (31–92%). Data from controlled trials showed that approximately 50% of patients with a baseline positive tilt-table test became negative when the test was repeated with placebo.

7.3.1 Active Standing Test

Initial and classical forms of orthostatic hypotension may often be diagnosed by this simple method in the clinic. A frequently used protocol is the short, bedside orthostatic test. In this test the patient's blood pressure is measured after a few minutes of rest in the supine position; the patient then arises and the measurements are then repeated while the patient is standing motionless for 3–5 min with the cuffed arm supported at heart level. The principal advantages of this test are that it corresponds to real-life situations and is simple to perform, the required equipment is available, and minimal patient cooperation is needed. The sphygmomanometer is adequate for routine clinical testing because of its ubiquity and simplicity. Automatic arm-cuff devices, as they are programmed to repeat and confirm measurements when discrepant values are recorded, may be a disadvantage due to the possibility that blood pressure may fall rapidly during orthostatic hypotension. With a sphygmomanometer more than four measurements per minute cannot be obtained without venous obstruction in the arm. When more frequent values are required, continuous beat-to-beat noninvasive blood pressure measurement (e.g., Finometer®, TaskForce®, Nexfin®) should be used. Tilt-table testing may also be used instead of active standing as an orthostatic challenge. The results are similar.[11]

7.3.1.1 Indications

The active standing test is part of the initial evaluation. Due to the marked day-to-day variability of postural response, active standing test may need to be repeated on different days when orthostatic hypotension is suspected but not yet proven in patients being investigated for syncope of uncertain etiology.[3]

7.3.1.2 Interpretation of Results

Orthostatic syncope is diagnosed when, with the active standing test, there is documentation of posturally triggered hypotension associated with syncope or near syncope. An asymptomatic abnormal fall in systolic blood is less specific, and competing diagnoses should be evaluated before the diagnosis of orthostatic syncope is made.[3]

Initial orthostatic hypotension is characterized by a blood pressure decrease >40 mmHg immediately on standing, it then spontaneously and rapidly returns to normal; the period of hypotension and symptoms is short (<30 s) (Fig. 7.3).

Classical orthostatic hypotension is a physical sign defined as a decrease in systolic blood pressure >20 mmHg (>30 mmHg in hypertensives) or <90 mmHg within 3 min of standing (Fig. 7.4).[13]

7.3.2 Tilt-Table Testing

Vasovagal syncope triggered by prolonged standing and delayed (progressive) orthostatic hypotension are both subject to diagnostic evaluation with tilt-table testing. However, the vast majority of published tilt-table experience deals with vasovagal syncope.

Tilt testing not only enables the reproduction of both of these syndromes in a laboratory setting but also may be helpful in diagnosing reflex syncope mediated by emotional distress and in patients with sick sinus syndrome. In patients without structural heart disease, tilt testing can be considered diagnostic, and no further tests are needed when syncope is reproduced as attested to by the patient (assuming the

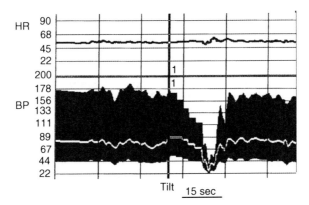

Fig. 7.3 "Initial" orthostatic hypotension during tilt-table testing. Beat-to-beat monitoring of heart rate (HR) and systolic, diastolic, and mean blood pressure (BP) are shown. Blood pressure decreases >40 mmHg immediately upon standing, then spontaneously and rapidly returns to normal; the period of hypotension and symptoms is short (<20 s). The heart rate does not show variations suggesting an impairment of cardiovascular adaptation reflexes. Recorded by Finapres device (Ohmeda, USA)

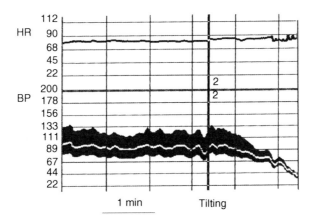

Fig. 7.4 "Classical" orthostatic hypotension during tilt-table testing. Beat-to-beat monitoring of heart rate (HR) and systolic, diastolic, and mean blood pressure (BP) are graphed throughout the time (*abscissa*) of the study. BP decreases progressively after tilting until hypotensive syncope occurs at approximately 3 min. The heart rate does not show variations suggesting an impairment of cardiovascular adaptation reflexes. Recorded by Finapres device (Ohmeda, USA)

medical history is supportive albeit not classical). In patients with structural heart disease, arrhythmia or other cardiac cause should be excluded prior to considering positive tilt test results to be definitive.

A positive tilt test response is observed in more than half of the patients with suspected vasovagal syncope. However, different methodologies and different protocols exist (see Chapter 18). In brief, the protocols that are most used are those that include a passive head-up tilt phase at 60°–70° followed, if negative, by a drug challenge with isoproterenol or nitroglycerin (the latter being the so-called Italian protocol).[14–16]

Orthostatic stress may induce two different abnormal responses: the first is a vasovagal reaction which is an expression of a reflex susceptibility leading to hypotension, while the second is progressive hypotension which is an expression of failure of the compensatory autonomic reflexes to provide appropriate vasoconstriction with standing (i.e., orthostatic hypotension). From a strictly pathophysiological point of view there is no overlap between reflex syncope (which requires a normal/hyperactive autonomic function) and autonomic failure (which implies impaired function). However, the clinical manifestations of the two conditions frequently do overlap. In fact, sometimes it is difficult to distinguish one from the other. Both conditions have a common trigger, namely blood pooling in the lower extremities and splanchnic bed and decrease in venous return due to orthostatic stress and immobilization. In both, the final effect, hypotension, is related to impaired vasoconstrictor capability. The absence of a bradycardic reflex (vagal overactivity) differentiates delayed orthostatic hypotension from reflex syncope, but even this difference may be subtle and not clear-cut.[3]

7.3.2.1 Responses to Tilt Testing

The endpoint of tilt-table testing is the induction of either reflex hypotension/bradycardia or delayed orthostatic hypotension, associated with syncope or presyncope. Positive responses can be classified into three main categories according to the various patterns of blood pressure and heart rate observed during the test[3] (Table 7.3).

The *vasovagal* pattern is characterized by an initial phase of rapid and full compensatory reflex adaptation to the upright position resulting in a stabilization of blood pressure and increased heart rate (which suggests normal baroreflex function) that may last for several minutes. Compared with the supine position, the heart rate increases during this phase. Patients are usually asymptomatic but may feel palpitation due to the increased rate. The onset of the syncopal vasovagal reaction can easily be determined at the time of an abrupt fall in blood pressure sometimes accompanied by a fall of heart rate. Vasovagal symptoms coincide with this phase.

Table 7.3 Classification of positive responses to tilt testing

- *Vasovagal.* Initially blood pressure stabilizes and heart rate may increase. Then blood pressure rapidly falls before the heart rate falls:
  - *Cardioinhibitory (asystolic) form*: heart rate falls and asystole >3 s coincides with syncope
  - *Mixed form*: heart rate falls, but asystole does not occur
- *Delayed (progressive) orthostatic hypotension.* Progressive decrease of systolic blood pressure for >3 min before syncope occurs. Heart rate progressively slightly increases
- *Delayed orthostatic hypotension plus vasovagal.* Blood pressure progressively decreases and heart rate increases for >3 min. Then blood pressure rapidly falls and heart rate falls; asystole may or may not occur

Once the vasovagal reaction starts, it leads to syncope within a few minutes (in general <3 min and on average 1 min after the onset of prodromal symptoms).

A decrease in systolic blood pressure to below 90 mmHg is associated with symptoms of impending syncope and to below 60 mmHg is associated with syncope. Prodromal symptoms are present in virtually all cases of tilt-induced vasovagal syncope (may be subtle in the elderly). During the prodromal phase, blood pressure falls markedly; this fall frequently precedes the decrease in heart rate, which may be absent at least at the beginning of this phase (Figs. 7.5 and 18.2). When a reflex is induced, according to the predominance of vasodepressor or cardioinhibitory components, the responses are classified as cardioinhibitory or mixed. The patients with these patterns are largely young and healthy with a history of several syncopal episodes; in many cases the first syncopal episodes occurred in the teenage years. Secondary trauma is infrequent. These responses are felt to represent a "hypersensitive" autonomic system that overresponds to various stimuli.

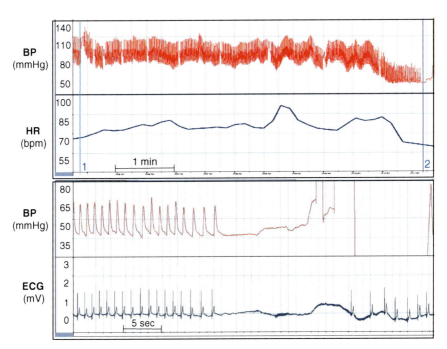

Fig. 7.5 Falling blood pressure (BP) and heart rate (HR) during a tilt-induced vasovagal pattern, cardioinhibitory type. *Upper panel.* The initial phase is characterized by a rapid and full compensatory reflex adaptation to the upright position (*vertical line 1*) (which suggests normal baroreflex function), which lasted for 4 min. The activation of adaptive mechanisms is evidenced by the slight oscillations in BP and HR, especially evident toward the end of this phase. The HR increases during this phase at a maximum of 100 bpm. The onset of the syncopal vasovagal reaction can easily be determined at the time of an abrupt fall in BP and HR. Vasovagal reaction leads to syncope in 1 min (*vertical line 2*). *Lower panel.* The expanded BP pressure and electrocardiographic tracing, recorded at the time of syncope, shows a progressive sinus bradycardia followed by an 18-s long asystolic pause. Recorded by Nexfin device (BMEYE, the Netherlands)

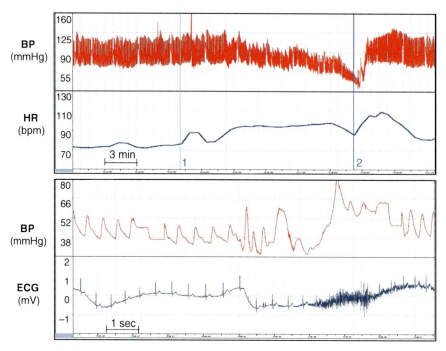

Fig. 7.6 Hemodynamic pattern of a patient with delayed orthostatic hypotension syndrome. Contrary to vasovagal pattern, there is inability to obtain a steady-state adaptation to the upright position (*vertical line 1*), and therefore, there is an early slow progressive decrease of blood pressure until symptoms occur (*vertical line 2*). Compared with the supine position, the heart rate increases during the test by a variable amount. Syncope occurs after 17 min, in the absence of bradycardia. Recorded by Nexfin device (BMEYE, the Netherlands)

Conversely, the pattern of *delayed (progressive) orthostatic hypotension* is characterized by inability to obtain a steady-state adaptation to the upright position, and therefore, there is an early slow progressive decrease of blood pressure until symptoms occur. Compared with the supine position, the heart rate increases during the test by a variable amount; the absence of bradycardia differentiates this form from the classical vasovagal response (Figs. 7.6 and 18.3). Typically these patients remain asymptomatic initially after standing and develop hypotensive symptoms that cause orthostatic intolerance a few minutes later. Symptoms are similar to those associated with other forms of orthostatic hypotension. Among these, dizziness, presyncope, weakness, fatigue, and palpitations are the most frequent; visual disturbances, syncope, hearing disturbances, and pain in the neck ("coat-hanger distribution") and in the chest are less frequently encountered. No clear vasovagal reaction is discerned.

The orthostatic response patients are predominantly in older age groups, and many have associated diseases; they have a short history of syncope with few episodes per patient and few and non-specific prodromes. Carotid sinus hypersensitivity is absent; syncopal episodes begin late in life, suggesting that they are due to the occurrence of some underlying autonomic dysfunction.

The pattern of *delayed orthostatic hypotension plus vasovagal reaction* combines the two patterns. In this form there is absence or impaired adaption to upright position. Initially the behavior of blood pressure and heart rate is similar to that of delayed orthostatic hypotension, but later a clear vasovagal reaction develops with the typical fall in heart rate of variable magnitude indicating a cardioinhibitory or a mixed response. Syncope occurs at the time of maximum bradycardia. The patients affected are predominantly older, and many have associated diseases. Their clinical features and medical history are intermediate between the previous two categories; history of typical vasovagal or situational syncopes and associated carotid sinus hypersensitivity are not infrequent and differentiate this form from that of pure orthostatic hypotension.

7.3.2.2 Role of Tilt-Table Test for Assessing the Effectiveness of the Treatment

The reproducibility of tilt testing limits its utility as a means of assessing therapy. The overall reproducibility of an initial negative response (85–94%) is higher than the reproducibility of an initial positive response (31–92%). In addition, data from controlled trials showed that approximately 50% of patients with a baseline positive tilt test became negative when the test was repeated with treatment or with placebo.[2,3] Moreover, the mechanism of tilt-induced syncope is frequently different from that of the spontaneous syncope recorded with the implantable loop recorder (ILR). The ISSUE 2 study [17] compared the response to tilt testing with spontaneous syncope recorded by ILR. While a positive cardioinhibitory response to tilt testing was able to predict with a high probability an asystolic spontaneous syncope, the presence of a positive vasodepressor or mixed response or even a negative response, did not exclude the presence of asystole during spontaneous syncope. These data show that the use of tilt testing for assessing the effectiveness of different treatments has important limitations.

Despite its apparent limitations, tilt test results may have some therapeutic utility in the following areas:[2,3]

- Differentiating reflex syncope from orthostatic hypotension is essential for a specific therapy.
- Tilt-table testing is widely accepted as a useful tool to demonstrate susceptibility of the patient to reflex syncope and thereby to allow the patient to better recognize onset of an episode and initiate treatment (e.g., physical counterpressure maneuvers).
- If the correlation between induced and spontaneous asystolic responses is confirmed by future trials, candidates for cardiac pacing could be selected based on tilt test results. Currently, however, this is not advocated.

7.3.2.3 Complications and Contraindications

Tilt-table testing is safe. There have been no reported deaths during the test. However, some rare life-threatening ventricular arrhythmias with isoproterenol in the presence of ischemic heart disease or sick sinus syndrome have been reported. No complications have been published with the use of nitroglycerin. Atrial fibrillation can be induced during or after a positive tilt test and is usually self-limited. Relative contraindications to the administration of isoproterenol include ischemic heart disease, uncontrolled hypertension, left ventricular outflow tract obstruction, and significant aortic stenosis. Caution should be used in patients with known arrhythmias.[2,3]

7.3.2.4 Indications

Tilt-table testing is indicated soon after the initial evaluation in patients with syncope of uncertain cause when either a neurally mediated vasovagal origin or an orthostatic hypotension is suspected.[2,3]

The main indication for tilt testing has been to support a diagnosis of reflex syncope in patients with an atypical presentation in whom such a diagnosis was suspected but not confirmed by initial evaluation (particularly the medical history). Tilt testing is not usually needed in patients whose reflex syncope is already diagnosed by clinical history and in patients with single or rare syncope unless justified by special situations (e.g., injury, anxiety, occupational implications such as aircraft pilots).

In patients with a high-risk profile for cardiovascular events or with data suggestive of arrhythmic syncope, tilt testing has been reported useful when a cardiovascular cause has been reasonably excluded by a comprehensive evaluation. Sometimes, tilt testing has been helpful in proving that an induced arrhythmia (usually a tachyarrhythmia) can lead to hypotension with the patient in the upright posture and for discriminating syncope from epilepsy. Tilt testing has been used in patients with frequent syncope and suspicion of psychiatric problems, even with traumatic injury, to investigate the reflex nature of the syncope. Similarly, tilt testing has been used in the elderly in order to distinguish syncope from falls.

Tilt-table testing is increasingly used in patients with suspected orthostatic hypotension when active standing test fails to show evidence of the diagnosis. About a quarter of all diagnoses of orthostatic hypotension that were undiagnosed at initial evaluation are made with tilt testing. Moreover, tilt testing should be considered to discriminate between reflex and delayed orthostatic hypotension.

Tilt-table testing has no value in assessing treatment efficacy. However, tilt testing is widely accepted as a useful tool to demonstrate susceptibility of the patient to reflex syncope and thereby to initiate an appropriate treatment strategy (e.g., salt/volume, physical manoeuvres; see Chapter 11)

7.3.2.5 Interpretation of Results

- *Reflex syncope with atypical presentation (vasovagal)* is diagnosed in patients without structural heart disease in whom the suspicion of a reflex cause is confirmed by tilt testing showing induction of reflex hypotension/bradycardia with reproduction of syncope.
- *Delayed (progressive) orthostatic hypotension* is diagnosed in patients without structural cardiovascular disease in whom the suspicion of orthostatic intolerance

syndrome is confirmed by tilt testing showing induction of progressive orthostatic hypotension.

Additional remarks:

– A negative tilt-table response does not exclude the diagnosis of reflex syncope; the latter is a frequent cause of syncope in tilt-negative patients.
– In patients with structural heart disease, arrhythmias or other cardiovascular cause of syncope should be excluded prior to considering positive tilt test results as diagnostic.
– Induction of syncope in the absence of hypotension and/or bradycardia should be considered diagnostic of psychogenic pseudosyncope.

7.4 ATP (Adenosine) Test

The test requires the rapid (<2 s) injection of a 20 mg bolus of ATP (or adenosine in countries where ATP is not available) during ECG monitoring [18,19] (Fig. 7.7). The induction of AV block with ventricular asystole lasting >6 s[19] or the induction of an AV block lasting >10 s[18] (for this second criterion "escape" beats are ignored) are considered abnormal (Fig. 7.8). ATP testing produced an abnormal response in 28% of patients with syncope of unknown origin (especially older women without structural heart disease), but not in controls, thus suggesting that paroxysmal AV block in such a population could be the cause of unexplained syncope.[19]

The clinical features of adenosine-sensitive patients are different from those of tilt-positive patients.[20] Adenosine-sensitive patients are older with a female predominance and have a shorter history of syncope and a higher prevalence of systemic hypertension. Low adenosine plasma levels are predictive factors for a positive ATP test while high adenosine plasma levels are predictive factor of positive tilt testing, thus supporting the observed clinical differences.[21,22] Low endogenous adenosine values have been found in patients affected by syncope due to otherwise unexpected paroxysmal AV block (so-called "idiopathic paroxysmal block").[22] Nevertheless, recent study showed no correlation between AV block induced by ATP and the ECG findings (documented by ILR) during spontaneous syncope.[17] Thus, while still a controversial point, the low predictive value of the test does not support its use in selecting patients for cardiac pacing. Further studies are needed.

7.4.1 Indications

The ATP test cannot as yet be recommended as a diagnostic test to select patients for cardiac pacing. Its use should for now be limited to research (to investigate the potential role of endogenous adenosine in the mechanisms of syncope).[2,3] Additional studies examining clinical correlations are needed.

The physiology of ATP test

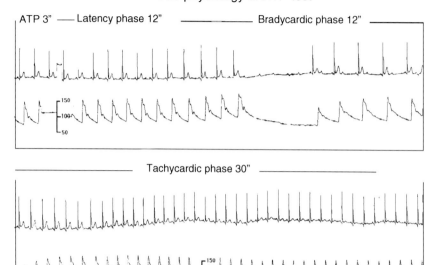

Fig. 7.7 Normal physiology of rapid (<3 s) i.v. injection of a bolus of 20 mg of adenosine with the patient in the supine position. Two continuous strips are shown. Each strip shows continuous electrocardiographic recording (*top*) and blood pressure monitoring (*bottom*). The maximum bradycardic effect after a bolus of ATP usually occurs after 10–20 s (the latency time necessary for the drug to reach the heart); this persists for up to 20 s and is followed by sinus tachycardia for up to 2 min. Hypotension occurs during and immediately after the bradycardic phase and is sometimes followed by moderate hypertension. Facial flushing, shortness of breath, and chest pressure are frequent side effects, but due to the rapid deactivation of the drugs, these are transient and well tolerated by the patient

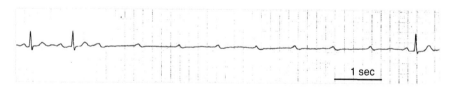

Fig. 7.8 Abnormal ATP (adenosine) test. An AV block with asystole longer than 6 s induced by the rapid injection of a bolus of 20 mg of adenosine in a patient with unexplained syncope. Note constant PP cycle interval

7.4.2 Interpretation of Results

Adenosine-sensitive patients are those who show an abnormal response to injection of a bolus of ATP (adenosine).

7.5 Electrophysiological Study

Electrophysiological study (EPS) is indicated in patients with structural heart disease when, at the initial evaluation, a cardiac arrhythmia (i.e., tachyarrhythmia, bradyarrhythmia, conduction disorder) is suspected to be the cause of syncope.[2,3] The methodology of performing EPS is described in Chapter 20.

The value of EPS in this setting is highly dependent not only on the likelihood of an abnormality (pretest probability) but also on the protocol and the criteria used for diagnosing clinically significant abnormalities. With the exception of patients with supraventricular tachycardias, positive results at EPS occur almost exclusively in patients with overt heart disease or conduction defects. Furthermore, normal EPS findings cannot completely exclude an arrhythmic cause of syncope. When an arrhythmia is likely, further evaluations (for example, long-term ambulatory loop recording) are recommended. Finally, depending on the clinical context, even apparently abnormal EPS findings (e.g., relatively long HV interval, inducible ventricular fibrillation with aggressive stimulation) may be nonspecific and may not be diagnostic of the cause of syncope in a given patient. For the above reasons, the appropriate selection of the patients is crucial. A guide for proper selection can be found in Chapter 5 (see Table 5.3) and in Chapter 6 (Tables 6.2 and 6.3).

EPS exhibits its best diagnostic accuracy in patients with ischemic heart disease, bundle branch block, or syncope preceded by sudden and brief palpitations. Consequently, careful patient selection for EPS evaluation is mandatory. Inappropriate indications increase the risk of false-positive results.

If appropriate indications are applied, EPS will be determined to be warranted in only a small percentage of syncope patients (probably <10% of those with uncertain syncope); in these patients the utility of EPS is good, being diagnostic in about one-third of patients (see Section 7.8).

There are four area conditions in which EPS may be helpful in the evaluation of syncope patients: suspected sinus node disease, bundle branch block (impending high-degree AV block), suspected supraventricular tachycardia, and suspected ventricular tachycardia.

7.5.1 Suspected Sinus Node Disease (SND)

The pretest probability of a transient symptomatic bradycardia as the cause of syncope is relatively high when there is asymptomatic sinus bradycardia (<50 bpm) or sinus pauses in the absence of negatively chronotropic medications (e.g., beta-adrenergic blockers, calcium channel blockers). In general, the diagnosis is most readily established by prolonged ambulatory ECG monitoring (e.g., wearable or insertable loop recorders); the end-point is a correlation between symptoms and bradycardia. EPS is only seldom necessary for this purpose.

A prolonged sinus node recovery time (SNRT) induced by periods of relatively rapid atrial pacing is associated with a higher likelihood of syncope due to sinus arrest or exit block (see also Fig. 20.3). The pause induced by atrial pacing has the same meaning as the spontaneous pause observed at the cessation of a paroxysmal atrial tachyarrhythmia in many SND patients (see also Fig. 20.2). Both indicate an impairment of the automatic properties of a diseased sinus node and therefore its ability to maintain a stable rhythm. In the presence of a prolonged SNRT (SNRT >2 s or corrected SNRT >800 ms), sinus node dysfunction may be the cause of syncope. However, the prognostic value of a prolonged SNRT is largely unknown.[2,3,23]

7.5.2 Bundle Branch Block

In patients with syncope and bifascicular block, documentation of a prolonged HV interval (i.e., >55 ms) denotes a conduction defect localized in the His–Purkinje system and predicts a higher likelihood of progression to high-degree AV block. However, only very prolonged HV intervals (i.e., ≥100 ms) are considered diagnostic, whereas intermediate values have a low specificity usually considered insufficient for diagnosis.[24] In order to increase the diagnostic yield, incremental atrial pacing and pharmacological provocation may be added.[25,26]

The development of intra- or infra-His block during incremental atrial pacing (see also Fig. 20.4) is highly predictive of impending AV block, but again is rarely observed and has low sensitivity. Acute intravenous pharmacological stress testing of the His–Purkinje system has been performed with several class IA antiarrhythmic substances: ajmaline, at a dosage of 1 mg/kg, procainamide at a dosage of 10 mg/kg, and disopyramide at a dosage of 2 mg/kg (see also Fig. 20.5). Provocation of high-degree AV block with drug challenge can be expected in 15% of patients. Overall, by combining the above-noted procedures, the positive predictive value of EPS is >80%. Nevertheless, development of permanent AV block was also observed in about 20% of patients with negative test within a few years, and paroxysmal AV block was documented by implantable loop recorder in 33% of patients within 15 months.[2] These latter results suggest that a negative EPS cannot be considered conclusive, and further investigations (i.e., implantable loop recorder) are likely to be needed (see Chapter 8).

Importantly, a high incidence of total deaths and sudden death is observed in patients with bundle branch block. However, neither syncope nor a prolonged HV interval is associated with a higher risk of death, and pacemaker therapy does not decrease this risk. The mechanism of sudden death is therefore supposedly due to a ventricular tachyarrhythmia or electromechanical dissociation rather than a bradyarrhythmia. A sustained ventricular tachyarrhythmia is frequently inducible in patients with bundle branch block by means of programmed ventricular stimulation. Nevertheless, clinical events during follow-up are not predicted by programmed ventricular stimulation, so such testing cannot be considered reliable to stratify the patients.[27]

7.5.3 Suspected Supraventricular Tachycardia

In patients with syncope preceded by sudden and brief palpitations, the induction during EPS of a rapid supraventricular arrhythmia reproducing hypotensive or spontaneous symptoms is usually considered diagnostic. Symptom reproduction may require induction of the arrhythmia with the patient in an upright posture on a tilt table. However, with modern ambulatory ECG monitoring, EPS is rarely necessary for diagnosis. EPS is primarily indicated if a therapeutic procedure, i.e., catheter ablation of the culprit-suspected arrhythmia, is being planned during the same session.

7.5.4 Suspected Ventricular Tachycardia

Inducibility of sustained monomorphic ventricular tachycardia and/or very depressed systolic function are the two strongest predictors of a life-threatening arrhythmia being the cause of syncope. Conversely, their absence suggests a more favorable etiology, but one which must be sought by other means such as long-term ECG recording.

EPS with programmed electrical stimulation (PES) to unmask ventricular tachyarrhythmias is an effective diagnostic test in patients with coronary artery disease, markedly depressed cardiac function (including bundle branch reentry in dilated cardiomyopathy), and unexplained syncope (see also Fig. 20.8). However, patients with heart failure and an established indication for ICD therapy according to current guidelines should receive this therapy before and independently of the evaluation of the mechanism of syncope. This is the case, for example, in patients with ischemic or dilated cardiomyopathy and low ejection fraction (<30% or 35% and NYHA class ≥ 2). Apart from these latter cases, the induction at EPS of monomorphic ventricular tachycardia is thought to be a specific finding that should guide therapy; conversely, noninducibility predicts a low risk of sudden death and ventricular arrhythmias. For example, in the ESVEM trial,[28] syncope, associated with induced ventricular tachyarrhythmias at EPS, indicated high risk of death, similar to that of patients with documented spontaneous ventricular tachyarrhythmias. The predictive value of EPS has been confirmed by studies in ICD patients which showed a good correlation between recurrent syncope and spontaneous ventricular tachyarrhythmias and an appropriate ICD discharge rate similar to that of the patients with documented spontaneous ventricular tachycardia.[29–31] On the other hand, the induction of polymorphic ventricular tachycardia and/or ventricular fibrillation has low specificity and is of no value in risk stratification and therapeutic decisions (see also Fig. 20.9).

EPS has a low predictive value in patients with non-ischemic dilated cardiomyopathy, and its use is discouraged.[32] Similarly, EPS studies appear unhelpful in identifying whether ventricular arrhythmia is the cause of syncope in patients with hypertrophic cardiomyopathy. For example, Kuck et al.[33] studied 54 consecutive patients with hypertrophic cardiomyopathy. The type and incidence of induced ventricular arrhythmias did not differ between the "symptomatic (syncope)" and the "asymptomatic (no syncope)" groups. Similarly, EPS was of no value in identifying patients at risk of tachyarrhythmias in patients with arrhythmogenic right ventricular dysplasia/cardiomyopathy (ARVC) and syncope (positive predictive value 49%, negative predictive value 54%).[34] On the other hand, although very controversial, EPS has been advocated for stratification of risk in patients affected by Brugada syndrome independently from the presence of syncope.[35–38] The inducibility of ventricular tachyarrhythmias is similar in patients with and without syncope. There are no data on its use for the diagnosis of unexplained syncope in Brugada syncope and in long QT syndrome.

In conclusion, EPS is indicated only in patients with undocumented syncope, coronary artery disease, and depressed systolic function. In these patients the inducibility of sustained monomorphic ventricular tachycardia is considered strong enough evidence to be diagnostic of the cause of the syncope; furthermore, inability to induce such a tachyarrhythmia predicts a more favorable outcome.

7.5.5 Indications

EPS is appropriate in patients in whom cardiac syncope seems likely and in whom there is evidence of[2,3]

- ischemic heart disease, unless there is already an established indication for an ICD,
- bundle branch block,
- (rarely) suspected sinus node dysfunction,
- (rarely) syncope is preceded by sudden and brief palpitations if prolonged ECG monitoring is inconclusive (i.e., probable paroxysmal supraventricular or ventricular tachycardia).

7.5.6 Interpretation of Results

Electrophysiological findings are able to establish the cause of syncope (and therefore to guide specific therapy) in case of[2,3]

- sinus bradycardia and very prolonged SNRT (SNRT >2 s or corrected SNRT >800 ms),
- bundle brunch block and either a baseline HV interval of ≥ 100 ms or second- or third-degree His–Purkinje block demonstrated during incremental atrial pacing or with pharmacological challenge,
- induction of sustained monomorphic VT in patients with previous myocardial infarction or bundle branch reentry in dilated cardiomyopathy,

- induction of rapid supraventricular tachycardia which reproduces hypotensive or spontaneous symptoms (often only observed if the patient is upright on a tilt table).

Other abnormal findings are of uncertain interpretation, and usually further tests (i.e., implantable loop recorder) are required for diagnosis. This is, for example, the case in

- bundle brunch block and HV interval between 70 and 100 ms,
- induction of polymorphic VT or ventricular fibrillation in patients with Brugada syndrome, arrhythmogenic right ventricular cardiomyopathy, or hypertrophic cardiomyopathy.

7.6 Exercise Testing

Exercise testing is indicated in patients who experience syncope during or shortly after exertion. The following two situations may be responsible for exercise-related syncope and should be separately considered.[39-41]

- Syncope occurring during exercise in the presence of structural heart disease (including preexcitation syndromes) is likely to have a cardiac cause. Tachycardia-related (phase 3), exercise-induced second- and third-degree AV block has been shown to be invariably located in the His–Purkinje system and is an ominous finding of progression to chronic AV block. The resting ECG frequently shows an intraventricular conduction abnormality. Myocardial ischemia is an important part of the differential diagnosis.
- Post-exertional syncope (either purely hypotensive or hypotensive and bradycardic) is almost invariably due to autonomic failure or to a neurally mediated reflex mechanism. Hypotensive syncope may rarely also occur during exercise as a manifestation of an exaggerated reflex vasodilatation in healthy subjects without structural heart disease. In this regard, syncope in athletes (including potential student athletes) is a particularly important problem. In the absence of structural heart disease, syncope occurring during or immediately after exercise in athletes is usually a benign condition, with a good long-term outcome. However, detailed evaluation is essential. The likely final diagnosis is neurally mediated reflex syncope.

Exercise-induced syncope, as defined above, is rare. As consequence exercise testing is only seldom needed in the evaluation of syncope, and even when it is used it is only infrequently diagnostic. Nevertheless, if exercise reproduces syncope, the finding can be a guide to direct specific therapy.

More often, such as in patients with symptoms suggesting angina, stress testing (and coronary angiography if appropriate) is recommended soon after the initial evaluation to assess underlying comorbidities that may directly or indirectly relate to the development of syncope. This indication (i.e., assessing comorbidities) is the most frequent indication for exercise testing in syncope patients. Used in this way, however, exercise testing is part of the evaluation of a comorbidity, and even if positive, such a test result cannot be considered diagnostic of the cause of the syncope; the evaluation should continue. Overall, exercise testing is appropriate in <10% of patients with uncertain syncope (see Section 7.8).

7.6.1 Indications

Exercise testing is indicated in patients who

- experience syncope during or shortly after exertion,
- in patients with preexcitation syndrome in whom the antegrade conduction properties of an accessory connection are in need of assessment, and
- in patients with chest pain suggestive of ischemic heart disease (e.g., coronary artery disease, congenital coronary anomalies).[2,3]

7.6.2 Interpretation of Results

- The development of a tachycardia-mediated Mobitz II second-degree or third-degree AV block during exercise, even if asymptomatic, is diagnostic of the cause of syncope.
- The development of a hypotension–bradycardia (pre-) syncope immediately after exercise is diagnostic of reflex syncope.
- Development of hypotension and syncope or presyncope with exercise but without bradycardia (often with a relatively "fixed" heart rate or only limited exercise-induced tachycardia) suggests autonomic failure as a cause of syncope.
- A positive ischemic response is not diagnostic of the cause of syncope (but provides direction for further evaluation).
- Evidence of a short antegrade refractory period of an accessory connection is not diagnostic of a syncope etiology, but may provide important supportive information.

7.7 Other Tests

Other (non-provocative) tests may be helpful to investigate the underlying substrate which may be responsible for or predispose to syncope. Their utility is in general limited to the evaluation of severe forms of syncope which, at initial evaluation, are suspected to be secondary to acute structural cardiac and cardiovascular disease. The most useful, echocardiography, is already part of the initial evaluation; the indications and interpretation of its results are reviewed in Chapter 5.

Transoesophageal echocardiography, computed tomography, magnetic resonance imaging, and pulmonary scintigraphy may be performed in selected cases when certain cardiac or vascular pathology is suspected of triggering syncope and transthoracic echocardiography alone has not been diagnostic. Such abnormalities include aortic dissection and hematoma, pulmonary embolism, cardiac masses, and pericardial and myocardial diseases. In particular, a suspected diagnosis of pulmonary embolism and syncope sometimes can only be confirmed by computed tomography or magnetic resonance imaging or pulmonary scintigraphy.

In patients with syncope suspected to be due, directly or indirectly, to myocardial ischemia, coronary angiography is recommended in order to confirm the diagnosis and stratify the risk of the patient. However, as was the case with exercise testing discussed above, even a positive response cannot be considered diagnostic of the exact mechanism of syncope in most cases; further assessment is usually needed. However, evidence of severe ischemia justifies the diagnosis of *cardiac ischemia-related syncope* and, if the anatomy is favorable, is an indication for revascularization therapy.

With the wider utilization of echocardiography, computed tomography, and magnetic resonance imaging, chest X-ray has very limited utility evaluation of syncope. Conversely, the role of genetic testing, while still ill-defined, is expanding and such testing will likely become a very important diagnostic tool.

Certain tests are not considered useful, and should only rarely be employed, in the syncope evaluation. The most notable of these are neurological studies such as head imaging (magnetic resonance [MR] or computed tomography [CT]) or electroencephalography (EEG). Of course, imaging may be needed if there is concern that a faint or fall may have resulted in an intracranial injury. Similarly, video-EEG monitoring may be valuable in rare cases in which differentiating syncope and seizure remains a problem. Abdominal ultrasound examination has no utility for the evaluation of syncope. Finally, abdominal echocardiography, vascular ultrasound, or abdominal CT/MR are not generally helpful in the evaluation of syncope. Nevertheless, such testing may be needed to assess pain syndromes that may trigger syncope in some patients (e.g., cholelithiasis, aortic dissection).

7.8 Diagnostic Yield of Laboratory Tests in Patients with Uncertain Syncope

About a half of the patients with uncertain syncope have a diagnosis established by laboratory tests. Most of these have reflex syncope diagnosed by tilt-table testing or carotid sinus massage. Only few patients are diagnosed with cardiac syncope by means of cardiac or vascular tests; the percentage depends on the setting, ranging from 2% of outpatients referred to a specialized syncope unit[42] to 9% of patients seen in the emergency department[43] and to 13% of patients referred to a cardiology department.[44] In any case, it seems that laboratory tests play a minor role in diagnosing cardiac syncope. When standardized criteria based on the appropriateness

Table 7.4 Diagnostic yield of the most used laboratory tests for diagnosis of uncertain etilology in two different clinical settings

	Emergency department (a) (175 pts)			Syncope unit (b) (673 pts)		
	Performed % patients	Diagnostic % tests	NND	Performed % patients	Diagnostic % tests	NND
Tilt testing	76 (43%)	46 (61%)	1.6	443 (66%)	237 (53%)	1.9
Carotid sinus massage	65 (37%)	18 (28%)	3.6	509 (76%)	62 (12%)	8.2
Exercise test	10 (6%)	3 (30%)	3.3	41 (6%)	1 (2%)	41
Electrophysiological study	15 (9%)	3 (30%)	3	40 (6%)	14 (35%)	2.9
Coronary angiography	8 (5%)	5 (62%)	1.6	14 (2%)	1 (7%)	14
Pulmonary computed tomography/Scintigraphy	5 (3%)	4 (80%)	1.2	–	–	–
Total (mean tests per patient)	181 (1.0)	79 (43%)	2.2	1,047 (1.6)	315 (30%)	3.3

NND, number needed for diagnosis
Source: (a) = Evaluation of Guidelines in Syncope Study 2 (EGSYS-2) study, (b) = Syncope Unit Project (SUP) study

Table 7.5 Case mix of diagnoses obtained with laboratory tests in two different clinical settings

	Emergency department (a) (175 pts)	Syncope unit (b) (673 pts)
Patients with a diagnosis established by laboratory tests:	79 (45%)	315 (47%)
–Reflex: tilt induced	38 (22%)	231 (34%)
–Reflex: carotid sinus syndrome	18 (10%)	61 (9%)
–Orthostatic hypotension	8 (5%)	7 (1%)
–Cardiac (arrhythmic, structural)	15 (9%)	16 (2%)

Source: (a) = Evaluation of Guidelines in Syncope Study 2 (EGSYS-2) study, (b) = Syncope Unit Project (SUP) study

of indications are used, only a few selected cardiac tests need to be performed in a minority of patients (Tables 7.4 and 7.5). The most helpful are those that provide long-term ECG monitoring such as insertable loop recorders (ILRs) and mobile cardiac outpatient telemetry (MCOT) capability.

7.9 Clinical Perspectives

In this chapter we describe the indications for and the interpretation of the most commonly performed laboratory tests for the diagnosis of syncope. When needed, these tests are usually performed shortly after the initial evaluation, as discussed in Chapter 5 (see Table 5.2).

Provocative tests are aimed at reproducing syncope or related abnormalities in an artificial setting (i.e., laboratory). Tilt-table testing and carotid sinus massage are probably the best examples of such testing. The assumption is that the positive response to the test reproduces the mechanism of spontaneous episode. Nevertheless, the sensitivity and specificity of any of these tests are difficult to measure due to the lack of a reference or "gold standard" in most cases. Since false-positive responses are not uncommon, the interpretation of a positive response requires the knowledge of the clinical context in which spontaneous syncope occurred; in more scientific terms, the pretest probability largely influences the interpretation of a positive response. In other words, some uncertainty on the cause of syncope still remains even after a positive test.

Many other tests are available to investigate the underlying substrate which is thought to be responsible for or predisposes to loss of consciousness. Their utility is in general limited to the evaluation of severe forms of syncope secondary to acute structural cardiac and cardiovascular diseases.

In Chapter 8 we describe the indications for and the interpretation of ambulatory ECG monitoring (Holter, external loop recorders, remote at-home telemetry, and implantable loop recorders) in the syncope assessment. Diagnosing syncope by means of ECG monitoring requires the documentation of a spontaneous event. Such documentation provides reliable evidence of diagnostic accuracy. Nevertheless, this strategy has two important disadvantages. First, diagnosis (and therapy) is delayed, often for a long time (months or even years), until an event can be documented; this implies that the patients remain at risk of injury or on occasion even life-threatening events until a convincing cause is documented. Second, since current technology allows only ECG signal recording, an ECG monitoring strategy is of diagnostic value only to patients in whom an arrhythmia is the likely cause of syncope. Vasodepressor syncope, absent any concomitant ECG changes, cannot yet be confirmed by monitoring strategies.

Neurological laboratory tests are almost never useful for establishing a basis of syncope, but may be needed in non-syncope T-LOC patients (i.e., epilepsy, dysautonomic syndromes). These tests are part of the neurological evaluation and will be described in Chapter 14.

References

1. Thomas JE. Hyperactive carotid sinus reflex and carotid sinus syncope. *Mayo Clin Proc.* 1969;44:127–139.
2. Brignole M, et al. Guidelines on management (diagnosis and treatment) of syncope: Update 2004. *Europace.* 2004;6:467–537.
3. Moya A, et al. Guidelines for the diagnosis and management of syncope (Version 2009). *Eur Heart J.* 2009;30:2631–2671.
4. Kerr SR, et al. Carotid sinus hypersensitivity in asymptomatic older persons: implications for diagnosis of syncope and falls. *Arch Intern Med.* 2006;166:515–520.
5. Puggioni E, et al. Results and complications of the carotid sinus massage performed according to the 'methods of symptoms. *Am J Cardiol.* 2002;89:599–601.

6. Brignole M, et al. Long-term outcome of paced and non paced patients with severe carotid sinus syndrome. *Am J Cardiol.* 1992;69:1039–1043.

7. Claesson JE, et al. Less syncope and milder symptoms in patients treated with pacing for induced cardioinhibitory carotid sinus syndrome: a randomized study. *Europace.* 2007;9: 932–936.

8. Menozzi C, et al. Follow-up of asystolic episodes in patients with cardioinhibitory, neurally mediated syncope and VVI pacemaker. *Am J Cardiol.* 1993;72:1152–1155.

9. Maggi R, et al. Cardioinhibitory carotid sinus hypersensitivity predicts an asystolic mechanism of spontaneous neurally-mediated syncope. *Europace.* 2007;9:563–567.

10. Davies AG, Kenny RA. Neurological complications following carotid sinus massage. *Am J Cardiol.* 1998;81:1256–1257.

11. Naschitz J, Rosner I. Orthostatic hypotension: Framework of the syndrome. *Postgrad Med J.* 2007;83:568–574.

12. Ward C, Kenny RA. Reproducibility of orthostatic hypotension in symptomatic elderly. *Am J Med.* 1996;100:418–422.

13. The Consensus Committee of the American Autonomic Society and the American Academy of Neurology. Consensus statement on the definition of orthostatic hypotension, pure autonomic failure, and multiple system atrophy. *Neurology.* 1996;46(5):1470.

14. Almquist A, et al. Provocation of bradycardia and hypotension by isoproterenol and upright posture in patients with unexplained syncope. *N Engl J Med.* 1989;320:346–351.

15. Benditt DG, et al. Tilt table testing for assessing syncope. ACC expert consensus document. *J Am Coll Cardiol.* 1996;28:263–275.

16. Bartoletti A, et al. The Italian Protocol': a simplified head-up tilt testing potentiated with oral nitroglycerin to assess patients with unexplained syncope. *Europace.* 2000;2:339–342.

17. Brignole M, et al. Lack of correlation between the responses to tilt testing and adenosine triphosphate test and the mechanism of spontaneous neurally mediated syncope. *Eur Heart J.* 2006;27:2232–2239.

18. Flammang D, et al. Contribution of head-up tilt test and ATP testing in assessing the mechanisms of vasovagal syndrome: preliminary results and potential therapeutic implications. *Circulation.* 1999;99:2427–2433.

19. Brignole M, et al. Adenosine-induced atrioventricular block in patients with unexplained syncope. The diagnostic value of ATP test. *Circulation.* 1997;96:3921–3927.

20. Brignole M, et al. Clinical features of adenosine sensitive syncope and tilt induced vasovagal syncope. *Heart.* 2000;83:24–28.

21. Saadjian A, et al. Role of endogenous adenosine as a modulator of syncope induced during tilt testing. *Circulation.* 2002;106:569–574.

22. Brignole M, et al. Syncope due to idiopathic paroxysmal AV block: long-term follow-up of a distinct form of AV block. *J Am Coll Cardiol.* 2011(in press).

23. Benditt DG, et al. Indications for electrophysiological testing in diagnosis and assessment of sinus node dysfunction. *Circulation.* 1987; 75(suppl III):93–99.

24. Scheinman MM, et al. Value of the H-Q interval in patients with bundle branch block and the role of prophylactic permanent pacing. *Am J Cardiol.* 1982;50:1316–1322.

25. Kaul U, et al. Evaluation of patients with bundle branch block and "unexplained" syncope: a study based on comprehensive electrophysiologic testing and ajmaline stress. *Pacing Clin Electrophysiol.* 1988;11:289–297.

26. Gaggioli G, et al. Progression to second or third-degree atrioventricular block in patients electrostimulated for bundle branch block: a long-term study. *G Ital Cardiol.* 1994;24: 409–416.

27. Englund A, et al. Diagnostic value of programmed ventricular stimulation in patients with bifascicular block: a prospective study of patients with and without syncope. *J Am Coll Cardiol.* 1995;26:1508–1515.

28. Olshansky B, et al. Clinical significance of syncope in the electrophysiologic study versus electrocardiographic monitoring (ESVEM) trial. *Am Heart J.* 1999;137:878–886.

29. Link MS, et al. High incidence of appropriate implantable cardioverter-defibrillator therapy in patients with syncope of unknown etiology and inducible ventricular tachycardia. *J Am Coll Cardiol*. 1997;29:370–375.

30. Pires L, et al. Comparison of event rates and survival in patients with unexplained syncope without documented ventricular tachyarrhythmias versus patients with documented sustained ventricular tachyarrhythmias both treated with implantable cardioverter-defibrillator. *Am J Cardiol*. 2000;85:725–728.

31. Andrews N, et al. Implantable defibrillator event rates in patients with unexplained syncope and inducible sustained ventricular tachyarrhythmias. *J Am Coll Cardiol*. 1999;34: 2023–2030.

32. Brilakis E, et al. Role of programmed ventricular stimulation and implantable cardioverter defibrillators in patients with idiopathic dilated cardiomyopathy and syncope. *Pacing Clin Electrophysiol*. 2001;24:1623–1630.

33. Kuck KH, et al. Programmed electrical stimulation in hypertrophic cardiomyopathy. Results in patients with and without cardiac arrest or syncope. *Eur Heart J*. 1988;9:177–185.

34. Corrado D, et al. Implantable cardioverter-defibrillator therapy for prevention of sudden death in patients with arrhythmogenic right ventricular cardiomyopathy/dysplasia. *Circulation*. 2003;108:3084–3091.

35. Antzelevitch C, et al. Brugada syndrome: report of the second consensus conference: endorsed by the heart rhythm society and the European heart rhythm association circulation. 2005;111:659–670.

36. Paul M, et al. Role of programmed ventricular stimulation in patients with Brugada syndrome: a meta-analysis of worldwide published data. *Eur Heart J*. 2007;28:2126–2133.

37. Sacher F, et al. Outcome after implantation of a cardioverter-defibrillator in patients with Brugada syndrome: a multicenter study. *Circulation*. 2006;114:2317–2324.

38. Probst V, et al. Long-term prognosis of patients diagnosed with Brugada syndrome: Results from the FINGER Brugada Syndrome Registry. *Circulation*. 2010;121:635–643.

39. Woeifel AK, et al. Exercise-induced distal atrio-ventricular block. *J Am Coll Cardiol*. 1983;2:578–582.

40. Colivicchi F, et al. Exercise-related syncope in young competitive athletes without evidence of structural heart disease: clinical presentation and long-term outcome. *Eur Heart J*. 2002;23:1125–1130.

41. Sakaguchi S, et al. Syncope associated with exercise, a manifestation of neurally mediated syncope. *Am J Cardiol*. 1995;75:476–481.

42. Brignole M, et al. Prospective multicentre systematic guideline-based management of patients referred to the Syncope Units of general hospitals. *Europace*. 2010;12:109–118.

43. Brignole M, et al. A new management of syncope: prospective systematic guideline-based evaluation of patients referred urgently to general hospitals. *Eur Heart J*. 2006;27:76–82.

44. Croci F, et al. The application of a standardized strategy of evaluation in patients with syncope referred to three syncope units. *Europace*. 2002;4:357–360.

Chapter 8
Prolonged Ambulatory ECG Diagnostic Monitoring . . . Current and Evolving Indications

Contents

Key points: Identifying the mechanism of syncope of uncertain cause by means of prolonged ECG monitoring

- Holter monitors, external loop recorders, remote telemetry (mobile cardiac outpatient telemetry, MCOT), and implantable loop recorders (ILRs) are currently the available prolonged ambulatory monitoring systems used

M. Brignole, D.G. Benditt, *Syncope*, DOI 10.1007/978-0-85729-201-8_8,
© Springer-Verlag London Limited 2011

for diagnosis of uncertain syncope. The diagnostic criteria are the same; the expected duration of monitoring needed for diagnosis determines the choice of the system.

- Be aware that the pretest selection of the patients influences the subsequent findings. Consequently, the most cost-effective application of ambulatory ECG monitors is in patients with a high likelihood of arrhythmic events.
- Exclude high-risk patients, i.e., those with a clear indication for ICD, pacemaker, or other treatments independent of a definite diagnosis of the cause of syncope.
- Include patients with a high probability of recurrence of syncope during the expected duration of monitoring and select the monitoring system (i.e., the duration of monitoring) according to the probability that a symptom recurrence will occur during the monitoring period.
- Due to the unpredictability of syncope recurrences, be prepared to wait for a substantial time before obtaining an ECG–symptom correlation.
- The ideal goal should be to obtain a correlation between ECG findings and syncope relapse. Weaker end-points are non-syncopal arrhythmias.
- While Holter monitoring and external loop recorders (with the exception of MCOT systems) have limited value in diagnosing syncope, the ILR with its ease of use and long recording duration (currently up to 3 years) has the potential to become the reference standard for establishing a diagnosis in patients with syncope of uncertain etiology. MCOT and ILRs offering wireless transmission of data are particularly desirable.
- ILRs seems to be largely underused in current clinical practice.

8.1 Introduction

In this chapter we describe the role of various prolonged ambulatory ECG monitoring systems (i.e., Holter monitor, external loop recorders [ELR], remote telemetry – mobile cardiac outpatient telemetry [MCOT], and implantable loop recorders [ILR]) in the diagnostic evaluation of patients with syncope of uncertain cause (i.e., syncope that remains of uncertain nature after the initial evaluation).

Diagnosing syncope by means of ECG monitoring requires the documentation of a spontaneous event. The correlation of ECG recordings with symptoms provides the strongest evidence of a relationship between syncope and a recorded arrhythmia; conversely, syncope absent a recorded arrhythmia eliminates an arrhythmic etiology. In either case the evidence is stronger than can be obtained by any laboratory tests. As a consequence, the knowledge of the probabilities of syncope recurrence within the operational duration of the devices (in general 1–7 days for

Table 8.1 Diagnostic power of different monitoring systems used in patients with syncope

	Average operational duration of monitoring (days)	
In-hospital monitoring	1–7	Same diagnostic criteria
Holter monitoring	1–7	
External loop recorder	30	
Remote (MCOT) telemetry	30	
Implantable loop recorder	1,000	

Holter monitoring, 4 weeks for external ELR/MCOT devices, and up to 3 years for implantable loop recorders [ILRs]) is crucial for appropriate selection of the monitoring device (Table 8.1).

As the name suggests, ECG loop recorders have a retrospective (loop) memory which continuously records and deletes one or two channels of ECG rhythm recording (first in–first out) in such a way that several minutes of recording is preserved and can be retrieved to document onset of a symptom episode. The patient activates the loop recorder once he/she recovers from loss of consciousness; the loop memory allows retrieval of ECG data from prior to onset of symptoms provided that the time of activation is within the "looping" memory duration of the device. The retrospective memory differentiates loop recorders from prospective-only *external event recorders.*

Event recorders are external devices which may be applied by the patient when symptoms occur or may be worn continuously, but recording is only triggered by the patient when symptoms begin. While event recorders have some usefulness in patients with intermittent palpitations, they have little value in the syncope assessment as most patients are unable to trigger the device in a timely fashion before they faint. Recently, newer technological advances offer certain external ambulatory ECG systems that are able to provide continuous ECG recording – i.e., remote telemetry. This so-called mobile cardiac outpatient telemetry (MCOT; Cardionet Inc., PA, USA, and Nuvant, Corventis Inc., San Jose, CA, USA) offers loop memory with wireless transmission (real time) to a service center. The service center reviews all recordings and immediately contacts the responsible physician if certain worrisome ECG criteria are exceeded. Otherwise, the physician receives a report during usual business hours.

As a general rule prolonged ambulatory ECG monitoring is indicated only when there is a high pretest probability of identifying an arrhythmia responsible for syncope. Short-term monitoring (usually several days) is warranted in patients at high risk of potentially life-threatening arrhythmias and in those who are likely to have early event recurrence. Conversely, patients at low risk with very infrequent syncope, recurring over months or years, are suitable candidates for longer term ECG monitoring such as MCOT or ILR.[1,2]

8.2 Interpretation of Results

Since an ECG diagnosis in a syncope patient requires the documentation of a spontaneous event, the diagnostic criteria are the same whichever monitoring system is used. There is general consensus that[1,2]:

- ECG monitoring is diagnostic when a correlation between syncope and an arrhythmia (brady- or tachyarrhythmia) is detected.
- Even in the absence of such correlation, ECG monitoring is diagnostic if:
    - periods of Mobitz II or third-degree AV block or a ventricular pause > 3 s are detected; possible exceptions are the cases of young physically well-trained persons, during sleep, medicated patients, or rate-controlled atrial fibrillation,
    - rapid prolonged paroxysmal SVT or VT (arbitrarily defined as ≥ 160 bpm for > 30 beats) are detected.

- ECG monitoring excludes an arrhythmic cause when there is no correlation between syncope and rhythm variation (i.e., typical syncope occurs and no arrhythmia is present at the time) as is often the case in vasodepressor form of reflex syncope. Though not properly diagnostic in this case, this finding provides a basis for terminating further arrhythmia investigations and instituting investigation of non-arrhythmic causes including vasodepressor forms of the neurally mediated reflex faints. On the other hand, ECG documentation of presyncope (near syncope) without any relevant arrhythmia is not an accurate surrogate for syncope and should not be used to definitively exclude an arrhythmic event; thus, in this case, in these latter cases ECG monitoring should be continued.
- Episodes of sinus bradycardia (in absence of syncope) and asymptomatic arrhythmias (other than those listed above) are not a surrogate for syncope; indeed, several studies have shown only a weak correlation with the mechanism of syncope when syncope was subsequently documented in the same patients. Thus, monitoring should also be continued in these cases. Admittedly, in real-world practice, there is occasionally the need to make a therapeutic decision even with weaker diagnostic criteria. Physicians should be aware that effectiveness of therapy is not well documented in such cases.

8.3 In-Hospital Monitoring

In-hospital monitoring (in bed or telemetric) is warranted, as part of the initial evaluation, when the patient is considered, by risk stratification techniques, to be at high risk of life-threatening arrhythmias (see also Chapter 5). A few days of ECG monitoring may be of value in patients with clinical features or ECG abnormalities suggesting a potentially life-threatening form of arrhythmic syncope such as those listed in Tables 5.3 and 5.6, especially if the monitoring is applied immediately after a syncopal faint. Furthermore, it is general experience that syncope is more likely to recur within a few hours or days after the index event either in patients affected by primary cardiac arrhythmias or when reflex syncope occurs in a cluster. The above situations justify early usage of prolonged in-hospital monitoring in few selected patients (Table 5.7).

8.3.1 Indications

Immediate in-hospital monitoring (in bed or telemetric) is warranted, as part on the initial evaluation, when patients have clinical features suggesting an arrhythmic cause that is potentially life-threatening.[1,2]

8.4 Holter Monitoring

The vast majority of patients have a syncope-free interval measured in weeks, months, or years, but not in days; therefore, symptom–ECG correlation is only rarely achieved with conventional 24- or 48-h Holter monitoring. In an overview[3] of the results of eight studies of ambulatory ECG monitoring in syncope patients, only 4% of patients had correlation of symptoms with arrhythmia. The true yield of conventional ECG monitoring in syncope may be as low as 1–2% in an unselected population. Furthermore, since many of these "diagnoses" were based on the documentation of asymptomatic minor arrhythmias it was likely that the basis of syncope was not correct and that the proposed therapy was inappropriate and ineffective, e.g., pacemaker implantation in a patient with neurally mediated reflex syncope due to detection of bradycardia on Holter monitoring. Thus, extensive utilization of Holter monitoring yields a very low diagnostic power and should be discouraged.

Conversely, Holter monitoring in syncope may be of more value if symptoms are very frequent, especially if it is applied soon after the index episodes as well as during in-hospital monitoring in the absence of a "full disclosure" in-hospital recording system (Table 8.2). There are consistent data from some studies which show that Holter yields a good diagnostic power when applied to few cases selected according to criteria like those listed in Tables 5.3 and 5.6.

8.4.1 Indications

- One to seven days of full disclosure ECG monitoring using a Holter system is useful, soon after the index episode, in selected patients at low risk who have very frequent syncopes or presyncopes ($\geq$1/week) or have a history suggesting syncopes occurring in clusters.
- A generalized use of Holter monitoring is not useful, owing to the low probability to detect a diagnostic episode during the operational period of recording.

Table 8.2 Diagnostic yield of different systems for prolonged ECG monitoring for diagnosis of uncertain syncope in two different clinical settings

	Emergency department (a) (175 pts)			Syncope unit (b) (673 pts)		
	Performed % patients	Diagnostic % tests	NND	Performed % patients	Diagnostic % tests	NND
24-h Holter monitoring (%)	12 (7%)	3 (25%)	4	166 (25%)	15 (9%)	11
External loop recorder (%)	4 (2%)	2 (50%)	2	9 (1%)	0 (0%)	na
Implantable loop recorder	3 (2%)	Delayed	na	30 (4%)	Delayed	na
Total (mean tests per patient)	19 (11%)	na	na	205 (30%)	na	na

NND = number needed for diagnosis (number of patients tested every one patient diagnosed)
Source: (a) = Evaluation of Guidelines in Syncope Study 2 (EGSYS-2) study[29], (b) = Syncope Unit Project (SUP) study[30]
na, not available.

8.5 External Loop Recorder (ELR) and Remote At-Home Telemetry

The ELR appears to have its greatest role in motivated patients with frequent syncope or pre-syncope where spontaneous symptoms are likely to recur within 4–6 weeks. This time frame is usually the maximum that a patient can comply with wearable ELRs; shorter duration results in a lower diagnostic yield. Even if ELRs are indicated in selected patients, they are probably underused in the clinical practice; unfortunately physicians still tend to order (or are forced to order based on cost considerations) Holter recordings, although they are in fact of lesser cost-effectiveness (Table 8.2). In a randomized comparison study, ELRs proved to yield a higher diagnostic value than Holter monitoring (Table 8.3); indeed, only 21% of diagnoses were made within 48 h (i.e., the usual time frame of Holter), whereas 50% were made by 15 days and 90% by 33 days (the latter periods being well within the capability of ELRs and MCOT).[4]

Since palpitations recur more frequently than syncopes, ELRs are much more useful for palpitation evaluation than for syncope evaluation. In a consecutive series of 125 patients referred to the syncope unit of Ospedali del Tigullio, affected by recurrent palpitations or pre-syncope or syncope, all with an inter-symptom interval ≤4 weeks, ELRs were applied in 86%, 8%, and 6% of cases, respectively. The ECG–symptom correlation rate was similar in those with palpitations, pre-syncope, and syncope, being 73%, 50%, and 60%, respectively.

Since true syncope usually recurs unpredictably over months or years, the indications for ELR and MCOT are limited to patients with high probability of recurrence in that time period. The diagnostic yield in such patients is quite low. In one study,[5]

Table 8.3 Diagnostic yield of external ambulatory monitoring systems

Author	System	Target	Arrhythmia excluded* (%)	Arrhythmia identified (%)
Schuchert et al.[5]	ELR	Syncope recurrence	4	0
Sivakumaran et al.[4]	Holter	Patient-activated symptoms	22	0
Sivakumaran et al.[4]	ELR	Patient-activated symptoms	56	1
Linzer et al.[6]	ELR	Patient-activated symptoms	16	9
Rothman et al.[7]	ELR	Patient-activated symptoms	25	15
Rothman et al.[7]	MCOT	Patient-activated symptoms and auto-triggered arrhythmias	14	27
Olson et al.[8]	MCOT	Patient-activated symptoms and auto-triggered arrhythmias	24	24

MCOT, mobile cardiac outpatient telemetry (remote at-home telemetry)
[a] No arrhythmia documented at the time of symptom recurrence

among 24 patients with a mean of three episodes during the previous 6 months and no structural heart disease, only one syncopal episode could be recorded by ELR and that recording showed only sinus tachycardia (Table 8.3).

ELRs proved to be more useful when frequent pre-syncopal symptoms were considered in addition to true syncopal episodes and less specific positivity criteria are used, mainly in order to exclude an arrhythmic cause of symptoms (Table 8.3). Indeed, while an arrhythmia was identified as a possible cause of syncope in 1–15% of patients, an arrhythmia could be excluded in 22–56% of patients.[4–6]

There is less experience with the newer auto-triggered ELRs and with remote MCOT systems. The MCOT systems provide automatic ECG detection (and transmission) of predefined events or even continuous or 24-h loop memory, thus potentially increasing the diagnostic power of the traditional ELRs. MCOT systems usually offer a central diagnostic center to overview the recording before notifying the physician.

With the new auto-triggered devices, many asymptomatic arrhythmias are usually recorded (Table 8.3). It should be stressed that, in absence of correlation with syncopal events, the positive predictive value of most asymptomatic arrhythmias is unknown in terms of establishing a syncope diagnosis; whenever possible monitoring should be continued until a diagnosis is confirmed by symptom documentation.

8.5.1 Indications

- ELR and MCOT systems are useful and more effective alternatives to Holter monitoring in most syncope evaluations. They are recommended for application soon after the index episode, in selected patients at low risk who have frequent syncope or presyncope (≥1/week) or have a history suggesting syncope occurring in clusters. More specifically, ELR and MCOT may be best indicated in selected patients at low risk with recurrent syncopes who have inter-symptom interval ≤4 weeks.

• MCOT is particularly recommended for patients who may not be able to trigger their monitor or who may not recognize that an arrhythmia has occurred (e.g., arrhythmias that trigger "falls," arrhythmias during sleep, arrhythmias in cognitively impaired patients). With MCOT, detected arrhythmias are not only saved but are transmitted automatically to the service center for review on a 24/7 basis.

8.6 Implantable Loop Recorder (ILR)

Patients with infrequent syncope (i.e., less than once per month) are unlikely to be diagnosed by the ambulatory ECG monitoring systems described above. In such circumstances, consideration should be given to placement of an ILR. ILRs are easily implanted and can be monitored remotely in the same manner as pacemakers and ICDs. However, current ILRs do not provide an intermediary service center. Consequently, the physician and medical staff are responsible for reviewing the recordings and correlating them with patient symptoms.

8.6.1 Natural History of Syncope (Probability of Recurrence of Syncope) in Patients at Low Risk

The knowledge of the probabilities of syncope recurrence within the operational duration of the ILR (in general up to 3 years) becomes crucial for an appropriate selection of the candidates for this type of diagnostic evaluation. Figure 8.1 provides

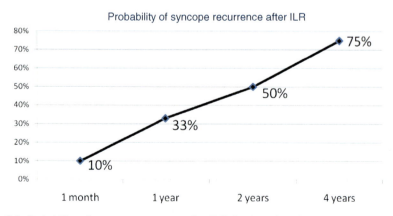

Fig. 8.1 Probability of syncope recurrence after ILR implantation. Source: pooled data from ISSUE 1 and ISSUE 2 studies (unpublished)

Table 8.4 Prognosis of patients with syncope of uncertain diagnosis and low risk >40 years according to the number of syncopes during last 2 years

Number of syncopes during last 2 years	Risk of recurrence of syncope after the index episode		
	Actuarial risk 1 year (%)	Actuarial risk 2 years (%)	Estimated risk 4 years[a] (%)
1–2	22.8	27.5	37.1
3	29.1	35.7	48.9
4–6	43.0	50.8	66.3
7–10	43.2	48.8	59.9
>10	85.6	98.1	100

[a] Assuming a linear increase

recurrence rates in a pooled population of 590 patients > 40 years, at low risk according to ESC classification, who participated in the ISSUE 1 and 2 studies due to having been diagnosed with unexplained syncope or suspected neurally mediated syncope.[2] The number of previous episodes of syncope are the strongest predictors of recurrence (Tables 8.4 and 16.4). Conversely, age, sex, tilt test response, severity of presentation, and presence or absence of structural heart disease have minimal or absent predictive value on probability of syncope recurrence and therefore are not useful for the selection of the patients. However, the presence of structural heart disease increases the likelihood of documentation of an arrhythmia with therapeutic implications.

8.6.2 Value of ILR in Diagnosis of Syncope

Data from nine studies[9–17] were pooled together in Table 8.5 for a total of 506 patients with unexplained syncope at the end of a complete conventional

Table 8.5 Correlation between syncope and ECG in patients with unexplained syncope at the end of conventional workup

	Asystole (%)	Brady (%)	Normal SR (%)	Tachy (%)	Total diagnoses
Pilot study[9]	na	47	40	13	15/16 (94%)
Khran et al.[10]	na	69	30	9	23/85 (27%)
Nierop et al.[11]	na	29	43	29	14/35 (40%)
Boersma et al.[12]	47	0	40	13	15/43 (35%)
Lombardi et al.[13]	67	0	22	11	9/34 (26%)
ISSUE-1 pooled[14–16]	63	5	26	5	57/198 (29%)
Pierre et al.[17]	49	na	37	14	43/95 (45%)
Average	56		33	11	176/506 (35%)

na, not available.

investigation. A correlation between syncope and ECG was present in 176 patients (35%); of these 176 individuals, 56% had asystole (or bradycardia in few cases) at the time of the recorded event, 11% had tachycardia, and 33% had no arrhythmia. ILR proved particularly useful in patients with bundle branch block and negative EPS to confirm or exclude the suspicion of a paroxysmal AV block and guide subsequent specific therapy, i.e., pacemaker implantation.

The diagnostic yield was higher in older patients. In one study,[18] patients >65 years had a higher syncope recurrence rate (56% versus 32%) than those <65 years and were more likely to have an arrhythmia at time of syncope (44% versus 20%). On the other hand, the diagnostic yield was similar in patients with and without structural heart diseases (including abnormal ECG). However, the patients with structural heart disease more frequently had paroxysmal AV block and tachyarrhythmias and patients without heart disease more frequently had sinus bradycardia/sinus arrest or no arrhythmia.[19] Similar findings were observed when an ILR was inserted in patients with suspected neurally mediated syncope in an early phase after the initial evaluation[20] (Fig. 8.2 and Table 8.6). In both cases a prolonged asystole (due to either sinus arrest or AV block) on average 10–15 s in duration was the most frequently observed event. In these patients, ILR implantation was useful in order to understand the exact mechanism and to guide specific therapy.

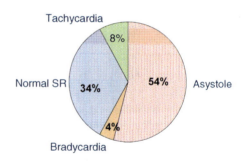

Fig. 8.2 Correlation between syncope and ECG in patients with suspected neurally mediated syncope when ILR was implanted in an early phase after the initial evaluation

Table 8.6 Diagnostic yield of ILR in patients with unexplained syncope (implanted after complete workup) and in patients with suspected neurally mediated syncope (implanted earlier after the initial evaluation)

	Performed no. of patients	Diagnostic % patients	NND
Unexplained syncope	506	176 (35%)	2.9
Suspected neurally mediated syncope	392	106 (27%)	3.7

Modified from EHRA Position Paper, 2009[2]
NND, number needed for diagnosis (number of patients tested every one patient diagnosed)

Table 8.7 ILR findings in patients with documented pre-syncopal events

	Asystole (%)	Brady (%)	Normal SR (%)	Tachy (%)	Number of events
Khran et al.[10]	15		81	4	27
Nierop et al.[11]	0	0	63	37	19
Boersma et al.[12]	10	20	70	0	10
Lombardi et al.[13]	0	43	43	14	7
ISSUE-1 pooled[14–16]	0	18	54	27	46
Total events(%)	21 (19%)		67 (61%)	21 (19%)	109

Presyncope was much less likely to be associated with an arrhythmia than syncope, indicating that pre-syncope is not an accurate surrogate for syncope in establishing a diagnosis. Data from seven studies[10–16] were pooled together in Table 8.7. Asystole was only seldom observed suggesting that asystole is quite specific for syncope.

Finally, ILR has been used in selected "difficult" cases of patients with transient loss of consciousness in whom the syncopal nature remains uncertain; the objective was to exclude definitely an arrhythmic mechanism. Examples of this latter situation include patients in whom epilepsy was suspected but the treatment has proven ineffective, patients with major depressive diseases and frequent recurrent unexplained episodes, or older patients with non-accidental falls of uncertain nature.[21]

8.6.3 ILR in Syncope – Where in the Workup?

The role of ECG monitoring cannot be defined in isolation. Physicians will be guided by the results of the initial evaluation. In some situations, where the clinical evidence strongly suggests a diagnosis of reflex syncope, and especially when syncope occurs only occasionally, ECG monitoring may be deemed unnecessary. In those patients with frequent symptoms or in those in whom arrhythmic syncope is suspected, but who are not at high risk, an ILR can be useful.

Initially, the ILR was used as a last resort in the evaluation of syncope after all investigations were negative. Subsequently, in one study[22] 60 patients with unexplained syncope were randomized to "conventional" testing (i.e., external loop recorder, and tilt and EPS testing) or to prolonged monitoring with the ILR. The ILR strategy proved more likely to provide a diagnosis than did conventional testing (52% versus 20%) during a 12-month follow-up period. However, patients at high risk of life-threatening arrhythmias, as were those with an ejection fraction < 35%, were excluded. These results were confirmed in another study[23] in 201 patients who, following a basic clinical workup, were randomized to receive the ILR versus conventional investigation and management. The ILR group patients had a 6.5-fold higher probability of achieving a diagnosis compared to the conventional group

Table 8.8 Safety of the ILR strategy in patients at low risk. Adverse events observed during the follow-up in the overall 590 patients enrolled in ISSUE studies

Sudden death	2 (0.3%)
Non-cardiac death	5 (0.8%)
Transient ischemic attack (TIA)	5 (0.8%)
Myocardial infarction	1 (0.2%)
Secondary severe trauma	8 (1.4%)
ILR explants for pocket infection	8 (1.4%)

(43% versus 6%) during a follow-up of 17 months. There were eight deaths in the ILR and nine in the conventional group.

An early ILR implantation immediately after the initial evaluation was also performed in the ISSUE 2 study in 392 patients with suspected neurally mediated syncope.[20] Patients with severe structural heart disease were excluded. A diagnosis was achieved in 26% of the patients during a median follow-up of 9 months. During the study period seven patients died, none of these for arrhythmic causes (two strokes and five non-cardiovascular). Severe trauma secondary to syncope relapse occurred in 2% and mild trauma in 4% (Table 8.8). Consequently, based on these data and due to the limited diagnostic value of laboratory tests and short-term ECG monitoring, it appears that early use of an ILR in the diagnostic workup may well be the reference standard to be adopted when an arrhythmic cause of syncope is suspected, provided that patients at risk of life-threatening events are carefully excluded.

According to the ESC syncope practice guidelines,[1] high-risk patients who require immediate hospitalization and intensive evaluation can be identified after the initial evaluation (see Chapter 6). These include in particular:

– patients with an established indication for ICD implantation according to guidelines. ICD therapy should be offered upfront. The monitoring function of the defibrillator can subsequently be used to study the mechanism of syncope
– patients with previous myocardial infarction and non-sustained ventricular tachycardia should undergo electrophysiological study which includes premature ventricular stimulation; ILR should be considered only at the end of a negative complete workup
– patients with clinical or ECG features that suggest an intermittent bradycardia should undergo in-hospital prolonged telemetric monitoring and eventually an electrophysiological evaluation; ILR should be considered at the end of a non-diagnostic complete workup

When features suggesting "high risk" are absent, an ILR strategy can safely be undertaken in patients suspected of having arrhythmic syncope; this includes those patients who had a "severe" presentation of syncope (i.e., high risk of trauma or high frequency of episodes) who can benefit of a mechanism-specific therapy. In less severe forms of syncope presentation, clinical evaluation is sufficient to establish a likely mechanism of syncope in the majority of patients and no further investigation is usually necessary.

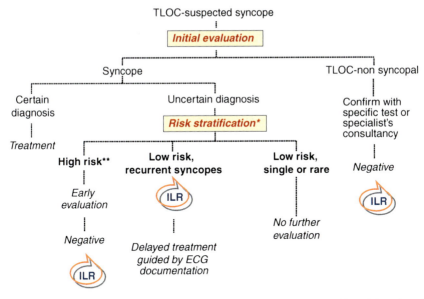

Fig. 8.3 Indications of ILR for diagnosis of syncope. ILR is indicated in high-risk patients in whom a comprehensive evaluation did not demonstrate a cause of syncope or lead to a specific treatment and who have clinical or ECG features suggesting arrhythmic syncope and in an initial phase of the workup instead of the completion of conventional investigations in patients with recurrent syncope of uncertain origin and absence of high-risk criteria. This is particularly the case for patients with recurrent syncope of uncertain origin who have a likely recurrence within battery longevity of the device (i.e., three or more episodes of syncopes during last 2 years). Moreover, ILR may be indicated in selected "difficult" cases of patients with T-LOC in whom the syncopal nature remains uncertain in order to exclude an arrhythmic mechanism

Patients at low risk for arrhythmic syncope are not candidates for ILR monitoring. Although the estimation of the usefulness of ILR implantation is largely individual, as a general rule, ILR is not indicated when the probability of syncope recurrence during the longevity of the battery is low (see Table 8.4) and when the knowledge of a precise ECG–symptom correlation is not required for therapeutic decisions. A schematic flowchart is provided in Fig. 8.3.

8.6.4 *Indications*

ILR is indicated in:

- an initial phase of the workup instead of the completion of conventional investigations in patients with recurrent syncope of uncertain origin and absence of high-risk criteria. This is particularly the case for patients with recurrent syncope of uncertain origin who are likely to have a likely recurrence within battery longevity of the device (i.e., three or more episodes of syncopes during last 2 years)

- high-risk patients in whom a comprehensive evaluation did not demonstrate a cause of syncope or lead to a specific treatment and who have clinical or ECG features suggesting arrhythmic syncope
- in patients with suspected or certain reflex syncope presenting with frequent or traumatic syncopal episodes in order to assess the contribution of bradycardia before embarking on cardiac pacing
- in selected "difficult" cases of patients with transient loss of consciousness (e.g., those who were thought to have had seizures, but antiepileptic treatment has been unsuccessful) in whom the syncopal nature remains uncertain in order to exclude an arrhythmic mechanism

8.6.5 Classification of Responses

Because of the heterogeneity of findings and the wide variety of rhythm disturbances recorded with the ILR at the time of syncope, the ISSUE investigators [24] have proposed a classification that attempts to group the observations into homogeneous patterns in order to define an acceptable standard useful for future studies and clinical practice (Table 8.9):

- Type 1 (asystole) was the most frequent finding and was observed in 63% of patients,
- Type 2 (bradycardia) was observed in 5% of patients,
- Type 3 (no or slight rhythm variations) was observed in 18% of patients, and
- Type 4 (tachycardia) was observed in 14% of patients.

The ISSUE classification has pathophysiological implications that may be helpful to distinguish among various types of arrhythmic syncope and have potential different diagnostic, therapeutic, and prognostic implications. For the present, however, the classification is primarily a research tool.

In types 1A, 1B (see Table 8.9), and 2 the findings of progressive sinus bradycardia, most often followed by ventricular asystole due to sinus arrest, or progressive tachycardia followed by progressive bradycardia, and, eventually, ventricular asystole due to sinus arrest suggest that the syncope is probably reflex in origin. In type 1C, the finding of prolonged asystolic pauses due to sudden-onset paroxysmal AV block with concomitant increase in sinus rate suggests another mechanism, namely intrinsic disease of the His–Purkinje system as observed in Stokes–Adams attacks. In types 4B, 4C, and 4D (Table 8.9) a primary cardiac arrhythmia is typically responsible for syncope. In the other types (3 and 4A), in which no arrhythmia is detected, the exact nature of syncope remains uncertain because of the lack of contemporaneous recording of blood pressure; however, the finding of progressive heart rate increase and/or decrease at the time of syncope suggests a (primary or secondary) activation of the cardiovascular system and a possible hypotensive mechanism. Chapters 18 and 19 review illustrative cases.

Table 8.9 Classification of ECG recordings obtained with ILR, with their probable related mechanism (adapted from ISSUE classification)

Classification	Description	Suggested mechanism
Type 1, asystole	R–R pause ≥3 s	
• Type 1 A, sinus arrest	Progressive sinus bradycardia or initial sinus tachycardia followed by progressive sinus bradycardia until sinus arrest	Probably reflex
• Type 1B sinus bradycardia plus AV block	Progressive sinus bradycardia followed by AV block (and ventricular pause/s) with concomitant decrease in sinus rate	Probably reflex
• Type 1C, AV block	Sudden-onset AV block (and ventricular pause/s) with concomitant increase in sinus rate	Probably intrinsic
Type 2, bradycardia	Decrease of heart rate >30% or <40 bpm for >10 s	Probably reflex
Type 3, no or slight rhythm variations	Variations of heart rate <30% and heart rate >40 bpm	Uncertain
Type 4, tachycardia	Increase of heart rate >30% or >120 bpm	
• *Type 4A*	Progressive sinus tachycardia	Uncertain
• *Type 4B*	Atrial fibrillation	Cardiac arrhythmia
• *Type 4C*	Supraventricular tachycardia (except sinus)	Cardiac arrhythmia
• *Type 4D*	Ventricular tachycardia	Cardiac arrhythmia

bpm = beats per minute; s = seconds

8.6.6 Therapy Guided by ILR

Since prolonged asystole is the most frequent finding at the time of syncope recurrence, cardiac pacing was the specific therapy used most often in the ILR-evaluated populations: pacemaker implantation ranged from 12% in patients with neurally mediated syncope to 44% in patients with bundle branch block. On average, pooling together the data from nine studies,[14–18,20,23,25,26] a pacemaker was finally implanted in 219/1,217 patients (18%), corresponding to 42% of those who had had an ILR-documented syncope (Table 8.10). ICD and catheter ablation were also consistently used in about 1% of patients. Finally, about one-third of the patients, those with a non-arrhythmic cause of syncope, received other therapies.

Few data are available on the subsequent outcome of the patients treated with pacing. In general, ILR-guided cardiac pacing reduces syncope burden in patients with asystole, but does not prevent all syncopes. ILR does not alter the course of non-arrhythmic syncope. In the ISSUE 2 study[20] the 1-year burden of syncope decreased from 0.83 ± 1.57 episodes per patient/year in the control group of patients without any ILR-guided specific therapy to 0.05 ± 0.15 episodes per patient/year in

Table 8.10 ILR-guided specific therapy

	Total patients	Diagnosis	Pacemaker	ICD	Catheter ablation	Case mix: % SHD
Sud et al.[25]	122	na	33 (27%)	na	na	64
Brignole et al.[18]	103	53 (51%)	28 (27%)	1 (1%)	1 (1%)	38
Pierre et al.[17]	95	43 (45%)	20 (21%)	3 (3%)	0 (0%)	43
ISSUE-1 pooled[14-16]	198	57 (29%)	40 (20%)	2 (1%)	1 (0.5%)	44
EaSyAS[23]	101	43 (43%)	16 (16%)	0 (0%)	1 (1%)	48
ISSUE-2[20]	392	106 (27%)	47 (12%)	1 (0.2%)	4 (1%)	14
Krahn et al.[26]	206	142 (69%)	35 (17%)	na	na	33
Total	1,217	444/1095 (41%)	219 (18%)	7/889 (1%)	7/889 (1%)	–

SHD, structural heart disease

na, not available.

the patients treated with a pacemaker (87% relative risk reduction, $p = 0.001$). In the study by Sud et al.[25] after the insertion of a cardiac pacemaker, syncope burden decreased from 2.17 to 0.45 per year in patients with 1A or 1B ECG pattern (Table 8.9) of the ISSUE classification ($p = 0.02$) and from 4.57 per year to 0 per year in the type 1C syncope ($p = 0.001$) patients.

8.6.7 Technical Aspects

The diagnostic yield of ILR monitoring was hampered by the failure to document a syncopal relapse despite the manual and automatic features of the device and by false-positive arrhythmia detection even in the most recent devices. This happens, on average, in 5–9% of the patients (16% of the events).[2]

Although an auto-activation feature increases the diagnostic yield, this feature can be compromised by false over-detections and missed detection of true arrhythmias.[27] Documented causes of false arrhythmia storage in ILRs include undersensing related to sudden reductions in R-wave signal amplitude during both normal sinus rhythm and arrhythmias and undersensing by transient loss of ECG signal related to device amplifier saturation, T-wave, and myopotential oversensing. A systematic analysis of a large series of 2,613 previously recorded, automatically detected episodes from 533 patients with the Reveal Plus model ILR (Medtronic Inc., Minneapolis, MN, USA) showed that a total of 71.9% of episodes were inappropriately detected by the original ILR and at least 88.6% of patients had one or more inappropriate episodes. Even if most of these misdetections can easily be recognized, they can potentially lead to misdiagnosis with consequent administration of useless therapies. The prevalence of misdiagnosis is unknown. Corresponding data concerning the new generations of ILR are still missing. However, avoidance of misdetection is clearly a priority for future research and device development.

Finally, like all implanted devices, ILRs also carry the risk of pocket infections; these readily resolve with device explantation. This complication, which can occur either in the periprocedural phase or late during the follow-up, was reported in 1–5% of patients.[2] Fortunately, however, since current ILRs do not require intravascular leads, device removal is relatively straightforward.

8.7 Diagnostic Yield of Prolonged Diagnostic Monitoring in Patients with Uncertain Syncope

While laboratory tests, especially carotid sinus massage (CSM) and tilt testing, provide a good diagnostic yield for reflex syncope, relatively few patients with cardiac syncope are diagnosed by means of cardiac laboratory tests (see Chapter 7). Prolonged ambulatory ECG monitoring has become the most effective strategy for diagnosis of arrhythmic syncope, either of intrinsic cardiac or of extrinsic reflex nature. MCOT recording systems are the next most effective tool; these devices offer automatic detection and transmission of detected arrhythmias as well as an opportunity for patients to transmit concomitant (or recent) symptoms.[7] MCOT is only limited by the ability of patients to tolerate skin-mounted ECG electrodes for a long period of time. On the other hand, a conventional event recorder is not useful for syncope evaluation as it offers no backward-looking "loop" capability and must be activated by the patient who in fact may have been disabled by the faint. In-hospital monitoring, Holter monitoring, and ELR, all together, are diagnostic in no more than 5% of the patients with uncertain syncope. However, since they are appropriately indicated in a minority of patients, the resulting diagnostic value is acceptable, with a diagnosis made in every 2–10 patients evaluated (Tables 5.7 and 8.2). In the end, ILR is probably substantially underused in clinical practice.[28] Despite this, it is diagnostic in about one-third of patients when restrictive diagnostic criteria (i.e., documentation of syncopal relapse) are used (Table 8.6). If less restrictive endpoints are used (i.e., pre-syncope or asymptomatic arrhythmias), its diagnostic value rises to 50% or more. In other words a diagnosis can be achieved every two or three ILRs implanted.

8.8 Clinical Perspectives

While Holter monitoring and ELR have limited value in diagnosing syncope, and MCOT is currently unavailable in most countries (other than the USA), ILR has the potential to become the reference standard for diagnosis in patients with recurrent syncope of uncertain etiology. ILR seems to be largely underused in current clinical practice. In two recent large multicenter studies it was employed in only 2% and 4% of the patients with uncertain syncope[29,30] (Table 8.2). The SUP investigators estimated that appropriate indications should be four times higher than those actually observed (16% instead of 4% of patients with syncope of undetermined cause); the corresponding need for ILR implantation in the general population was estimated to be 120 ILRs per million inhabitants per year instead of the observed 30 per million inhabitants per year.

It is likely that ILRs will become increasingly important and their use will be appropriately positioned before many other current conventional investigations. The ultimate goal of therapy guided by ILR should be to improve the clinical outcome of the patients, i.e., prevention of syncopal recurrences, severe injuries, and death. To what extent an ILR-guided strategy is superior to a conventional evaluation strategy remains largely to be demonstrated.

Continuous long-term ECG telemetry monitoring (particularly MCOT) is becoming a widely accepted diagnostic methodology. Data are transmitted through a standard telephone line or via the Internet to a secure network, such as in the current technology for remote monitoring of pacemakers and defibrillators. New generation monitors may be used to identify various arrhythmias automatically, particularly atrial fibrillation episodes. For this purpose, R–R cycle analysis algorithms and advanced discrimination criteria similar to those implemented in ICDs have been introduced into these monitoring systems.

Remote monitoring through advanced telecommunications technology of not only ECG recordings but other physiological measures as well will potentially be useful for the management of patients with chronic disease. It will be possible to obtain nearly continuous assessment ECG and other physiological signals automatically (e.g., blood flow or pressure and electroencephalography). In addition, when symptomatic or otherwise concerned, patients will be able to self-transmit diagnostic information stored in the device memory for later scheduled follow-up or post-event follow-up.

Blood pressure recording is crucial for the majority of clinical T-LOC situations and will add important information for therapy of syncope. Unfortunately current long-term blood pressure (or surrogate) recording systems are not optimal for diagnostic use in the syncope evaluation setting.

References

1. Moya A, et al. Guidelines for the diagnosis and management of syncope (version 2009). *Eur Heart J.* 2009;30:2631–2671.
2. Brignole M, et al. EHRA position paper. Indications for the use of diagnostic implantable and external ECG loop recorders. *Europace.* 2009;11:671–687.
3. Linzer M, et al. Diagnosing syncope. Part II: Unexplained syncope. *Ann Intern Med.* 1997;127:76–86.
4. Sivakumaran S, et al. A prospective randomized comparison of loop recorders versus Holter monitoring in patients with syncope or presyncope. *Am J Med.* 2003;115:1–5.
5. Schuchert A, et al. Diagnostic yield of external loop recorders in patients with recurrent syncope and negative tilt table test. *Pacing Clin Electrophysiol.* 2003;26:1837–1840.
6. Linzer M, et al. Incremental diagnostic yield of loop electrocardiographic recorders in unexplained syncope. *Am J Cardiol.* 1990;66:214–219.
7. Rothman S, et al. The diagnosis of cardiac arrhythmias: a prospective multicenter randomized study comparing mobile cardiac outpatient telemetry versus standard loop event monitoring. *J Cardiovasc Electrophysiol.* 2007;18:241–247.

8. Olson JA, et al. Utility of mobile cardiac outpatient telemetry for the diagnosis of palpitations, presyncope, syncope and the assessment of therapy efficacy. *J Cardiovasc Electrophysiol.* 2007;18:473–477.

9. Krahn A, et al. The etiology of syncope in patients with negative tilt table and electrophysiologic testing. *Circulation.* 1995;92:1819–1826.

10. Krahn AD, et al. Use of an extended monitoring strategy in patients with problematic syncope. Reveal Investigators. *Circulation.* 1999;26(99):406–410.

11. Nierop P, et al. Heart rhythm during syncope and presyncope. *Pacing Clin Electrophysiol.* 2000;23:1532–1538.

12. Boersma L, et al. Value of implantable loop recorder for the management of patients with unexplained syncope. *Europace.* 2004;6:70–76.

13. Lombardi F, et al. Utility of implantable loop recorder (Reveal Plus) in the diagnosis of unexplained syncope. *Europace.* 2005;7:19–24.

14. Moya A, et al. Mechanism of syncope in patients with isolated syncope and in patients with tilt-positive syncope. *Circulation.* 2001;104:1261–1267.

15. Menozzi C, et al. Mechanism of syncope in patients with heart disease and negative electrophysiologic test. *Circulation.* 2002;105:2741–2745.

16. Brignole M, et al. The mechanism of syncope in patients with bundle branch block and negative electrophysiologic test. *Circulation.* 2001;104:2045–2050.

17. Pierre B, et al. Implantable loop recorder for recurrent syncope: influence of cardiac conduction abnormalities showing up on resting electrocardiogram and of underlying cardiac disease on follow-up developments. *Europace.* 2008;10:477–481.

18. Brignole M, et al. The usage and diagnostic yield of the implantable loop-recorder in detection of the mechanism of syncope and in guiding effective antiarrhythmic therapy in older people. *Europace.* 2005;7:273–279.

19. Solano A, et al. Incidence, diagnostic yield and safety of the implantable loop-recorder to detect the mechanism of syncope in patients with and without structural heart disease. *Eur Heart J.* 2004;25:1116–1119.

20. Brignole M, et al. Early application of an implantable loop recorder allows effective specific therapy in patients with recurrent suspected neutrally-mediated syncope. *Eur Heart J.* 2006;27:1085–1092.

21. Pezawas T, et al. Implantable loop recorder in unexplained syncope: classification, mechanism, transient loss of consciousness and role of major depressive disorder in patients with and without structural heart disease. *Heart.* 2008;94:17–24.

22. Krahn A, et al. Randomized Assessment of Syncope Trial. Conventional diagnostic testing versus a prolonged monitoring strategy. *Circulation.* 2006;104:46–51.

23. Farwell D, et al. The clinical impact of implantable loop recorders in patients with syncope. *Eur Heart J.* 2006;27:351–356.

24. Brignole M, et al. Proposed electrocardiographic classification of spontaneous syncope documented by an Implantable Loop Recorder. *Europace.* 2005;7:14–18.

25. Sud S, et al. Implications of mechanism of bradycardia on response to pacing in patients with unexplained syncope. *Europace.* 2007;9:312–318.

26. Krahn A, et al. Predicting the outcome of patients with unexplained syncope undergoing prolonged monitoring. *Pacing Clin Electrophysiol.* 2002;25:37–41.

27. Brignole M, et al. Improved arrhythmia detection in implantable loop recorders. *J Cardiovasc Electrophysiol.* 2008;19:928–934.

28. Vitale E, et al. Discrepancy between clinical practice and standardized indications for ILR in patients with unexplained syncope. A SUP substudy. *Europace.* 2010;12:1475–1479.

29. Brignole M, et al. A new management of syncope: prospective systematic guideline-based evaluation of patients referred urgently to general hospitals. *Eur Heart J.* 2006;27:76–82.

30. Brignole M, et al. Prospective multicentre systematic guideline-based management of patients referred to the Syncope Units of general hospitals. *Europace.* 2010;12:109–118.

Chapter 9
Syncope Facilities: Background and Current Standards

Contents

Key points: A proposed model of organization for the evaluation of the T-LOC/syncope patient in a community

- Despite the implementation of several clinical guidelines, current strategies for assessment of T-LOC/syncope are not standardized and vary widely among physicians and among hospitals and clinics. The results are an inappropriate use of diagnostic tests, a high number of misdiagnoses, a high number of patients in whom diagnosis remains unexplained, and excessive cost.
- Multiple experiences with specialized syncope diagnostic and treatment facilities have shown improvement in diagnostic yield and cost effectiveness (i.e., cost per reliable diagnosis).
- The European Society of Cardiology (ESC) Task Force on Syncope recommended that a cohesive, structured care pathway – either delivered within a single syncope facility or as a more multi-faceted service – is desirable to optimize quality service delivery.

M. Brignole, D.G. Benditt, *Syncope*, DOI 10.1007/978-0-85729-201-8_9,
© Springer-Verlag London Limited 2011

- Physician(s) in charge of the T-LOC/syncope facility lead the process of comprehensive management from diagnosis, risk stratification, therapy, and, if necessary, follow-up. They perform the core laboratory tests and have access to hospitalization, diagnostic tests, and therapeutic procedures.
- The facility should be multidisciplinary with physicians and nurses experienced in key components of cardiology, neurology, emergency, and geriatric medicine.
- Core equipment for the facility include surface ECG recording, continuous blood pressure monitoring, tilt-table testing equipment, external (including MCOT where available) and internal (Implantable) ECG loop recorder (ILR) systems, 24 h ambulatory blood pressure monitoring, 24 h ambulatory ECG and autonomic function testing, and electrophysiological testing.
- Preferential access to other tests or therapy for T-LOC/syncope should be available.
- The majority of patients should be investigated as outpatients or day cases.

9.1 Background: Why Should We Need a Dedicated Facility?

Currently, the strategies for assessment for T-LOC/syncope vary widely among physicians and among hospitals and clinics. In the case of syncope, patients are not adequately stratified according to risk, and more often than not the evaluation and treatment is haphazard. The result is an excessive number of hospital admissions, wide variation in the diagnostic tests applied, and the proportion and types of attributable diagnoses and the proportion of syncope patients in whom the diagnosis remains unexplained.[1]

A prospective observational registry from a sample of 28 general hospitals was performed in Italy in order to evaluate the impact of the guidelines of the European Society of Cardiology (ESC) on usual management of syncope admitted emergently. The Evaluation of Guidelines in Syncope Study 1 (EGSYS-1)[2] enrolled 996 consecutive patients referred to emergency rooms from November 5, 2001 to December 7, 2001 who were affected by transient loss of consciousness as the principal symptom. The findings of each of the 28 hospitals participating in the survey were evaluated separately. The authors observed substantial inter-hospital and inter-department heterogeneity regarding the incidence of emergency admission, in-hospital pathways, the examinations performed, and the final assigned diagnosis. For example, carotid sinus massage was performed in 0–58% (Fig. 9.1) and head-up tilt tests in 0–50% syncopal patients. Prolonged ECG monitoring was performed in 3–90% of patients (Fig. 9.2). Consequently the final diagnosis for neurally mediated syncope ranged from 10 to 79%.

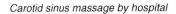

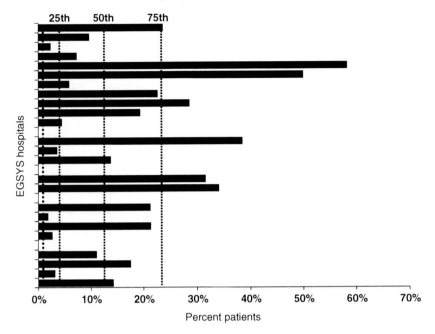

Fig. 9.1 Observations from the EGSYS-1 study.[2] Incidence of the performance of carotid sinus massage (expressed as percentage of total patients admitted) among 28 participating hospitals in Italy. Each bar represents one hospital. The vertical *dotted lines* are those corresponding to the 25th, 50th, and 75th percentiles of distribution

The disparate patterns of syncope assessment, exemplified in the EGSYS-1 experience, explain why there are substantial differences in terms of the effectiveness of syncope assessment and treatment. For instance, pacing rates for carotid sinus syndrome vary, even within countries, from 1 to 25% of implants, depending on whether carotid sinus hypersensitivity is systematically assessed in the investigation profile. As a consequence of the great inter-hospital variability, the EGSYS-1 authors were unable to identify a uniform strategy for the management of syncope. The observed heterogeneity could not be adequately accounted for by a difference in the clinical characteristics of the population referred to the hospitals participating in the study. Indeed, the proportion of explained variability was calculated to be less than 10% of total variance. Thus, the authors concluded that the main determinant of the different behaviors lay in different attitudes and knowledge levels of the medical staff.

A comparative analysis of several other population-based studies shows similarly great heterogeneity. For example, the diagnosis of neurally mediated syncope ranged between 13% and 49% of patients and the diagnosis of cardiac syncope ranged between 6% and 46% of patients; syncope remained unexplained in 13%–54% of patients.[3-13]

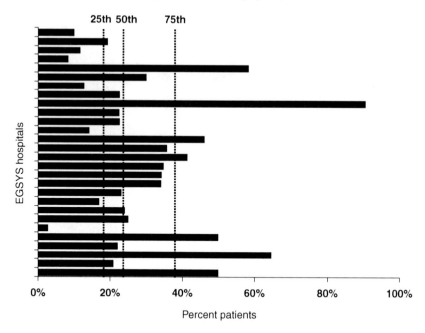

Fig. 9.2 Observations from the EGSYS-1 study.[2] Incidence of the performance of Holter/ECG monitoring (expressed as percentage of total patients admitted) among the 28 participating hospitals. Each bar represents one hospital. The vertical *dotted lines* are those corresponding to the 25th, 50th, and 75th percentiles of distribution

There are several possible explanations for heterogeneity among published reports. First, a major issue in the use of diagnostic tests is that the causal relationship between a diagnostic abnormality and syncope in a given patient is often presumptive. Further, test sensitivity cannot be measured, as there is no reference or "gold standard" for most of these tests; therefore, usually decisions have to be made on the basis of the patient's history or abnormal findings during asymptomatic periods. Second, uncertainty is compounded by the wide variation in the manner with which physicians take a history and perform a physical examination, and the types of tests requested and how they are interpreted. The choice of procedures seems to be unduly influenced by the specialty and department to which the patient is referred. Third, guidelines are often drawn up by specialists in one field and are not well known or accepted by those of other specialties. Multidisciplinary recommendations are essential.

If the status quo for the evaluation of syncope is unchanged, diagnostic and treatment effectiveness is unlikely to improve substantially. Furthermore, the implementation of the published syncope management guidelines will be diverse and incomplete. Thus, to maximize implementation of the guidelines, it is essential that models of care for assessment and management of syncope are in place and that information about the models within each organization is adequately communicated to all parties involved in the care of these patients.

It was the view of the ESC Syncope Task Force that a cohesive, structured care pathway – delivered either within a single syncope facility (i.e., "syncope unit" or "syncope management unit") or as a more multi-faceted service – is needed to optimize quality service delivery.[1] Furthermore, considerable improvement in diagnostic yield and cost effectiveness (i.e., cost per reliable diagnosis) can be achieved by focusing skills and following well-defined, up-to-date diagnostic guidelines.

9.2 Some Existing T-LOC/Syncope Facility Models

Recent data support the notion that a designated T-LOC/syncope facility, in either the emergency department (ED) or hospital, can provide more efficient and effective triage and evaluation of patients than is accomplished by conventional approaches. In this regard, after the pivotal experience in Newcastle,[14] various models of care have been developed. Most of these were restricted to patients referred urgently for evaluation of T-LOC/syncope to the ED.[15–18] In general, a considerable improvement in diagnostic yield and cost effectiveness (i.e., cost per reliable diagnosis) was achieved in comparison to the usual practice. Nevertheless, these models have not been widely adopted. A comprehensive model of management of patients referred with T-LOC/syncope to ED is shown in Fig. 9.3.[19] The model is based on the results of two controlled studies; however, this model has not been validated with a formal prospective study.

9.2.1 Newcastle, UK

The *Rapid Access Falls and Syncope Service* (FASS) adopted by the Newcastle group[14,20] is a rapid access, multidisciplinary approach to the evaluation of T-LOC/syncope. FASS operation is based on application of standardized algorithms to referrals with syncope and falls for adults of all ages, but with particular expertise in the evaluation of older patients with these overlapping problems. There is a rapid access pathway for inpatients and for those attending the ED with as many investigations as possible completed at the initial assessment. FASS has a full range of tilt testing, beat-to-beat BP monitoring, and ambulatory monitoring equipment as well as physiotherapy, occupational therapy, and specialist nursing expertise. All patients have an initial detailed assessment by a general physician, a geriatrician, or a general practitioner with falls and syncope expertise. Then the patients are either managed at the Service or referred to colleagues associated with the Service in neurology, neurophysiology, cardiology, or ear nose and throat surgery depending on the symptoms and the findings at the initial assessment. FASS operation showed a significant saving in emergency hospital costs. The savings were attributed to a combination of factors – reduced readmission rates, rapid access to day case facilities for ED staff and community physicians, and reduced recurrent event rates because of effective targeted treatment strategies for syncope and falls.

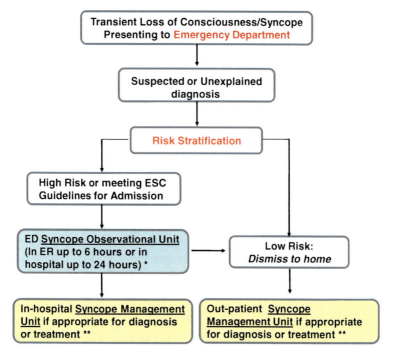

Fig. 9.3 Proposed model of comprehensive management of patients referred with syncope to the emergency department (ED)

9.2.2 Manchester, UK

The Manchester experience[21] is a model of *T-LOC Facility* where cardiologists (with an interest in syncope) and neurologists (with an interest in epilepsy) developed a multidisciplinary facility for a comprehensive evaluation of T-LOC with special emphasis on differential diagnosis between syncope, epilepsy, and psychogenic episodes. A Rapid Access "Blackout" Clinic is an element of the Manchester model.

9.2.3 Controlled Studies of Patients Presenting with Syncope to the Emergency Department

Two models of management of patients presenting with syncope have been developed in USA and in Italy. These models have been evaluated by means of controlled studies which were able to show a benefit in terms of diagnostic efficiency and cost effectiveness in comparison to usual practice. Nevertheless, both models were experimental; their results may not be readily reproduced in everyday clinical practice due to their special design and they have not been yet widely adopted. However, these models provided evidence of the superiority of specialized facilities in comparison to the usual practice. Further, the knowledge derived from these experiences has been useful to develop newer models, such as in use at present in several Italian hospitals that will be described in Chapter 10.

9.2.3.1 Syncope Observational Unit in Emergency Department

In the Syncope Evaluation in the Emergency Department Study (SEEDS),[15] investigators at the Mayo Clinic in Rochester, Minnesota, USA, examined the utility of a critical pathway for the evaluation and management of intermediate-risk patients with syncope presenting to the ED. It was hypothesized that a syncope unit equipped with diagnostic resources that target common causes of syncope would improve the diagnostic yield and reduce the hospital admission rate compared with standard care (controls) and that the reduction in hospital admission would not negatively affect patient outcomes in survival and recurrent symptoms of syncope. SEEDS was a prospective, single-center, un-blinded randomized study. After initial assessment with a complete history, physical examination, and routine laboratory studies (ECG and CBC), intermediate-risk patients were randomly assigned to standard care or to the syncope unit evaluation. Under the "standard care," patients received continuous cardiac monitoring, nasal oxygen, and intravenous fluid support. Any additional testing in the ED was performed at the discretion of the ED physician on the basis of the patient's initial evaluation. Because of the patient's risk profile, time, and resource constraints, most patients in the standard care group were triaged to hospital admission. Patients randomized to the syncope unit evaluation received continuous cardiac telemetry for up to 6 h, hourly vital signs and orthostatic blood pressure checks, and echocardiogram for patients with abnormal cardiovascular examination or ECG findings. Tilt-table testing, carotid sinus massage, and electrophysiology consultations were made available to the ED physician. After completion of syncope unit evaluation, follow-up appointment at one of the outpatient clinics could be arranged if needed within 72 h if the patient was not to be admitted to the hospital. The outpatient clinics available for referral included, but were not limited to cardiology, neurology, and general medicine.

The study found that: (1) in the ED, a presumptive diagnosis of the cause of syncope was significantly increased from 10% among the "standard care" patients to 67% among patients who underwent syncope unit evaluation; (2) hospital admission was reduced from 98% among the standard care patients compared to 43% among the syncope unit patients; (3) the total length of patient-hospital days was reduced by >50% for patients in the syncope unit group versus controls; and (4) during follow-up, all-cause mortality and recurrent syncope events were similar between the standard care patients and syncope unit patients. From these results, the investigators concluded that a designated syncope unit in the ED, with a multidisciplinary effort and appropriate resources, can provide effective and efficient care for a large and challenging group of patients seeking evaluation for syncope. However, one should be cognizant of the fact that the experience from a single-center study may not be generally applied to other hospitals and that the syncope unit has costs of staffing, training, testing, and hospital space.

9.2.3.2 Syncope Management Unit in Hospital (Cardiology Department)

The Evaluation of Guidelines in Syncope Study (EGSYS) 2[16] evaluated a model of a functional Syncope Management Unit (SMU) managed by cardiologists inside the department of cardiology, with dedicated personnel. Patients attending this SMU had preferential access to all other facilities within the department including admission to the intensive care unit. Patients were referred from the ED but the personnel of the unit were not usually involved in the initial evaluation of the patient. In EGSYS 2, implementation of this practice was facilitated by a combination of (1) decision-making software based on the ESC guidelines; (2) a designated physician trained in syncope evaluation; and (3) a central supervisor.

Among 19 Italian hospitals, the investigators demonstrated that 78% of study subjects were managed according to the guideline-based evaluation, resulting in lower hospitalization rate (39% versus 47%), shorter in-hospital stay (7.2+5.7 versus 8.1+5.9 days), and fewer tests performed per patient (median 2.6 versus 3.4) compared to historical controls. More standardized care patients had a diagnosis of reflex (65% versus 46%) or orthostatic syncope (10% versus 6%) than was the case in historical controls. The mean cost per patient and the mean cost per diagnosis were 19% and 29% lower in the SMU group, respectively.

Due to their experimental design, both SEEDS and EGSYS 2 results are probably difficult to reproduce in everyday clinical practice. Nevertheless, these studies showed that a guideline-based standardized approach to the management (i.e., diagnosis and treatment) of syncope is more effective both medically and financially than is the status quo.

9.3 The Standards Recommended by the ESC Guidelines

It is probably inappropriate to be dogmatic regarding standardized care of T-LOC/syncope patients. For this reason, ESC guidelines do not provide concrete recommendations but only a framework of general standards.[1] The model of care delivery should be that which is most appropriate to existing practice and resources.[22] With these caveats in mind, the following may provide useful direction for establishing a standardized care unit:

9.3.1 Referral

Referral can be directly from family practitioners, the ED, acute hospital inpatients, or from institutional settings after the initial screening and risk stratification (Fig. 9.4). In general, about a half of the patients with T-LOC are suitable for referral to a syncope unit for diagnosis and/or therapy.

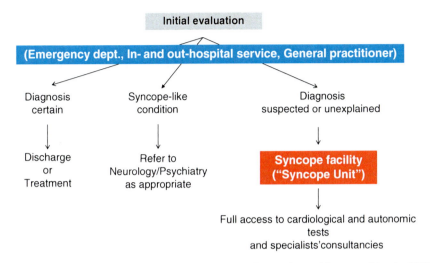

Fig. 9.4 Organizing the management of syncope according to the model proposed by the ESC guidelines[1]

9.3.2 Objectives

Each syncope (T-LOC) unit should target the following goals:

- *Provide continuity of care*. Physician(s) in charge of the syncope unit leads the process of comprehensive management from diagnosis, risk stratification, therapy, and, if necessary, follow-up. They perform the core laboratory tests and have ready access to hospitalization, diagnostic tests, and therapeutic procedures.
- *Reduce hospitalizations*. The majority of patients can be investigated as out-patients or day cases. A major objective of the syncope facility is to reduce the number of hospitalizations by offering the patient a well-defined, quick, alternative evaluation pathway.
- *Set standards for clinical excellence*. The role of a local integrated syncope service is to set standards for the following in keeping with the objectives of the ESC guidelines on syncope and other appropriate guideline publications:

    ○ diagnostic criteria for causes of T-LOC/syncope;
    ○ the preferred approach to the workup in subgroups of patients with syncope;
    ○ risk stratification of the patient with T-LOC/syncope;
    ○ treatment to prevent recurrences.

9.3.3 Professional Skill Mix for the Unit

In a single dedicated facility, the skill mix will depend on the specialty of the physician in charge of the unit. Cardiologists (with interest in pacing and electrophysiology), neurologists (with interest in autonomic disorders and epilepsy), general physicians, internists, and geriatricians (with interest in age-related cardiology and falls) have led syncope facilities without evidence of superiority of any model. If referrals hail directly from the community and/or from the ED, a broader skill mix is required.

Experience and training in key components of cardiology, neurology, emergency, and geriatric medicine are pertinent in addition to access to psychiatry and clinical psychology. Whatever be their specialization, physician(s) in charge of the syncope facility leads the process of comprehensive management from diagnosis, risk stratification, therapy, and, if necessary, follow-up. They perform the core laboratory tests and have ready access to hospitalization, diagnostic tests, and therapeutic procedures. Core medical and support personnel should be involved full time or most of the time in the management of the unit and should interact with other stakeholders within hospital and community.

9.3.4 Equipment

Core equipment for the syncope unit include ECG recorders, continuous blood pressure (BP) monitors, tilt table, external (including MCOT where available) and implantable ECG monitoring systems, 24 h ambulatory BP monitoring, and autonomic function testing. The facility should have access to echocardiography, electrophysiological study, coronary angiography, stress testing, and, when needed, computed tomography, magnetic resonance imaging, and electroencephalography. Easy access to hospitalization for dedicated therapeutic procedures – pacemaker and defibrillator implantation, catheter ablation, etc. – is essential. Dedicated rooms for assessment and investigation are desirable.

9.4 Clinical Perspectives

The diagnosis and treatment of T-LOC/syncope has been subject to sufficient study that it is now possible to provide recommendations favoring the use of standardized care protocols based on substantial scientific evidence. An unresolved problem is dissemination of these concepts in clinical practice. Indeed, the management of the patients with T-LOC/syncope requires organizational solutions that are probably quite different from those of the majority of other clinical situations.

Syncope is a frequent symptom that may be a manifestation of normal physiology gone awry or many different diseases. Therefore, virtually all physicians, including primary care, cardiology, internal and emergency medicine, geriatrics, neurology, psychiatry, and orthopedics, may need to be involved in the care of syncope patients, and depending on the circumstances each of these specialties may need to take a leading role. However, in practice, this degree of collaboration is virtually impossible to achieve. Several attempts have been made in the last two decades, all failed.

Based on pivotal experiences, the alternative solution proposed by the ESC Syncope Task Force was to promote the development of (functional) specialized facilities and to define a new professional skill, i.e., the "syncope specialists." In other words, relatively few T-LOC/syncope units and syncope specialists act as a "hub" where all stakeholders can refer their patients and participate in care delivery as appropriate to their expertise. Theoretically, this goal should be easier to achieve. Nevertheless, huge problems still need to be solved before this model can be broadly established. First, the model is largely experimental and its effectiveness needs to be verified and refined in clinical practice before it can be perceived as necessary by a large majority of physicians. Second, owing to the epidemiology and the heterogeneous clinical features of the patients with T-LOC/syncope, syncope units cannot be limited to very few tertiary centers, but rather they should be replicated in almost all district general hospitals. We anticipate that the T-LOC/syncope management unit concept will continue to evolve and be refined, as additional evidence is obtained, to eventually provide optimal care of the T-LOC/syncope patient.

References

1. Brignole M, et al. Guidelines on management (diagnosis and treatment) of syncope – Update 2004. *Europace*. 2004;6:467–537.
2. Disertori M, et al. Management of syncope referred for emergency to general hospitals (EGSYS 1). *Europace*. 2003;5:283–291.
3. Ammirati F, et al. The management of syncope in the hospital: the OESIL Study (Osservatorio Epidemiologico della Sincope nel Lazio). *G Ital Cardiol*. 1999;29:533–539.
4. Ben-Chetrit E, et al. Syncope: a retrospective study of 101 hospitalized patients. *Isr I Med Sci Med*. 1985;21:950–953.
5. Blanc JJ, et al. Prospective evaluation and outcome of patients admitted for syncope over 1 year period. *Eur Heart J*. 2002;23:815–820.
6. Day SC. Evaluation and outcome of emergency room patients with transient loss of consciousness. *Am J Med*. 1982;73:15–23.
7. Del Greco M, et al. The ECSIT study (Epidemiology and Costs of Syncope in Trento). Diagnostic pathway of syncope and analysis of the impact of guidelines in a district general hospital. *Ital Heart J*. 2003;4:99–106.
8. Eagle KA, Black HR. The impact of diagnostic tests in evaluating patients with syncope. *Yale J Biol Med*. 1983;56:1–8.
9. Farwell D, Sulke N. How do we diagnose syncope? *J Cardiovasc Electrophysiol*. 2002;13: S9–S13.
10. Kapoor W. Evaluation and outcome of patients with syncope. *Medicine*. 1990;69:169–175.
11. Oh JH, et al. Do symptoms predict cardiac arrhythmias and mortality in patients with syncope? *Arch Intern Med*. 1999;159:375–380.
12. Martin GJ, et al. Prospective evaluation of syncope. *Ann Emerg Med*. 1984;13:499–504.
13. Sarasin F, et al. Prospective evaluation of patients with syncope: a population-based study. *Am J Med*. 2001;111:177–184.

14. Kenny RA, et al. Impact of a dedicated syncope and falls facility for older adults on emergency beds. *Age Ageing.* 2002;31:272–275.
15. Shen WK, et al. Syncope evaluation in the emergency departments (SEEDS): A multidisciplinary approach to syncope management. *Circulation.* 2004;110:3636–3645.
16. Brignole M, et al. Standardized care pathway versus usual management of syncope referred in emergency to general hospitals (EGSYS 2). *Europace.* 2006;8:644–650.
17. Bartoletti A, et al. Hospital admission of patients referred to the emergency department for syncope: a single hospital prospective study based on the application of the European Society of Cardiology Guidelines on syncope. *Eur Heart J.* 2006;27:83–88.
18. McCarthy F, et al. Management of syncope in the Emergency Department: a single hospital observational case series on the application of European Society of Cardiology Guidelines. *Europace.* 2009;11:216–224.
19. Brignole M, Shen W. Syncope management from emergency department to hospital. *J. Am. Coll. Cardiol.* 2008;51:284–287.
20. Parry S, et al. Evidence-based algorithms and the management of falls and syncope presenting to acute medical services. *Clin Med.* 2008;8:157–162.
21. Fitzpatrick AP, Cooper P. Diagnosis and management of patients with blackouts. *Heart.* 2006;92:559–568.
22. Brignole M, et al. Prospective multicentre systematic guideline-based management of patients referred to the syncope units of general hospitals. *Europace.* 2010;12:109–118.

Chapter 10
Syncope (T-LOC) Management Units: The Italian Model

Contents

Key points: A proposed model of organization for the evaluation of the T-LOC/syncope patient in a community

- Several hospitals in Italy have adopted an organizational model for syncope management facilities (syncope unit) derived from that proposed by the ESC.
- This organizational model has been certified by a national multidisciplinary organization and its effectiveness in clinical practice has been documented in an observational study.
- Patients may be referred from the emergency room, or from in-hospital and out-of-hospital services.
- Each syncope unit is provided with a core equipment for syncope evaluation, on-site access to the usual investigations and therapy, and dedicated rooms for ambulatory examinations and tests.
- The unit is led by "syncope specialists". The syncope expert is a single physician or a team of physicians who lead/s the comprehensive management of the patient from risk stratification to diagnosis, therapy, and follow-up.

M. Brignole, D.G. Benditt, *Syncope*, DOI 10.1007/978-0-85729-201-8_10,
© Springer-Verlag London Limited 2011

- The objective of the unit is to assess the cause of transient loss of consciousness (T-LOC) spells and determine appropriate treatment strategy in a cost-effective manner.
- Most T-LOC/syncope units are located inside the department of cardiology; when it is outside, a formalized cooperation is established with the cardiology department.

10.1 Introduction

Various models of care have been developed in order to improve the management of transient loss of consciousness (T-LOC)/syncope (see Chapter 9). Guidelines have also been assessed in several studies. Most of these care models were restricted to patients referred urgently for T-LOC/syncope to the emergency department. In general, a considerable improvement in diagnostic yield and cost effectiveness (i.e., cost per reliable diagnosis) was achieved in comparison to conventional practice. Nevertheless, these models have not been widely adopted and their implementation in clinical practice and effectiveness are largely unknown.

A nationwide census taken in 2006 in Italy showed that there were 86 hospitals equipped with dedicated T-LOC/syncope facilities which partly or completely met the requisites of the European Society of Cardiology (ESC) as outlined in the ESC Syncope Task Force guidelines.[1] The model proposed by the ESC guidelines has been endorsed by the Associazione Italiana di Aritmologia e Cardiostimolazione (AIAC). By 2010, 21 T-LOC/syncope units have been certified as meeting the ESC and AIAC requisites by the Gruppo Italiano Multidisciplinare per lo studio della Sincope (GIMSI, www.gimsi.it), a multidisciplinary organization nominated by the national societies of arrhythmias, internal and emergency medicine, and geriatrics.[2]

This chapter describes the current practice of management of T-LOC/syncope in specialized facilities in Italy that have adopted the management model proposed by ESC.[3] The results may be useful for those who wish to replicate this model in other hospitals and provide all stakeholders (physicians, hospital and clinical governance managers, future research planners, etc.) with a frame of reference for their daily activity when dealing with T-LOC/syncope.

10.2 The Italian Syncope Management Unit

In accordance with the certification document by GIMSI, the syncope unit is intended as a functional facility located inside a general hospital endowed with 24-h emergency department and a cardiology ward with a coronary care unit. The referral districts of these hospitals typically have a median of 220,000 inhabitants (inter-quartile range 150,000–250,000).

The principal characteristics of patient flow and care in the hospitals with syncope units (the term "syncope unit" is commonly used as a short form for what is in reality a T-LOC/syncope management unit) are as follows:

- Patients are referred from the emergency department (ED) and from in-hospital and out-of-hospital services. Hospitalized patients are cared for directly by specialist physicians in the syncope unit during hospitalization. Patients considered to be at low risk of serious immediate injury or life-threatening arrhythmia when evaluated in the ED are offered delayed referral to the syncope unit clinic (so-called *protected discharge* with an appointment for early assessment), in order to reduce hospitalization rate. The patients are evaluated in the syncope facility benefit by formalized procedures for a preferential access to other investigations, therapies, and specialists' consultations as needed.
- Each unit is provided with
  1. core equipment for syncope evaluation (i.e., phasic blood pressure monitoring, tilt-table testing, external and implantable loop recorders, 24-h ambulatory blood pressure monitoring, 24-h ambulatory electrocardiographic (ECG) monitoring, and autonomic function testing);
  2. on-site access to the usual investigations (echocardiography, invasive electrophysiological testing, stress testing, cardiac imaging, computed tomography or magnetic resonance imaging, and electroencephalography) and on-site access to any therapy that may be required for syncope (i.e., pacemaker and ICD implantation, and catheter ablation of arrhythmias);
  3. dedicated room for ambulatory examinations and laboratory for the execution of core tests;
  4. a separate waiting list and schedules for follow-up visits.

- The unit is led by the "syncope specialist/consultant," formally appointed by the director of the department or by the director of the hospital. The syncope specialist/consultant is a single physician or a team of physicians (2–4 each who lead the unit in turn) who lead the comprehensive management of the patient from risk stratification to diagnosis, therapy, and follow-up. The absence of an individual or a group who takes such responsibility is a key factor leading to inappropriate use of diagnostic tests and therapies and of many misdiagnosed and/or unexplained T-LOC episodes.

  Many cardiology units within general hospitals already have the equipment necessary for the management of syncope. Thus, it is the creation of a well-identifiable facility and the appointment of the syncope leader/s – i.e., in essence, an organization – that characterizes the Italian model of syncope management unit.
- The syncope team includes part-time trained technical personnel. This team usually performs the core laboratory tests and takes care of the administrative issues.
- Of the 21 certified syncope units, 15 are located inside the cardiology department; their activity (and personnel and resources) is part of the daily non-invasive arrhythmia management activity of the department. One syncope unit is located

in dedicated rooms inside the ED Observation Unit and is run by an emergency physician; triage and initial evaluation of patients referred in an emergency are performed by different physicians; referral of the patient to the syncope unit, if necessary, may be either immediate or delayed ("protected discharge"), according to the initial risk stratification. Finally, three syncope units are located inside geriatric departments and two in internal medicine departments. When the syncope unit is outside the cardiology department, a formalized multidisciplinary cooperation in diagnostic/therapeutic procedures is established with the cardiology department. Moreover, almost all the syncope units have formalized multidisciplinary cooperation with the Neurology department.

10.2.1 Clinical Results

The volume of activity and the management of patients of nine certified syncope units have been documented in the Syncope Unit Project study.[3] This prospective study enrolled 941 consecutive patients from March 15, 2008 to September 15, 2008; patients were enrolled for one of the following reasons:

- they were affected by unexplained transient loss of consciousness (T-LOC) which, on initial evaluation, was believed to be syncope, or
- non-syncope T-LOC could not be excluded, or
- there was a need to evaluate the precise mechanism of syncope in order to administer the proper specific treatment.

Patients aged <18 years and those with a definite cause of syncope on initial evaluation were excluded. Specifically, patients with arrhythmia-related syncope diagnosed by 12-lead standard ECG (i.e., sinus bradycardia <40 beats/min or repetitive sinoatrial blocks or sinus pauses >3 s; second-degree Mobitz II or third-degree atrioventricular block; rapid paroxysmal supraventricular tachycardia or ventricular tachycardia; and pacemaker malfunction) were excluded because in these cases, the diagnosis is already certain and the proper therapy can be administered immediately. Of the 941 eligible patients, findings in 891 (95%) were able to be analyzed.

10.2.2 Volume of Activity

A median of 15 (interquartile range 12–23) patients per month were evaluated in each syncope unit during the 6 months of observation. The five oldest syncope units had a two-fold higher volume of activity compared to the four newest units (instituted <1 year before): median 23 (20–28) vs.12 (11–14), $p = 0.02$. This difference was mainly due to a higher rate of out-of-hospitals referrals for the older than for the newer units: 16 (13–18) vs. 7 (6–8), $p = 0.04$. These figures give an estimated volume of 163 (132–181) and 60 (54–65) patients per 100,000 inhabitants per year, respectively ($p = 0.03$) (Fig. 10.1).

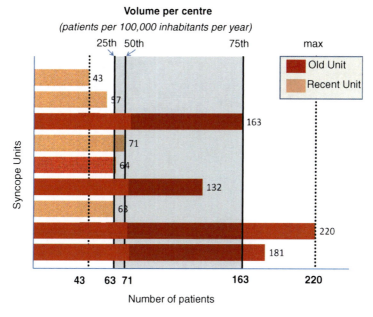

Fig. 10.1 Volume of activity. Each bar is a syncope unit. The syncope units assessed in SUP study are low-volume units. At least 1 year for the volume of activity to grow and stabilize

The syncope units assessed in this study are low-volume units. The preferred model seems to be that of "one hospital–one unit" rather than that of larger "hub" unit serving several hospitals. It seems to take at least 1 year for the volume of activity to grow and stabilize. Even after this stabilization period, we have estimated a relatively low average volume. Therefore, the syncope team cannot be involved full time in the management of T-LOC syncope and must therefore be part of a broader service. In the vast majority of cases, in Italy, the syncope unit as well as the Atrial Fibrillation Unit, the Remote Monitoring Unit, the Pacemaker Clinic, etc. is part of the Arrhythmia Service.

10.2.3 Referral

The majority of patients (60%) were referred from out-of-hospital services (general practitioners, other specialists, primary care, patients themselves), 11% had immediate referral and 13% delayed referral (so-called "protected discharge" with an appointment for early assessment) from the Emergency Department, and 16% were hospitalized patients (Fig. 10.2). Referral from out of hospitals was higher for the oldest than for the newest syncope units: 73% vs. 58%, $p = 0.001$.

Owing to established formal relationships with out-of-hospital services (general practitioners, other specialists, primary care, patients themselves), most referrals

Fig. 10.2 Source of referral
to the syncope units

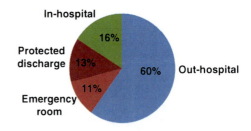

come from these sources. The majority of syncope patients are investigated as out-patients or day cases. The new units had a lower number of outpatient referrals as would be expected.

10.2.4 Diagnosis

A diagnosis was established on initial evaluation in 191 (21%) patients, early (within 45 days) through 2.9±1.6 diagnostic tests in 541 (61%) patients (Fig. 10.3) and remained unexplained in 159 (18%) patients. In 102 (11%) patients, a different diagnosis was assigned "post-hoc" by the Definition Committee according to the definitions reported in Table 10.1. Among these, 60 patients were reclassified as having unexplained syncope because they did not fully meet diagnostic criteria or had multiple possible causes of syncope and 33 patients were reclassified as likely having reflex rather than unexplained syncope (Fig. 10.4). The breakdown of diagnoses was (Fig. 10.5):

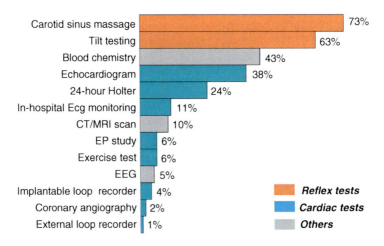

Fig. 10.3   Tests performed (after initial evaluation) in 700 patients enrolled in the SUP study[3]

Table 10.1 Diagnostic criteria (and their observed prevalence in 891 patients) for causes of syncope based on the classification of syncope of the ESC guidelines and adopted by Italian syncope units

Diagnosis	Prevalence (%)
– *Reflex (neurally mediated), classical vasovagal syncope* (VVS) if the syncope was precipitated by emotional distress (fear, severe pain, and instrumentation) or prolonged standing and was associated with typical prodromes	131 (15%)
– *Reflex (neurally mediated), atypical form* if the syncope occurred without apparent triggers and/or had an atypical presentation and the diagnosis was based on the reproduction of similar symptoms by means of tilt testing (and ATP test) and on the exclusion of other causes of syncope (absence of structural heart disease)	231 (26%)
– *Reflex (neurally mediated), carotid sinus syncope* if the syncope was reproduced by carotid sinus massage in the presence of asystole >3 s and/or fall in systolic blood pressure >50 mmHg and in the absence of competing diagnoses	61 (7%)
– *Reflex (neurally mediated), situational syncope* if the syncope occurred during or immediately after micturition, defecation, coughing, swallowing, laughing, meal, or immediately after the end of an exercise	38 (4%)
– *Likely reflex (neurally mediated)* if the history suggested a reflex cause, unconfirmed by tests, structural heart disease was absent and other causes could reasonably be excluded; or syncope was the first (or rare) episode, structural heart disease was absent and other causes could reasonably be excluded	139 (15%)
– *Orthostatic hypotension* if syncope occurred after standing up and symptomatic orthostatic hypotension was documented. The *classical form* was diagnosed if orthostatic hypotension occurred within 3 min after active standing up, while *progressive (delayed) form* was diagnosed – usually by means of tilt testing – if progressive orthostatic hypotension occurred more than 3 min after standing up	32 (4%)
– *Cardiac arrhythmia* if the class I diagnostic criteria of the ESC guidelines [1, 2] were met during prolonged ECG monitoring or by means of electrophysiological study; cardiac arrhythmia also included the case of patients with severely depressed EF who had a definite indication for ICD regardless of the mechanism of syncope	50 (5%)
– *Structural cardiac or cardiopulmonary disease* if the patient was affected by acute cardiac ischemia or other acute cardiopulmonary diseases or prolapsing atrial myxoma or severe aortic stenosis	8 (1%)
– *Non-syncopal attacks* if the episode of transient loss of consciousness was initially attributed to a syncopal condition but the subsequent evaluation demonstrated a non-syncopal mechanism [i.e., metabolic disorders (hypoxia, hypoglycemia), epilepsy, intoxication, vertebrobasilar ischemic attack, accidental fall, or psychogenic (functional) pseudosyncope]	42 (5%)
– *Unexplained* in those patients without any of the above diagnosis	159 (18%)

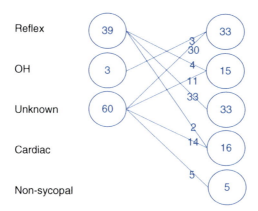

Fig. 10.4 In SUP study[3] a discrepancy between initial diagnosis and that assigned by the Definition Committee was observed in 11% of the patients. Finally, the study suggests some limitations and pitfalls of the current strategy of evaluation of the syncope patient, even if it is performed according to the standard provided by the guidelines. The most commonly observed inconsistency was between reflex and unexplained syncope. This finding underlines the difficulty of reaching a diagnosis based mainly on pathophysiological reasoning and testifies the need for careful adoption of well-accepted standardized diagnostic criteria

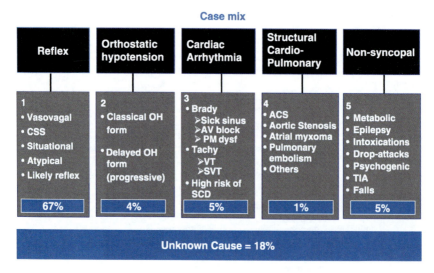

Fig. 10.5 Case mix by final assigned diagnosis according to the definition of Table 10.1

- "likely reflex cause" in 67%,
- orthostatic hypotension in 4%,
- cardiac in 6%,
- non-syncopal in 5% of cases,
- unexplained in 159 (18%) patients (despite a mean of 3.5 ± 1.8 tests per patient).

These latter "unexplained" subgroup of patients were older, more frequently had structural heart disease or ECG abnormalities, had unpredictable onset of syncope due to the lack of prodromes, and exhibited higher OESIL and EGSYS risk scores than did the other groups of patients. In the end, the evidence was insufficient to establish a definite diagnosis; nonetheless, several patients were suspected of having cardiac syncope because of the presence of bundle branch block (41 patients), moderate bradycardia (14 patients), or an EGSYS score ≥ 3 (71 patients). Only 4% of the patients with unexplained syncope received an implantable loop recorder.

Some general comments can be drawn. Fisrt, if investigations are appropriately selected, few ILRs are needed for diagnosis and their diagnostic value is in general very good and cost effective. However, despite thorough evaluation, the diagnosis may often remain presumptive. Thus, it is not surprising that we observed an 11% rate of contrasting diagnoses between the initial local hospital diagnosis and that resulting from strict application by the Definitions Committee of the ESC classification (Fig. 10.4). This finding underlines the difficulty of reaching a diagnosis based mainly on pathophysiological reasoning and provides support for the need for adoption of well-accepted standardized diagnostic criteria (Table 10.1). Uncertainty regarding diagnostic definitions hampers comparison between different studies and the evaluation of treatments.

Second, one-fifth of patients are referred to the syncope units, even though a diagnosis is already suggested by initial evaluation. In these patients, tilt-table testing and carotid sinus massage are performed most frequently, in order to train the patients to recognize reflex susceptibility and to start counterpressure maneuver therapy (biofeedback training). Thus, syncope units, apart from their diagnostic utility, have an important role as the starting point for treatments of reflex syncope, i.e., expert confirmation of diagnosis, patient education regarding awareness and possible avoidance of triggers (including discontinuation of vasodepressive drugs), reassurance, and training in maneuvers to abort syncope episodes.

10.2.5 Treatment

The treatment assigned at the end of the workup is summarized in Table 10.2. Physical counterpressure maneuvers were the most frequently used specific treatments for reflex syncope and orthostatic hypotension; vasoconstrictor drugs were only seldom used in these situations. Most patients with a diagnosis of cardiac syncope received a specific treatment. Overall, 100 patients received cardiac pacing therapy: 61 for asystolic reflex syncope, 29 for established primary arrhythmia, and 10 with unexplained syncope and bundle branch block. A cardioverter-defibrillator was implanted in nine patients.

Table 10.2 Treatment and measures prescribed according to the final diagnosis

Reflex (neurally mediated) and likely reflex[a]	600
Education, reassurance and avoidance of triggers alone (%)	253 (42%)
Physical maneuvers (counterpressure maneuvers) (%)	247 (41%)
Tilt training	69 (11%)
Cardiac pacing (%)	61 (10%)
Modification or discontinuation of hypotensive drugs (%)	53 (9%)
Implantable loop recorder (%)	2 (0%)
Vasoconstrictor drugs (%)	9 (1%)
Orthostatic hypotension[a]	32
Modification or discontinuation of hypotensive drugs (%)	21 (66%)
Education and avoidance of triggers (%)	20 (62%)
Physical maneuvers (counterpressure maneuvers, elastic stockings) (%)	18 (56%)
Volume expansion (%)	15 (47%)
Vasoconstrictor drugs (%)	1 (3%)
None	1 (3%)
Cardiac arrhythmias as primary cause[a]	50
Cardiac pacing (%)	29 (58%)
Cardioverter-defibrillator implantation (%)	8 (16%)
Modification or discontinuation of antiarrhythmic/hypotensive drugs (%)	5 (10%)
Antiarrhythmic drug therapy (%)	5 (10%)
Catheter ablation (%)	1 (1%)
Not specified	9 (18%)
Structural cardiac or cardiopulmonary disease	8
Cardiac surgery (%)	3 (37%)
Coronary revascularization (%)	2 (25%)
Antithrombotic drug therapy (%)	3 (37%)
Syncope of unknown origin	159
Implantable loop recorder (%)	28 (18%)
Physical maneuvers (counterpressure maneuvers) (%)	14 (9%)
Modification or discontinuation of hypotensive drugs (%)	4 (3%)
Cardiac pacing (%)	10 (6%)
Tilt training	4 (2%)
None of the above (%)	109 (68%)
Non-syncopal attacks	42
Anti-epileptic drugs (%)	6 (14%)
Antidepressant drugs (%)	2 (5%)
No therapy or referred to specialist (%)	36 (81%)

[a]More than one treatment was assigned to some patients of this group.

Treatment was in line with the ESC guidelines. Some results seem worthy of mention:

– In accordance with the lack of scientific evidence, pharmacological therapy had a very limited role for therapy of syncope.
– Although only recently developed, physical counterpressure maneuvers were widely accepted and were the cornerstone of active therapy of reflex syncope.
– The negative role of hypotensive drugs was recognized; discontinuation of such agents was recommended for patients with reflex syncope hypotension.
– Cardiac pacing was the most frequent device therapy and perhaps surprisingly was used more often in patients with reflex syncope than in those with cardiac syncope.

10.2.6 Hospitalization and Cost Analysis

The mean cost of the diagnostic tests and examinations (excluding treatment) of the 720 patients evaluated on an outpatient basis was €209 ±140 per patient. A total of 171 (19%) patients needed to be hospitalized: of these, 144 had already been hospitalized before referral to the syncope unit, whereas 27 were hospitalized upon request of the syncope specialist in order to perform invasive tests; the median in-hospital stay was 7 days (interquartile range 5–10). The median cost per hospital stay (excluding the costs of tests and treatments) was €2,990 (interquartile range 2,004–4,497). The mean cost of the diagnostic tests for hospitalized patients was €1,073 ± 716. The total cost of evaluating the study population was €1,034,511, which corresponds to a cost per patient of €1,161. In this study as in others, hospitalization costs per se (excluding tests) accounted for >75% of the total costs. The logical conclusion is that reducing the need for hospitalization would result in a substantial cost saving.

10.3   Clinical Perspectives

Current guideline-based management of T-LOC/syncope has limitations and pitfalls. Apart from the difficulty of reaching an accepted diagnosis and the subsequent need for careful adoption of well-accepted standardized diagnostic criteria, the principal limitation is the unacceptably high rate of unexplained T-LOC/syncope. It seems that the most complex (i.e. with competing possible causes) and potentially severe syncope cases – which therefore would require more specific treatment – remain undiagnosed by means of in-hospital investigations. Indeed, the patients with unexplained syncope tended to be older, more frequently had structural heart disease or ECG abnormalities and unpredictable onset of syncope due to the lack of prodromes compared to the other groups of patients. Many of these were suspected of having cardiac syncope, though this was not confirmed definitively; further, they were at higher risk of death and cardiac syncope than were the other patients as predicted by the significantly higher OESIL and EGSYS risk scores. Conversely, a diagnosis was more easily obtained in healthy young patients without structural heart disease, who are known to have a favorable outcome. *The paradox is that the more we need a precise diagnosis, the more difficult it is to obtain one.*

The patients with unexplained syncope in syncope units are probably different from those with unexplained T-LOC/syncope in epidemiological studies or in other settings who show a relatively good outcome. The patients referred to the syncope unit are, not surprisingly, the most difficult cases because they have been selected as needing specialized care. The finding that 18% of patients potentially at high risk remain without a diagnosis cannot be considered satisfactory for a specialized facility and emphasizes the need for new management strategies. A strategy of extensive utilization of prolonged ECG monitoring, i.e., implantable loop recorders, is likely to be helpful, but it is matter for future research (see Chapter 8). In this SUP (Syncope Unit Project) study, ILRs were used in only a minority of patients. As pointed out in Chapter 8, more aggressive ILR use is advocated in the future. By illustrating the limitations and pitfalls of the current standard of T-LOC/syncope evaluation summarized by the most recent ESC guidelines,[1] the findings summarized in this chapter support the need for future research aimed at improving diagnostic accuracy in patients with syncope.

References

1. Brignole M, et al. Guidelines on management (diagnosis and treatment) of syncope – Update 2004. *Europace*. 2004;6:467–537.
2. Gruppo Italiano Multidisciplinare per lo Studio della Sincope (GIMSI)/Area Syncope Unit/ Syncope Unit certificate GIMSI. www.gimsi.it
3. Brignole M, et al. Prospective multicentre systematic guideline-based management of patients referred to the syncope units of general hospitals. *Europace*. 2010;12:109–118.

Section IC
Current Evidence-Based Knowledge: Clinical Syndromes – Diagnosis and Therapy

Chapter 11
Reflex Syncope (Neurally Mediated Syncope)

Contents

M. Brignole, D.G. Benditt, *Syncope*, DOI 10.1007/978-0-85729-201-8_11,
© Springer-Verlag London Limited 2011

Key points: Diagnosing and treating reflex syncopes

- Reflex (neurally mediated) syncope has a unique pathophysiological mechanism (i.e., a reflex response that, when triggered, gives rise to vasodilatation and/or bradycardia), but there are various clinical presentations, mostly age related.
- There are two diagnostic goals: (1) to identify the etiology (i.e., differentiate reflex from other forms of syncope) and (2) to identify the mechanism of the reflex (i.e., to measure the relative contributions of vasodepression and bradycardia/asystole in causing syncope).
- Therapy consists of general measures which are in common with all forms of reflex syncope, as well as specific therapies which are guided by the knowledge of the mechanism of the reflex.
- In general, education and reassurance are sufficient for most patients. Modification or discontinuation of hypotensive drug treatment (if medically possible) for concomitant conditions is another first-line measure for the prevention of syncope recurrences. Treatment is not necessary for patients who have sustained a single/rare syncope/s and are not having syncope in a high-risk setting (i.e., commercial drivers, pilots).
- Non-pharmacological "physical" treatments (counterpressure maneuvers and so-called tilt or standing training) are now the new first-choice therapies for neurally mediated reflex syncope.
- There is evidence and general agreement that cardiac pacing is useful in cardioinhibitory or mixed carotid sinus syndrome and in some older patients with documented asystolic reflex syncope of the vasovagal type.
- Advice to encourage increased fluid and salt intake for recurrent reflex fainters seems to be well supported clinically and by one randomized study, but has not yet been subjected to rigorous outpatient evaluation.
- The evidence fails to support the efficacy of beta-blocking drugs. Beta-blocking drugs may aggravate bradycardia in some cardioinhibitory cases.
- The role of fludrocortisone is currently undergoing randomized controlled study.
- To date there are not sufficient data to support the use of any other pharmacological therapy for vasovagal syncope, although vasoactive agents such as midodrine have found some support in the literature.

11.1 The Wide Clinical Spectrum of a Unique Disorder

Reflex syncope (synonym: *neurally mediated syncope*) refers to a reflex response that, when triggered, gives rise to vaso-/venodilatation and/or bradycardia; however, the contribution of each of these two factors to systemic hypotension and cerebral hypoperfusion may differ considerably among affected individuals and may even differ in the same patient at different times. Since all forms of reflex syncope share essentially the same basic pathophysiology (i.e., they basically represent the same disorder as best we currently understand), the apparent clinical differences only reflect primarily which specific trigger elicits the reflex.[1,2]

There is an overabundance of names for reflex syncope, and this has proved confusing.[1,2] For example, *"neurogenic"* has been used as a synonym for "reflex syncope," but there is no compelling utility to this term. *"Vasovagal syncope"* is best reserved for a specific form of reflex syncope (see later), but some sources appear to consider it as a synonym for the broad range of reflex faints. We do not believe that the latter is appropriate and would prefer that the term "vasovagal" be reserved for the specific form of reflex faint that occurs in the setting of emotional distress or that occurs in the absence of a specific identifiable trigger. The descriptor *common faint* is appropriate as a synonym of vasovagal as it has an epidemiological basis, since vasovagal syncope is the most frequent form of syncope in the population up to the age of 60 (i.e., the word "common" refers to frequency in this case and does not imply simplicity). Other names that are commonly used in publications to depict "reflex syncope" include *neurocardiogenic* and *neurally mediated cardiac*. *Neurocardiogenic*, as a synonym for reflex syncope, has the disadvantage that it emphasizes cardiac effects while ignoring the vasodepressor contribution. *Vasodepressor* has also been used as an alternative for vasovagal syncope, but has the disadvantage of emphasizing the fall in systemic vascular resistance that, while important, overlooks the cardiac element. The terminology in children is particularly confusing, in that *pallid breath holding spells* and *reflex anoxic seizures* concern reflex syncope in infants with pronounced cardioinhibition often leading to asystole. Neither name conveys that the entity in question is a form of reflex syncope. In the end, the Task Force on Syncope of the European Society of Cardiology recommended that the broad condition be termed reflex or neurally mediated syncope. Specific subsets can then be specifically identified (e.g., vasovagal and carotid sinus syndrome).

The presence of a trigger of a recognizable type is important for the diagnosis of reflex syncope (in which case the general term "situational syncope" is often employed)[1,2] (Table 11.1). Most variants are in fact named for their triggers, such as cough syncope, micturition syncope, and swallow syncope. The exception is vasovagal syncope, a name focusing on efferent mechanisms. Except for the presence of a trigger, autonomic activation is an important clue to diagnose vasovagal syncope in adolescents and most adults (with the exception of the elderly in whom the autonomic activation is less noticeable and therefore causes fewer warning symptoms).

Table 11.1 Classification of reflex (neurally mediated) syncope

---

- Vasovagal syncope (common faint)
  - Mediated by emotional distress: fear, pain, instrumentation, blood phobia
  - Mediated by orthostatic stress
- Situational syncope
  - Cough, sneeze
  - Gastrointestinal stimulation (swallow, defecation, visceral pain)
  - Micturition (post-micturition)
  - Post-exercise
  - post-prandial
  - Others (e.g., laughing, brass instrument playing, and weightlifting)
- Carotid sinus syncope
- Atypical forms (without apparent triggers and/or atypical presentation)

Often, reflex syncope has an *atypical* presentation. The term *atypical form* is used to describe those situations in which reflex syncope occurs with uncertain or even apparently absent triggers. The diagnosis then rests less on history taking alone and more on the exclusion of other causes of syncope (absence of structural heart disease) and on reproducing similar symptoms with carotid sinus massage, tilt-table testing, or other tests. Eye-witness accounts should also be sought as they can be very helpful.

The spectrum of reflex syncope demonstrates much overlap among the clinical forms. Frequently, patients with recurrent syncope have their episodes triggered by different stimuli. In this regard, age is an important determinant of the clinical presentation of reflex syncope[3-5] (Fig. 11.1). Situational syncope and tilt-induced

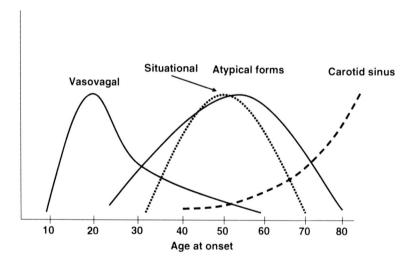

Fig. 11.1 Schematic representation of age-related presentation of reflex syncope

syncope are observed at all ages. By contrast, typical vasovagal syncope is observed in youth but only rarely in old age. Since the elderly are not immune to emotional stimuli (fear, severe pain, and strong emotion), the difference between young and older patients suggests that in older age the responsiveness to afferent neural signals located in cortical sites is decreased or altered. By contrast, positive responses to carotid sinus massage increase with age; indeed, patients with carotid sinus syncope and those with so-called atypical presentation are usually elderly. Since autonomic responses tend to decrease with advancing age, a positive response to carotid sinus massage probably implies a reduction in compensatory mechanisms in a part of the reflex arc. At present, the pathophysiological substrate responsible for the increase in positive responses to carotid sinus massage in older age is unknown (although one report associates this with age-related concomitant deafferentation of neck muscles).

The prevalence of the various forms of reflex syncope is also influenced by the setting in which patients are evaluated. In Table 11.2, the prevalence observed in the emergency departments (EDs)[6] and in syncope units[7] is shown.

Vasovagal syncope usually starts in young subjects, is not generally associated with cardiovascular, neurological, or other diseases, and, therefore, represents an isolated manifestation of transient autonomic dysfunction.[5] Isolated vasovagal syncope cannot be regarded as a disease, but rather as a relatively frequent transient aberration of normal physiology (it may affect sporadically a large proportion of the general population during their life). Isolated vasovagal syncope should be distinguished from those forms, usually with an atypical presentation, that start in older age and which are often associated with cardiovascular or neurological disorders and other dysautonomic disturbances such as carotid sinus hypersensitivity, postprandial hypotension, and persistent disturbances of autonomic function. In these latter subjects, the reflex syncope appears to be expression of a pathological process, mainly related to impairment of the autonomic nervous system to activate compensatory reflexes; the result appears to be an overlap with autonomic failure[5] (Table 11.3).

An abnormal reflex plays a role in causing syncope in different clinical settings where more than one pathophysiological factor may contribute to the symptoms.

Table 11.2   Prevalence of different forms of reflex syncope in two different clinical settings

	Emergency department (a) (309 pts)	Syncope unit (b) (602 pts)
– Vasovagal	101 (33%)	131 (22%)
– Situational	71 (23%)	38 (6%)
– Carotid sinus syncope	18 (6%)	61 (10%)
– Atypical	38 (12%)	231 (38%)
– Likely reflex	81 (26%)	139 (23%)

Source: (a) = Evaluation of Guidelines in Syncope Study 2 (EGSYS-2) study[6]; (b) = syncope unit project (SUP) study[7]

Table 11.3 Differences in clinical features of isolated vasovagal syncope and the atypical forms of reflex syncope occurring in the elderly

Isolated vasovagal syncope	Other forms (atypical)
• Onset at a young age • Otherwise healthy people • Typical vasovagal prodromes/triggers ("classical" form) • Affects about 50% of all individuals • 70% of population predisposed • Strong stressor • No genetic basis • No evidence of autonomic involvement or hormonal disorders • Low risk of trauma • Frequent spontaneous disappearance in advanced age	• Onset in old age • Patients with cardiovascular or neurological disease • Presentation without prodromes/atypical triggers ("non-classical" form) • Often diagnosed only after a positive head-up tilt test • Overlap with carotid sinus syndrome • Overlap with situational syncope • Overlap with orthostatic hypotension or other dysautonomic symptoms • High risk of trauma • Sometimes progressively worsening over time
• Similar hypotension–bradycardia mechanism • Similar rate of positive responses during tilt testing • Similar rate of cardioinhibitory and vasodepressor forms during spontaneous syncope	

For instance, in the setting of valvular aortic stenosis or left ventricular outflow tract obstruction, syncope is not solely the result of restricted cardiac output, but is in part due to inappropriate neurally mediated reflex vaso-/venodilatation and/or primary cardiac arrhythmias. Similarly, a neural reflex component (preventing or delaying vasoconstrictor compensation) appears to play an important role when syncope occurs in association with certain brady- and tachyarrhythmias.[8-10]

11.2 Diagnosis

There are two diagnostic goals: (1) identify the etiology (i.e., differentiate reflex from other forms of syncope) and (2) identify the mechanism of the reflex (i.e., to measure the relative contribution of vasodepression and bradycardia/asystole in causing syncope).

11.3 Identifying the Etiology of Syncope

Diagnosis of reflex syncope is made by typical history or positive response to tests and exclusion of other competing diagnosis.[1,2] The starting point for the evaluation is a careful detailed medical history. In many patients without heart disease a definite diagnosis can be made by the history alone without further testing. This is the case in "classic" forms of vasovagal and situational syncope. Under such circumstances, the diagnosis is readily established and treatment, if any, can be planned. However, the diagnostic value of the history decreases with advancing age of the patient. For example, in one study,[3] history alone was able to define the diagnosis in 38% of patients aged <65 years but only in 9% of patients aged >65 years.

More commonly, the initial evaluation leads to a suspected diagnosis when one or more of the features listed in Table 5.3 are present. A suspected diagnosis needs to be confirmed by directed testing (Table 11.4). Tests are often more essential to confirm suspected diagnoses in the elderly. For a detailed description of indications and interpretation of diagnostic tests for reflex syncope, refer to Chapters 7 and 8. The diagnostic criteria are summarized in Table 11.5.

Table 11.4 Investigations for neurally mediated syncope (see also Chapters 7 and 8)

More useful
- History and physical exam
- Carotid sinus massage
- Tilt-table testing
- Implantable loop recorder (ILR)

Less useful
- ATP test (adenosine test)
- Eyeball compression test (especially useful in teenagers)
- Valsalva maneuver
- External loop recorder and mobile cardiac outpatient telemetry [MCOT (USA)]
- Echocardiogram (if structural heart disease is a serious concern)

Minimal or no value
- Holter monitoring
- Head CT/MRI
- EEG

Table 11.5 Diagnostic criteria of the different forms of reflex (neurally mediated) syncope

- *Vasovagal syncope* is diagnosed if syncope is precipitated by emotional distress (fear, severe pain, instrumentation, or blood phobia) or prolonged standing and is associated with typical prodromes due to autonomic activation. Under such circumstances, no further evaluation of the disease or the disorder may be needed
- *Situational syncope* is diagnosed if syncope occurs during or immediately after micturition, defecation, coughing, swallowing, laughing, meal, or immediately after the end of an exercise. Under such circumstances, no further evaluation of the disease or disorder may be needed
- *Carotid sinus syncope* is diagnosed if syncope is reproduced by carotid sinus massage in the presence of asystole >3 s and/or fall in systolic blood pressure >50 mmHg and in the absence of competing diagnoses
- *Atypical form* is diagnosed if syncope occurs without apparent triggers and/or has an atypical presentation and the diagnosis is based on the reproduction of similar symptoms by means of tilt testing (and ATP test) and on the exclusion of other causes of syncope (absence of structural heart disease)
- *Likely reflex (neurally mediated)* is diagnosed if the history suggests a reflex cause, unconfirmed by tests, structural heart disease was absent, and other causes can reasonably be excluded; or syncope is the first (or rare) episode, structural heart disease is absent, and other causes can reasonably be excluded

11.3.1 Vasovagal Syncope

Vasovagal syncope is characterized by its triggers and by autonomic activation before (and sometimes after) attacks.[1,2,11–14]

11.3.1.1 Triggers

There are two main triggers for vasovagal syncope: (1) central and (2) peripheral. Among the central triggers, emotion, pain, and instrumentation are the most frequent. With respect to the peripheral triggers, standing is particularly important, especially when it is associated with a hot/crowded environment, exercise, dehydration, illness, or excessive alcohol consumption. However, prolonged standing alone may provoke vasovagal syncope (i.e., even in the absence of other contributing factors), especially if the individual is standing very still (e.g., guards in front of prominent buildings). Most vasovagal episodes are probably triggered by peripheral triggers.

In some subjects, the range of triggers varies widely, including syncopal attacks without any trigger at all. In such cases the presence of typical vasovagal attacks in the same individual's history allows atypical attacks to be accepted as vasovagal, more so than when no typical attacks have ever occurred. In orthostatic vasovagal syncope, the triggering pattern differs from that in orthostatic hypotension due to autonomic failure. In the first, syncope or presyncope occurs very rarely compared to the number of times the subjects stand; syncope may occur after a highly variable time of standing and sets in quickly when it occurs. In autonomic failure, blood pressure usually drops immediately and consistently after standing up; the blood pressure drop may be measured, even though symptoms may not occur at the time.

11.3.1.2 Autonomic Activation

Vasovagal syncope is usually preceded by autonomic activation: intense pallor ("white as a sheet"), sweating, and nausea are most common. Prodromal symptoms usually start 30–90 s before syncope. A feeling of warmth, an odd sensation in the abdomen, and light-headedness or dizziness may be mentioned in addition to nausea and sweating. Eyewitnesses may notice pallor and wide pupils. After syncope, autonomic activation may continue a while, and vasovagal syncope may reoccur if the triggers are not removed. Although consciousness recovers quickly without confusion in adults, patients may be upset and experience pronounced fatigue after syncope (often lasting many hours).

As a consequence of the above findings, vasovagal syncope can be diagnosed if the syncope is precipitated by emotional distress (fear, severe pain, instrumentation, or blood phobia) or prolonged standing and is associated with typical prodromes due to autonomic activation. No further evaluation is needed unless there are other clues to important concomitant conditions that on rare occasion may be responsible for triggering a vasovagal faint (e.g., inferior wall myocardial infarction, temporal lobe epilepsy).

11.3.2 Situational Syncope

Situational syncope traditionally refers to reflex syncope associated with certain specific circumstances, which act as the trigger. The various forms have the efferent reflex syncope pathway in common, but obviously differ in terms of the afferent triggers. Several authors compared situational syncope with vasovagal syncope; people with situational syncope tended to be older and more often had pronounced prodromal symptoms and signs.

Situational syncope is less common than vasovagal syncope. Specific forms are diagnosed if syncope occurs during or immediately after micturition, defecation, coughing, swallowing, laughing, eating, or immediately after vigorous exercise.[1,2] Under such circumstances, no further evaluation is needed.

11.3.2.1 Cough (Tussive Syncope)

Cough (tussive syncope) is evoked by coughing.[15,16] Cough syncope occurs during bouts of intense coughing without prodromal symptoms, usually in heavy-built, obese, middle-aged smoking men with chronic obstructive pulmonary disease. Attacks may occur not only while standing and sitting (e.g., driving) but also while lying down. The pathophysiology remains incompletely understood. Consequently, it is uncertain whether cough syncope should be considered a form of syncope mostly due to mechanical factors (high intra-thoracic pressure transmitted to veins resulting in such a high intracranial pressure that there is no longer a pressure gradient, i.e., no perfusion pressure) or to a reflex (baroreflex hypotensive response to very high transient blood pressures induced by the cough or the stimulation of pulmonary or atrial receptors during coughing).

11.3.2.2 Swallow (Deglutition Syncope)

Swallow (deglutition) syncope, as the name suggests, is induced by swallowing.[17] Presyncope and syncope follow swallowing almost immediately in this condition. Swallow syncope may occur at any age, although most case reports concern those of middle age or older. It may occur only after specific foods, which may be solids, liquids, or carbonated drinks; either hot or cold drinks can elicit syncope. In others, syncope can occur independently of the nature of the food item. In reported cases the mechanism is almost always through either cardioinhibition with sinus bradycardia or asystole, or AV block. Swallow syncope occurs either in healthy subjects or in patients suffering from esophageal or cardiac disease; how esophageal pathology triggers the reflex is not known, but bradycardia following balloon inflation of the esophagus implicates mechanoreceptors. Atropine can block bradycardia, making it clear that the efferent arc is vagal in nature.

11.3.2.3 Micturition (Post-micturition)

Syncope occurs during or immediately after emptying the bladder. It typically occurs in men who get up from sleep at night to go to the bathroom. They faint either at the toilet or shortly after leaving the bathroom. It is much less common in women. Micturition syncope probably represents a reflex "helped along" by various circumstances: subjects may arise from sleep, suggesting low nocturnal blood pressure and peripheral vasodilatation due to lying in a warm bed. Standing still during micturition allows pooling of blood without counteraction by the leg muscle pump. Finally, voiding the bladder triggers the syncopal reflex. A complex mechanism entailing a balance between the hypertensive effect of a full bladder and the compensating vasodilatory baroreceptor action has been hypothesized. When the bladder is abruptly emptied, the hypertensive reflex is terminated but the vasodilation persists just long enough to trigger a collapse.

11.3.2.4 Defecation Syncope

Defecation syncope occurs during or shortly after defecation.[18] It is likely that defecation syncope results from multiple influences. One factor may be getting up out of a warm bed. Additionally, straining at stool involves multiple repeated Valsalva maneuvers which may impede cardiac venous return and cerebral blood flow. Finally, pressure in the colon may evoke a true reflex syncope, evidenced by bradycardia and low blood pressure during colonoscopy.

11.3.2.5 Post-exercise Syncope

Post-exertional syncope[19,20] is almost invariably due to autonomic failure or to a neurally mediated mechanism and is characterized by hypotension which can be associated with marked bradycardia or asystole; it typically occurs in subjects without heart disease, especially in athletes. Rarely, as has been discussed earlier in this volume, reflex syncope can also occur during exercise; in this latter case, it is caused by marked hypotension without bradycardia. It has been supposed that epinephrine plays an important role in the mechanisms leading to neurally mediated syncope associated with exercise. A failure of reflex vasoconstriction in splanchnic capacitance vessels and in forearm resistance vessels has been shown during exercise in patients with vasovagal syncope. Tilt-table testing has been used to diagnose neurally mediated syncope, which may manifest as post-exertional syncope; however, it is not a very reliable way of reproducing the phenomenon in these very select and physically fit patients.

11.3.2.6 Post-prandial Syncope

Post-prandial hypotension is a prevalent condition in the elderly population and seems to be more common in frail elderly individuals who may be particularly susceptible to complications such as syncope.[21,22] The diagnosis is based on the measurement of meal-induced blood pressure changes. The precise relationship between symptoms and post-prandial reductions in blood pressure is unclear. Blood pressure maintenance after a meal may depend on the interaction of sympathetic function, baroreceptor function, and vasoactive peptide release to compensate for the increase in bowel blood volume. The impairment of one or more of these mechanisms could result in inadequate compensation that leads to hypotension and syncope. The presence of symptoms depends on the individual patient's ability to develop adequate compensatory cerebral autoregulation. A hypertensive elderly patient may experience symptoms with only a small reduction in blood pressure. Thus, the mechanism of post-prandial syncope could be similar to that of vasovagal syncope triggered by orthostatic stress.

11.3.2.7 Laughter (Gelastic) Syncope

Laughter (gelastic) syncope is elicited by laughter.[23] Very few cases have been described and the differentiation from cataplexy attacks (which are also often associated with laughter) is important (but difficult). Prolonged hearty laughter triggers the episode, without prodromal symptoms. In one case, Valsalva maneuver showed a drop in blood pressure at the end of the maneuver with unconsciousness. In some cases, tilt-table testing resulted in a vasovagal response, suggesting susceptibility to reflex syncope. The mechanism could be similar to that of cough syncope. The triggering by laughter may suggest cataplexy, but laughter syncope causes amnesia for the event, which is not typically the case in cataplexy.

11.3.2.8 Sleep Syncope

In *sleep syncope*, sleep is the circumstance which characterizes this form of reflex syncope, but is not its trigger.[24,25] The patients, mostly middle-aged women, give a history of waking from sleep with either abdominal discomfort or the urge to defecate followed by syncope. In some, syncope occurs in bed, in others while trying to get to the toilet. Some patients remember nightmares before the episode. Most patients also have daytime episodes, which sound vasovagal in nature. Tilt-table testing is frequently positive. When ECG documentation could be obtained, a typical vasovagal pattern has been observed. In the differential diagnosis of nocturnal syncope, epilepsy is probably the foremost alternative diagnosis, but cardiac arrhythmias need careful consideration as well.

11.3.3 Carotid Sinus Syncope

The prevalence of carotid sinus syndrome (CSS) increases with age, ranging from 4% in patients <40 years to 41% in patients >80 years among those referred to a specialized facility for syncope of uncertain origin. It is more frequent in men than in women with a 4:1 ratio.[26,27]

In its rare spontaneous form, CSS is believed to be triggered by mechanical manipulation of the carotid sinuses, either by external stimuli (e.g., tight collar) or by masses in the neck close to the sinuses (e.g., tumor and lymph nodes). Previous neck surgery and/or irradiation markedly increases susceptibility to CSS. In the more common form of CSS, no evident mechanical trigger is identified; the condition is diagnosed by carotid sinus massage and it is called *induced* carotid sinus syndrome.[1,2] *Spontaneous* carotid sinus syncope should therefore be considered as a form of situational syncope as, by definition, a specific trigger has been identified.

Unlike vasovagal syncope, in CSS there are no clear signs of autonomic activation. Prodromes are usually absent or non-specific and of short duration; recovery is usually prompt. CSS occurs mostly while the patients are standing. Owing to its unpredictability and its occurrence in the elderly, major trauma (defined as bone fracture, intracranial hemorrhage, internal organ lesions requiring urgent treatment, and retrograde amnesia or focal neurologic defect) is more frequent than in other patients with syncope.

There are several diseases that predispose to carotid sinus syndrome. These are atherosclerosis, coronary artery disease, head and neck surgery/irradiation, acute biliary tract disturbances, diabetes, and some drugs such as digitalis and beta-blockers. Moreover, carotid sinus syndrome is frequently associated with sinus node dysfunction (from 21 to 56% in various surveys) and with AV conduction abnormalities (from 21 to 37% in various surveys). Patients affected by CSS are expected to have recurrence of syncope (about 50% at 2 years) and minor symptoms (about 2/3 of affected individuals at 2 years). Carotid sinus syndrome is associated with a high mortality (about 35% at 5 years) but this mortality seems to be related to associated comorbidities and older age rather than to the syndrome itself.[28]

In practice, the diagnosis of induced CSS virtually coincides with that of positive carotid sinus massage. Carotid sinus hypersensitivity is present in many subjects who have not yet manifested the clinical syndrome, i.e., syncope. It is well known, for example, that abnormal responses are frequently observed in 17–20% of asymptomatic patients affected by various types of cardiovascular diseases and in 38% of asymptomatic patients with severe narrowing of the carotid arteries. However, in asymptomatic subjects, the induction of syncope is much less frequent so that the specificity of the test increases if reproduction of spontaneous syncope during carotid massage is required. In other words, the potential number of patients who might suffer from CSS is higher than those who have actually manifested it. Nevertheless, from a practical point of view, a positive response to carotid massage should be considered diagnostic of the cause of syncope only in patients with a high likelihood of CSS as identified in the initial evaluation. Indeed, when competitive diagnoses for the cause of syncope are still present, the finding of a positive carotid sinus massage must be viewed with caution. In these cases, other tests are needed to confirm the mechanism of syncope (i.e., ECG documentation by prolonged monitoring). Therefore, CSS is diagnosed only if syncope is reproduced by carotid sinus massage in the presence of asystole >3 s and/or fall in systolic blood pressure >50 mmHg and in the absence of competing diagnoses[1,2] (see Chapter 7).

11.3.4 Atypical Forms (Without Apparent Triggers and/or Atypical Presentation)

Atypical forms of reflex syncope are diagnosed if syncope occurs without apparent triggers and/or has an otherwise unusual presentation. The diagnosis is based on the reproduction of similar symptoms by means of tilt-table testing[29] and/or ATP test (the atypical form diagnosed by carotid sinus massage is classified as carotid sinus syncope) and on the exclusion of other causes of syncope (e.g., absence of structural heart disease) (see Chapter 7). Atypical forms are the most frequent cause of reflex syncope among the elderly and patients referred to specialized syncope facilities (Table 11.2). Atypical forms are frequently associated with cardiovascular or neurological disorders and other dysautonomic disturbances (Table 11.3). The absence of a clear history and the possibility of multiple etiologies make the diagnosis difficult to establish. Documentation of a spontaneous event by means of prolonged ECG monitoring is frequently necessary either for confirming the diagnosis or for starting mechanism-specific treatment.

In patients without structural heart disease, tilt-table testing can be considered diagnostic, and no further tests are needed when syncope is reproduced.[1,2] In patients with structural heart disease, arrhythmias or other cardiac causes should be excluded prior to considering the positive tilt test results to be diagnostic. ATP testing produces an abnormal response in some patients with syncope of unknown origin, but only infrequently in controls. ATP testing identifies a group of patients (usually older women) with otherwise unexplained syncope with definite clinical features and benign prognosis but possibly heterogeneous mechanism of syncope. The clinical feature of adenosine (ATP)-sensitive patients is different from that of tilt-positive patients. Adenosine-sensitive patients are older with a female predominance, have a shorter history of syncope, and have a higher prevalence of systemic hypertension.

11.3.5 Likely Reflex (Neurally Mediated)

Reflex (neurally mediated) syncope is considered likely if the history suggests but is not definitive for a reflex cause (see historical features discussed above), the diagnosis has not been confirmed by tests, structural heart disease is absent, and other causes can reasonably be excluded; or syncope has occurred only one time or very rarely, structural heart disease is absent, and other causes can reasonably be excluded.[1,2] These two situations are very frequent in clinical practice (Table 11.2). Since a certain diagnosis has not been made, syncope in these cases should be classified as "unexplained." In general, these forms have a clinical presentation characterized by one or few episodes of syncope, usually preceded by warnings, not accompanied by trauma, and a benign outcome. For the above reasons, intensive evaluation (e.g., loop recorder implantation) is usually not justified unless the patient and/or the family is very concerned or there is a worrisome family history (i.e., unexplained sudden death). In the latter circumstance, an insertable loop recorder (ILR) is probably the best choice in order to ultimately capture a spontaneous episode.

11.4 Identifying the Mechanism of Syncope

Determining the relative contribution of vasodilatation and bradycardia/asystole to the hypotension causing syncope is of practical importance when the severity of the clinical presentation (because of high frequency or high risk of the episodes) justifies a specific treatment (i.e., cardiac pacing when the cardioinhibitory reflex is dominant and vasoactive measures when the vasodepressor reflex is dominant). Apart from this situation, the knowledge of the precise mechanism is less important as the two forms have similar outcome and share common preventive basic measures.

In terms of evaluating the vasodepressor versus cardioinhibitory contributions, the ECG documentation of a spontaneous syncopal episode by prolonged ambulatory monitoring is the current reference standard. However, ultimately it would be better to record both ECG and blood pressure simultaneously. Provocative tests (carotid sinus massage, tilt testing, and ATP) provide results more quickly but are less reliable than ECG-syncope correlation (Table 11.6).

11.4.1 ECG Monitoring

ECG monitoring is diagnostic when a correlation between syncope and ECG abnormality (brady- or tachyarrhythmia) is detected. Conversely, ECG monitoring excludes an arrhythmic cause (but not a vasodepressor cause) when syncope

Table 11.6 Value of different examinations in predicting the mechanism of the spontaneous reflex

	Predicting value	Notes
Prolonged ECG monitoring	Excellent	No documentation in about a half of patients up to a 2-year period
Carotid sinus massage	Good	Only if syncope is reproduced by massage
Tilt-table testing	Low	With the possible exception of asystole occurring during tilt testing
ATP test (adenosine test)	Uncertain	Further study is needed. May play a role in patients with idiopathic paroxysmal AV block

occurs in the absence of a clinically significant rhythm variation; in this case a dominant vasodepressor form can be hypothesized but cannot be said to be established. Pseudosyncope is still a consideration. Even in the absence of syncope–ECG correlation, ECG monitoring is currently deemed diagnostic if major arrhythmias are detected (periods of Mobitz II- or III-degree AV block or a ventricular pause >3 s, rapid prolonged paroxysmal atrial or ventricular tachyarrhythmias). Conversely, presyncope may not be an accurate surrogate for syncope in establishing a diagnosis in the absence of such arrhythmias and, therefore, therapy should not be guided by presyncopal findings. See also Chapter 8.

11.4.2 Carotid Sinus Massage

The relationship between induced carotid sinus syndrome (i.e., reproduction of syncope during the massage) and spontaneous, otherwise unexplained syncope was derived from one study[30] using a pacemaker designed to detect asystolic episodes. Long pauses ($\geq$6 s) were detected in 53% of the patients with CSS during 2 years of follow-up, suggesting that a positive response to carotid massage predicts the occurrence of spontaneous asystolic episodes. This correlation was recently confirmed by means of documentation of spontaneous episodes by an implantable loop recorder (ILR) in 18 patients affected by cardioinhibitory carotid sinus syndrome in whom carotid sinus massage was positive (maximum pause of 5.5 ± 1.6 s [range 3.6–8.5 s]).[31] Asystole >3 s (average longest pause of 9 [8–18]s) was observed at the time of the spontaneous syncope in 16 (89%) patients. Sinus arrest was the most frequent finding and was observed in 72% of these cases. Moreover, the relationship between induced carotid sinus syndrome and spontaneous syncope is indirectly supported by the results of the studies on cardiac pacing in patients with cardioinhibitory forms which generally showed a reduction of syncopal relapses. Finally, when performed with a proper protocol, carotid sinus massage showed an excellent reproducibility. Thus, the type of response to carotid sinus massage is usually considered a good predictor of the spontaneous forms of the reflex syncope and consequently is in general sufficient to guide therapy (usually cardiac pacing) unless competing diagnoses are present. See also Chapter 7.

11.4.3 Tilt-Table Testing

The clinical significance of the type of response to tilt-table testing in predicting the behavior of blood pressure and heart rate during spontaneous syncope has recently been questioned. The reproducibility of a positive tilt test is low. The reproducibility of an initial positive response ranges in the literature from 31 to 92%. The relative contributions of vasodilatation and cardioinhibition components of hypotension during tilt-induced syncope are frequently different from those of spontaneous syncope recorded with the implantable loop recorder. In the ISSUE 2 study,[32] while a positive cardioinhibitory response to tilt testing predicted an asystolic spontaneous syncope in a few cases, the presence of a positive vasodepressor or mixed response, or even a negative response, did not exclude the presence of asystole during spontaneous episodes. Thus, the type of response to tilt-table testing does not adequately predict the spontaneous forms of the reflex syncope; therefore, other tests (i.e., prolonged monitoring) are usually required before embarking on cardiac pacing therapy (the possible exception, as noted above, may be a tilt test that results in prolonged asystole in older patients). See also Chapter 7.

11.4.4 ATP (Adenosine) Test

The role of the ATP (Adenosine) test is controversial and there is substantial difference of opinion regarding its place in the evaluation of syncope patients. Initial studies supported potential pacing benefit if the test was positive, a recent study showed no correlation between AV block induced by ATP and ECG findings (documented by ILR) during spontaneous syncope. Thus, finding to date do not support its use as a solitary diagnostic test for selecting patients for cardiac pacing. ATP may, however, have a role to play in assessing syncope in middle-aged and older patients (especially women) with suspected paroxysmal AV block. See also Chapter 7.

11.5 Therapy

Although there are different forms of reflex syncope, the strategies for prevention of syncope apply to most causes (carotid sinus syndrome may be an exception). Owing to its benign nature, the goal of therapy is primarily prevention of recurrence and associated injuries and improvement in quality of life but not prolongation of survival.

11.5.1 Lifestyle Measures

The cornerstone of the non-pharmacological management of patients with reflex syncope is education and reassurance regarding the benign nature of the condition. In this context, the term "benign" means "not directly life threatening." However, recurrent faints may lead to injury and accidents. Consequently, it is crucial that the importance of preventive treatment be emphasized in discussion with patients, family members, and other caregivers.

In general, initial treatment comprises education regarding awareness and possible avoidance of triggers (e.g., hot crowded environments, volume depletion) and early recognition of prodromal symptoms.[1,2] Eliminating exposure to triggers may be difficult, but the response may be attenuated by maintenance of central volume, protected posture, and slower changes in posture. Careful avoidance of agents that lower blood pressure (including beta-blockers, angiotensin-converting enzyme inhibitors, alpha-blockers, calcium antagonists, diuretics, antidepressant agents, and alcohol) is important. In younger patients, increased salt and volume intake is encouraged. Often, young persons restrict their salt intake excessively, and while this may have theoretical long-term health benefits, it may increase risk of reflex faints.

11.5.2   Additional Treatments

Additional treatment may be necessary in unpredictable and frequent syncope. This is particularly the case when

- very frequent syncope alters quality of life,
- recurrent syncope without or with very short prodrome exposes patients to risk of trauma,
- syncope occurs during high-risk activity (e.g., driving, machine operation, flying, and competitive athletics).

11.5.3   Physical Counterpressure Maneuvers (PCM)

Non-pharmacological "physical" treatments are emerging as a new frontline treatment of reflex syncope (with the exception of carotid sinus syndrome). Two clinical trials[33,34] have shown that isometric PCM of the legs (leg crossing) or of the arms (hand grip and arm tensing) are able to induce a significant blood pressure (BP) increase during the phase of impending reflex syncope that allows the patient to avoid or delay losing consciousness in most cases. The results have been confirmed in a multicenter prospective trial,[35] which assessed the effectiveness of PCM in daily life in 223 patients, aged 38 ± 15 years, with recurrent reflex syncope and recognizable prodromal symptoms: 117 patients were randomized to standardized conventional therapy alone, and 106 patients received conventional therapy plus training in PCM. The median yearly syncope burden during follow-up was significantly lower in the group trained in PCM than in the control group ($p < 0.004$); overall 51% of the patients with conventional treatment and 32% of the patients trained in PCM experienced recurrence of syncope ($p < 0.005$). Actuarial recurrence-free survival was better in the treatment group (logrank $p < 0.018$), resulting in a relative risk reduction of 39% (95% confidence interval, 11–53%). No adverse events were reported.

Tilt-table testing can be employed to teach the patient to recognize early prodromal symptoms. All patients should be taught PCM, which now forms the cornerstone of therapy together with education and reassurance. However, this therapy is hampered by the fact that patients sometimes do not have recognizable prodromal symptoms or these are of too short duration to allow the activation of PCM. Moreover, the maneuvers are much less effective in female and in older patients because of diminished muscle strength and slower response time, and associated diseases.

As a rule, syncope burden dramatically decreases after starting PCM, but syncope sometimes recurs in a substantial percentage of patients, approximately 20% per year.[36,37] A practical description of how to train patients is given in Chapter 21. In patients who continue to faint despite adequate lifestyle measures and PCM, "tilt training" (also known as "standing training") may be considered, particularly in younger, very symptomatic, well-motivated patients. Despite controversy regarding efficacy, tilt training may prove useful and at the very least helps by reassuring the patient that they are active participants in the treatment.

11.5.4 Tilt Training (Standing Training) Method

In highly motivated young patients with recurrent vasovagal symptoms triggered by orthostatic stress, the prescription of progressively prolonged periods of enforced upright posture may reduce susceptibility to syncope recurrence.[37] However, this treatment is hampered by the low compliance of patients in continuing the training program for a long period and four small randomized controlled trials failed to confirm short-term effectiveness of tilt training.[38–41]

11.5.5 Pharmacological Therapy

Many drugs have been tested in the treatment of reflex syncope; for the most part the results have been disappointing.[42–46] The list includes beta-blockers, disopyramide, scopolamine, theophylline, ephedrine, etilefrine, midodrine, clonidine, and serotonin reuptake inhibitors. While results have been satisfactory in uncontrolled trials or short-term controlled trials, several long-term placebo-controlled prospective trials have been unable to show a benefit of the active drug over placebo with some exceptions.

Beta-blockers have been advocated in vasovagal syncope based on presumed lessening of ventricular mechanoreceptor activation owing to their anti-sympathetic and negative inotropic effects in reflex syncope. This theory has not been supported by the outcome of one major clinical trial (POST[45]). A rationale for use of beta-blockers in other forms of neurally mediated syncope is lacking. They may enhance bradycardia in carotid sinus syndrome. Beta-blockers have failed to be effective in five of six long-term follow-up studies.[42–46]

Since failure to achieve proper vasoconstriction of the peripheral vessels is common in reflex syncope, alpha agonist vasoconstrictors (etilefrine and midodrine) have been used. Two double-blind, acute tilt studies have shown apparent contrasting effects. Moya et al.[47] administered etilefrine for 1 week, then repeated the test and found no difference between active and placebo treatment. On the contrary, Kaufman et al.[48] administered a single dose of midodrine just 1 hr before tilt testing and found a significant reduction in syncope during tilt with active treatment. Etilefrine was studied in a large randomized placebo-controlled, double-blind clinical trial.[49] During follow-up, patients treated with etilefrine 25 mg twice daily or placebo showed no difference in frequency or time to recurrent syncope. Thus, the evidence fails to support the use of etilefrine. Midodrine was studied in three small, open-label, randomized trials in patients affected by very frequent "hypotensive" symptoms (>1 syncope/month).[50–52] Even if defined as "neurally mediated," there is overlap in clinical features of patients in these studies with other forms of orthostatic intolerance rendering the results difficult to interpret. The major limitation of midodrine is frequent dosing (2–3 times daily), which may limit long-term compliance. Caution must be taken in the use of midodrine in older males because of adverse effects on urinary outflow. Overall, these data suggest that chronic pharmacological treatment with alpha agonists alone may be helpful but inadequate in reflex syncope; further, long-term treatment cannot be advised for occasional symptoms. Even if not proven, a self-administered single dose of midodrine, for example, 1 dose 1 h before prolonged standing or performing an activity that usually triggers syncope (the so-called pill in the pocket strategy), may be useful in selected patients when added to lifestyle measures and PCM.

Fludrocortisone has been shown to be ineffective in a small, randomized double-blind trial in children.[53] Fludrocortisone has been widely used in adults with reflex syncope, but there is no trial evidence to support this. It is, however, currently being evaluated in a large randomized trial in adults (POST 2).

Paroxetine was shown to be effective in one placebo-controlled trial, which included highly symptomatic patients from one institution.[54] This has not been confirmed by other studies. Paroxetine may reduce anxiety, which precipitates events. Paroxetine is a psychotropic drug requiring caution in use in patients without severe psychiatric disease.

11.5.6 Cardiac Pacing

11.5.6.1 Carotid Sinus Syndrome (CSS)

Pacing has been considered as the most important therapeutic option for CSS since the early 1970s when case reports demonstrated that recurrences of syncope were abolished after implantation of a pacemaker.[55] Subsequent case series then confirmed that pacing in patients with CSS could significantly reduce the number of syncope episodes.[56] Non-randomized comparative studies supported these preliminary results and in the mid-1980s, pacing became the recognized treatment of CSS.

The first randomized trial which compared in 60 patients pacing and no pacemaker was reported in 1992.[57] After a mean follow-up of 36 ± 10 months, syncope recurred in 9 and 57% of the patients in pacing and control group, respectively ($p < 0.0002$). There was a trend for a better outcome of patients with dominant cardioinhibitory form compared to those with mixed form (Fig. 11.2). A recent randomized trial[58] confirmed the results. Sixty patients with CSS were randomized to receive a permanent pacemaker ($n = 30$) or no pacing ($n = 30$). At 12 months, the rate of syncope was 40% in non-treated patients compared with 10%

Fig. 11.2 Main results of the first randomized trial of comparison between pacing and no pacing therapy on long-term follow-up in carotid sinus syndrome[57]

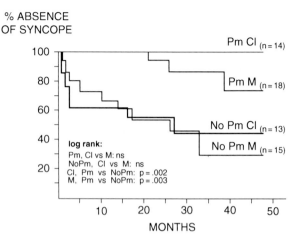

in the paced patients ($p = 0.008$). Finally, in the already mentioned ILR study,[31] after ILR documentation, 14 patients with asystole received dual-chamber pacemaker implantation; during 35 ± 22 months of follow-up, two syncopal episodes recurred in two patients (14%) and presyncope occurred in another two patients (14%). Syncope burden decreased from 1.68 (95% confidence interval 1.66–1.70) episodes per patient per year before to 0.04 (0.038–0.042) after pacemaker implant (98% relative risk reduction).

Thus, cardiac pacing appears to be effective in CSS and is acknowledged to be the treatment of choice when bradycardia has been documented. Dual-chamber pacing is generally preferred over single-chamber ventricular pacing. There are as yet no randomized studies examining treatment of dominant vasodepressor CSS; this same limitation also pertains for other vasodepressor conditions.

11.5.6.2 Other Forms of Reflex Syncope

Pacing for reflex vasovagal syncope has been the subject of five major multicenter, randomized controlled trials, which gave contrasting results.[59-63] In all the patients, the pre-implant selection was based on tilt-table testing response. Adding together the results of the five trials, 318 patients were evaluated: syncope recurred in 21% of the paced patients and in 44% of unpaced patients ($p < 0.001$). A recent meta-analysis of all studies suggested a non-significant 17% reduction in syncope from the double-blinded studies and an 84% reduction in the studies where the control group did not receive a pacemaker.[64] The results are not surprising if we consider that pacing may affect the cardioinhibitory component of the vasovagal reflex, but will have no effect on the vasodepressor component, which is often dominant.

Two non-randomized trials evaluated the efficacy of pacing by selecting patients with documented asystole during spontaneous syncope by ILR. In the study of Sud et al.,[65] after the insertion of a cardiac pacemaker, syncope burden decreased from 2.7 per year to 0.45 per year ($p = 0.02$). The ISSUE 2 study[32] hypothesized that spontaneous asystole and not tilt test results should form the basis for patient selection for pacemaker therapy. This study followed 392 patients with presumed reflex syncope with an ILR. Of the 102 patients with a symptom–rhythm correlation, 53 underwent loop recorder-guided therapy, predominantly pacing for asystole. These patients experienced a striking reduction in recurrence of syncope compared with non-loop recorder-guided therapy (10% versus 41%, $p = 0.002$). It must be stressed that ISSUE 2 was not a randomized trial. It merely provides the basis for such a trial, now ongoing (ISSUE 3, the enrollment of which is complete but the follow-up phase in ongoing).

In conclusion, pacing plays only a small role in therapy for reflex syncope, unless severe spontaneous bradycardia is detected during prolonged monitoring (especially in older individuals).

11.5.7 Conclusion

Evidence for effectiveness of therapy of neurally mediated syncope is in general weak. Few randomized controlled trials have been undertaken, especially in terms of evaluating physical maneuvers and drug therapy options. Nevertheless, combining together the knowledge derived from several less rigorous studies and that derived from the epidemiology and the pathophysiology of syncope, the European Society of Cardiology Syncope Task Force[2] was recently able to draw some recommendations. These recommendations are summarized in Table 11.7.

11.6 Clinical Perspectives

Clear criteria for diagnosis of reflex syncope have been recently established in the ESC syncope practice guidelines. Application of these guideline recommendations should provide practicing physicians a solid basis for establishing whether a reflex faint underlies their patients' symptoms. On the other hand, the therapeutic strategies for reflex syncope (especially vasovagal syncope), despite the advances of recent years, are still not completely satisfactory. Syncope recurrence rate remains high, being approximately 10% per year in the general population and even up to 40% in selected populations (see also Fig. 6.3). New therapeutic options are needed.

The efficacy of therapy is hampered by difficulty identifying the relative contributions of vasodepression and bradycardia/asystole in causing syncope in a given patient at a particular time; this distinction is important as it forms the basis for a mechanism-specific therapy. Whether a diagnostic strategy of extensive utilization of prolonged ECG monitoring, i.e., implantable loop recorders, could provide more insight in this regard is a matter for future research.

Cardiac pacing seems to be effective when a dominant cardioinhibitory reflex is documented (the best example being carotid sinus syndrome), but the coexistence of a vasodepressor reflex accounts for the failure of pacing to prevent all symptoms in some cases. In this regard, the difficulty of documenting blood pressure during spontaneous syncope is a major diagnostic problem and a challenge for future technological developments. On the other hand, no predictably effective therapies

Table 11.7 Treatment of reflex syncope

Recommendations of the 2009 ESC Task Force on Syncope	Class[a]	Level[b]
• Explanation of the diagnosis, provision of reassurance, and explanation of risk of recurrence are indicated in all patients	I	C
• Isometric PCM are indicated in patients with prodrome	I	B
• Cardiac pacing should be considered in patients with dominant cardioinhibitory CSS	IIa	B
• Cardiac pacing should be considered in patients with frequent recurrent reflex syncope, age > 40 years, and documented spontaneous cardioinhibitory response during monitoring	IIa	B
• Midodrine may be indicated in patients with VVS refractory to lifestyle measures	IIb	B
• Tilt training may be useful for education of patients but long-term benefit depends on compliance	IIb	B
• Cardiac pacing may be indicated in patients with tilt-induced cardioinhibitory response with recurrent frequent unpredictable syncope and age > 40 after alternative therapy has failed	IIb	C
• Triggers or situations inducing syncope must be avoided as much as possible	III	C
• Hypotensive drugs must be modified or discontinued	III	C
• Cardiac pacing is not indicated in the absence of a documented cardioinhibitory reflex	III	C
• Beta-adrenergic blocking drugs are not indicated	III	A

CSS, carotid sinus syndrome; PCM, physical isometric counterpressure maneuvers; VVS, vasovagal syncope
[a]Class of recommendation
[b]Level of evidence

for the vasodepressor reflex yet exist. Even physical counter maneuvers, which are probably the most effective among current acute treatments, often fail to abort the attack because the patients are unable to activate them with sufficient force, or at all. This limitation most frequently happens when prodromes are absent or are of very short duration and in older patients because they have diminished muscle strength and difficulty reacting rapidly. No pharmacological therapy has been proven to be totally effective. Midodrine, a vaso-/venoconstrictor, is the most useful of currently available drugs but side effects often preclude aggressive dosing.

References

1. Brignole M, et al. Guidelines on management (diagnosis and treatment) of syncope: Update 2004. *Europace*. 2004;6:467–537.
2. Moya A, et al. Guidelines for the diagnosis and management of syncope (version 2009). *Eur Heart J*. 2009;30:2631–2671.

3. Del Rosso A, et al. Relation of clinical presentation of syncope to the age of patients. *Am J Cardiol.* 2005;96:1431–1435.
4. Alboni P, et al. Clinical spectrum of neurally-mediated reflex syncopes. *Europace.* 2004;6: 55–62.
5. Alboni P, et al. Is vasovagal syncope a disease? *Europace.* 2007;9:83–87.
6. Brignole M, et al. A new management of syncope: Prospective systematic guideline-based evaluation of patients referred urgently to general hospitals. *Eur Heart J.* 2006;27:76–82.
7. Brignole M, et al. Prospective multicentre systematic guideline-based management of patients referred to the syncope units of general hospitals. *Europace.* 2010;12:109–118.
8. Alboni P, et al. An abnormal neural reflex plays a role in causing syncope in sinus bradycardia. *J Am Coll Cardiol.* 1993;22:1130–1134.
9. Brignole M, et al. Role of autonomic reflexes in syncope associated with paroxysmal atrial fibrillation. *J Am Coll Cardiol.* 1993;22:1123–1129.
10. Leitch JW, et al. Syncope associated with supraventricular tachycardia: An expression of tachycardia or vasomotor response. *Circulation.* 1992;85:1064–1071.
11. Benditt DG. Neurally mediated syncopal syndromes: pathophysiological concepts and clinical evaluation. *Pacing Clin Electrophysiol.* 1997;20:572–584.
12. Hamer AWF, Bray JE. Clinical recognition of neurally mediated syncope. *Intern Med J.* 2005;35:216–221.
13. Mathias CJ, et al. Observations on recurrent syncope and presyncope in 641 patients. *Lancet.* 2001;357:348–353.
14. Ganzeboom KS, et al. Prevalence and triggers of syncope in medical students. *Am J Cardiol.* 2003;91:1006–1008.
15. Benditt DG, et al. Effect of cough on heart rate and blood pressure in patients with "cough syncope". *Heart Rhythm.* 2005;2:807–813.
16. Krediet CT, et al. Sharpey-Schafer was right: evidence for systemic vasodilatation as a mechanism of hypotension in cough syncope. *Europace.* 2008;10:486–488.
17. Omi W, et al. Swallow syncope, a case report and review of the literature. *Cardiology.* 2006;105:75–79.
18. Kapoor WN, et al. Defecation syncope. A symptom with multiple etiologies. *Arch Intern Med.* 1986;146:2377–2379.
19. Sakaguchi S, et al. Syncope associated with exercise, a manifestation of neurally mediated syncope. *Am J Cardiol.* 1995;75:476–481.
20. Colivicchi F, et al. Exercise-related syncope in young competitive athletes without evidence of structural heart disease: Clinical presentation and long-term outcome. *Eur Heart J.* 2002;23:1125–1130.
21. O'Mara G, Lyons D. Postprandial hypotension. *Clin Geriatr Med.* 2002;18:307–321.
22. Puisieux F, et al. Intraindividual reproducibility of postprandial hypotension. *Gerontology.* 2002;48:315–320.
23. Sarzi Braga S, et al. Laughter-induced syncope. *Lancet.* 2005;366:426.
24. Krediet CTP, et al. Vasovagal syncope interrupting sleep?. *Heart.* 2004;90:e25.
25. Jardine DL, et al. Fainting in your sleep? *Clin Auton Res.* 2006;16:76–78.
26. Thomas JE. Hyperactive carotid sinus reflex and carotid sinus syncope. *Mayo Clin Proc.* 1969;44:127–139.
27. Puggioni E, et al. Results and complications of the carotid sinus massage performed according to the "Methods of Symptoms". *Am J Cardiol.* 2002;89:599–601.
28. Brignole M, et al. Survival in symptomatic carotid sinus hypersensitivity. *Am Heart J.* 1992;123:687–692.
29. Livanis EG, et al. Situational syncope: response to head-up tilt testing and follow-up: comparison with vasovagal syncope. *Pacing Clin Electrophysiol.* 2004;27:918–923.
30. Menozzi C, et al. Follow-up of asystolic episodes in patients with cardioinhibitory, neurally mediated syncope and VVI pacemaker. *Am J Cardiol.* 1993;72:1152–1155.

31. Maggi R, et al. Cardioinhibitory carotid sinus hypersensitivity predicts an asystolic mechanism of spontaneous neurally-mediated syncope. *Europace*. 2007;9:563–567.

32. Brignole M, et al. Early application of an implantable loop recorder allows effective specific therapy in patients with recurrent suspected neurally mediated syncope. *Eur Heart J*. 2006;27:1085–1092.

33. Krediet P, et al. Management of vasovagal syncope: controlling or aborting faints by leg crossing and muscle tensing. *Circulation*. 2002;106:1684–1689.

34. Brignole M, et al. Isometric arm counter-pressure maneuvers to abort impending vasovagal syncope. *J Am Coll Cardiol*. 2002;40:2054–2060.

35. van Dijk N, et al. Effectiveness of physical counterpressure maneuvers in preventing vasovagal syncope: the Physical Counterpressure Manoeuvres Trial (PC-Trial). *J Am Coll Cardiol*. 2006;48:1652–1657.

36. Croci F, et al. Efficacy and feasibility of isometric arm counter-pressure manoeuvres to abort impending vasovagal syncope during real life. *Europace*. 2004;6:287–291.

37. Reybrouck T, et al. Long-term follow-up results of tilt training therapy in patients with recurrent neurocardiogenic syncope. *Pacing Clin Electrophysiol*. 2002;25:1441–1446.

38. Foglia-Manzillo G, et al. Efficacy of tilt training in the treatment of neurally mediated syncope. A randomized study. *Europace*. 2004;6:199–204.

39. Kinay O, et al. Tilt training for recurrent neurocardiogenic syncope: effectiveness, patient compliance, and scheduling the frequency of training sessions. *Jpn Heart J*. 2004; 45:833–843.

40. On YK, et al. Is home orthostatic self-training effective in preventing neurocardiogenic syncope? A prospective and randomized study. *Pacing Clin Electrophysiol*. 2007;30:638–643.

41. Duygu H, et al. The role of tilt training in preventing recurrent syncope in patients with vasovagal syncope: A prospective and randomized study. *Pacing Clin Electrophysiol*. 2008;31:592–596.

42. Flevari P, et al. Vasovagal syncope: a prospective, randomized, crossover evaluation of the effect of propranolol, nadolol and placebo on syncope recurrence and patients' well-being. *J Am Coll Cardiol*. 2002;40:499–504.

43. Madrid AH, et al. Lack of efficacy of atenolol for the prevention of neurally mediated syncope in a highly symptomatic population: A prospective, double-blind, randomized and placebo-controlled study. *J Am Coll Cardiol*. 2001;37:554–559.

44. Sheldon R, et al. Effect of beta blockers on the time to first syncope recurrence in patients after a positive isoproterenol tilt table test. *Am J Cardiol*. 1996;78:536–539.

45. Sheldon R, et al. Prevention of syncope trial (POST): a randomized, placebo-controlled study of metoprolol in the prevention of vasovagal syncope. *Circulation*. 2006;113:1164–1170.

46. Brignole M, et al. A controlled trial of acute and long-term medical therapy in tilt-induced neurally mediated syncope. *Am J Cardiol*. 1992;70:339–342.

47. Moya A, et al. Limitations of head-up tilt test for evaluating the efficacy of therapeutic interventions in patients with vasovagal syncope: results of a controlled study of etilefrine versus placebo. *J Am Coll Cardiol*. 1995;25:65–69.

48. Kaufman H, et al. Midodrine in neurally mediated syncope: a double-blind randomized crossover study. *Ann Neurol*. 2002;52:342–345.

49. Raviele A, et al. Effect of etilefrine in preventing syncopal recurrence in patients with vasovagal syncope: a double-blind, randomized, placebo-controlled trial. *Circulation*. 1999;99:1452–1457.

50. Ward CR, et al. Midodrine: a role in the management of neurocardiogenic syncope. *Heart*. 1998;79:45–49.

51. Samniah N, et al. Efficacy and safety of midodrine hydrochloride in patients with refractory vasovagal syncope. *Am J Cardiol*. 2001;88:80–83.

52. Perez-Lugones A, et al. Usefulness of midodrine in patients with severely symptomatic neurocardiogenic syncope: a randomized control study. *J Cardiovasc Electrophysiol*. 2001;12: 935–938.

53. Salim MA, et al. Effectiveness of fludrocortisone and salt in preventing syncope recurrence in children: a double blind, placebo-controlled, randomized trial. *J Am Coll Cardiol.* 2005;45:484–488.

54. di Girolamo E, et al. Effects of paroxetine hydrochloride, a selective serotonin reuptake inhibitor, on refractory vasovagal syncope: a randomized, double-blind, placebo-controlled study. *J Am Coll Cardiol.* 1999;33:1227–1230.

55. Voss DM. Demand pacing and carotid sinus syncope. *Am Heart J.* 1970;79:544–547.

56. Morley CA, et al. Carotid sinus syncope treated by pacing. Analysis of persistent symptoms and role of atrio ventricular sequential pacing. *Br Heart J.* 1982;47:411–418.

57. Brignole M, et al. Long-term outcome of paced and non paced patients with severe carotid sinus syndrome. *Am J Cardiol.* 1992;69:1039–1043.

58. Claesson JE, et al. Less syncope and milder symptoms in patients treated with pacing for induced cardioinhibitory carotid sinus syndrome: a randomized study. *Europace.* 2007;9: 932–936.

59. Connolly SJ, et al. The North American Vasovagal Pacemaker Study (VPS). A randomized trial of permanent cardiac pacing for the prevention of vasovagal syncope. *J Am Coll Cardiol.* 1999;33:16–20.

60. Sutton R, et al. Dual-chamber pacing in the treatment of neurally mediated tilt-positive cardioinhibitory syncope : pacemaker versus no therapy: a multicenter randomized study. *Circulation.* 2000;102:294–299.

61. Ammirati F, et al. Permanent cardiac pacing versus medical treatment for the prevention of recurrent vasovagal syncope: a multicenter, randomized, controlled trial. *Circulation.* 2001;104:52–57.

62. Connolly SJ, et al. Pacemaker therapy for prevention of syncope in patients with recurrent severe vasovagal syncope: Second Vasovagal Pacemaker Study (VPS II): A randomized trial. *JAMA.* 2003;289:2224–2229.

63. Raviele A, et al. A randomized, double-blind, placebo-controlled study of permanent cardiac pacing for the treatment of recurrent tilt-induced vasovagal syncope. The Vasovagal Syncope and Pacing Trial (SYNPACE). *Eur Heart J.* 2004;25:1741–1748.

64. Sud S, et al. The expectation effect and cardiac pacing for refractory vasovagal syncope. *Am J Med.* 2007;120:54–62.

65. Sud S, et al. Implications of mechanism of bradycardia on response to pacing in patients with unexplained syncope. *Europace.* 2007;9:312–318.

Chapter 12
Orthostatic Intolerance: Orthostatic Hypotension and Postural Orthostatic Tachycardia Syndrome

Contents

Key points: Orthostatic intolerance

- Orthostatic intolerance syndromes are common and comprise a range of often very disabling symptoms associated with postural change to a more upright position or with sustained upright posture.
- Orthostatic hypotension (OH), whether symptomatic or asymptomatic, is the most common clinically recognized manifestation of orthostatic intolerance.
- In the case of symptomatic OH, near-syncope or syncope may occur shortly (i.e., immediate to about 4–5 min) after movement from a

M. Brignole, D.G. Benditt, *Syncope*, DOI 10.1007/978-0-85729-201-8_12,
© Springer-Verlag London Limited 2011

gravitationally relatively "neutral" position (e.g., lying or sitting) to one that places greater gravitational stress on the cardiovascular system and overwhelms the vascular system's ability to maintain adequate cerebral blood flow.

- OH may be asymptomatic in many individuals, but nevertheless it can be the source of important clinical consequences. In this regard, OH is a serious concern in older and particularly institutionalized individuals in whom it may be responsible for triggering falls with considerable risk of injury.

- In younger persons, OH (particularly of the "immediate form") is usually less serious than in the elderly, but the transient "grey-out" of vision is often a worry for otherwise healthy young people.

- Postural orthostatic tachycardia syndrome (POTS) is the second most common form of orthostatic intolerance and tends to occur primarily in the young. This can be a prolonged disability, with multiple associated and difficult-to-assess symptoms including fatigue, palpitations, "dizziness and light-headedness," and weakness. The clinical course may last for years despite best treatment efforts.

- Treatment of these and other less well-defined orthostatic intolerance syndromes is imperfect; in most cases, treatment focuses on symptom relief rather than cure.

- The overall treatment strategy must focus on trying to improve venous return to the heart, and in the case of POTS, to diminish adrenergic hyperactivity. This entails non-pharmacologic and pharmacologic approaches.

- While treatment goals are clear and now widely accepted, they are often difficult to accomplish and the approach must be adapted to each individual.

12.1 Introduction

In health, movement from lying or sitting to standing is largely unassociated with evident change in well-being. However, in some individuals, especially those who are physically deconditioned, there may be a transient sense of increased heart rate. In others, a brief "grey-out" of vision may occur from time to time, but this sensation usually disappears quickly (perhaps <10 s) and does not occur consistently. On the other hand, if symptoms of near-syncope or syncope develop repetitively, or if patients begin to complain of symptoms suggestive of sympathetic autonomic hyperactivity (e.g., palpitations, heart racing, and anxiety) with movement to the upright posture, then they may be considered to be exhibiting orthostatic intolerance.

Orthostatic hypotension (OH), whether symptomatic or asymptomatic, is the most common clinically recognized manifestation of orthostatic intolerance.[1-3] In the case of symptomatic OH, near-syncope or syncope occurs shortly (i.e., immediate to about 4–5 min) after movement from a gravitationally relatively "neutral" position (e.g., lying or sitting) to one that places greater gravitational stress and overwhelms the vascular system's ability to maintain adequate cerebral blood flow. Frank syncope induced by moving from supine or seated to upright posture is an important problem in elderly or less physically fit individuals, or patients who are volume depleted.

Postural orthostatic tachycardia syndrome (POTS) is the second most common clinical manifestation of orthostatic intolerance.[4-6] In this condition, clinical features are often diverse and the apparent causes numerous, but the primary unifying factor is an apparent symptomatic sympathetic autonomic hyperactivity occurring either as a result of movement to upright posture or if the affected individual attempts to remain in an upright posture for prolonged periods of time.

Although they are usually considered as separate entities, OH and POTS may be related to several other conditions that are also believed to be due at least in part to abnormal or inappropriate autonomic nervous system function; these include inappropriate sinus tachycardia, neurally mediated syncope (in particular, vasovagal syncope which is discussed elsewhere in this volume), and chronic fatigue syndrome (Fig. 12.1). This chapter reviews the terminology associated with orthostatic intolerance, the essential pathophysiology of the clinical presentations, and approaches to therapy.

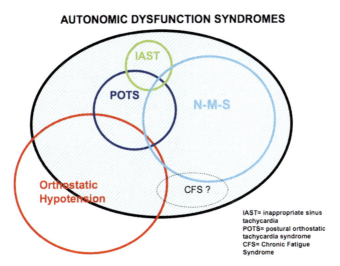

Fig. 12.1 Schematic Venn diagram illustrating the relationships among various conditions that are believed due, at least in part, to abnormal autonomic system function

12.2 Terminology

12.2.1 Orthostatic Intolerance

Orthostatic intolerance is a general descriptor of those conditions which occur as a result of the affected individual's moving to a more gravitationally "at–risk" position (e.g., lying to sitting, sitting to standing) or if the affected individual had been remaining in the upright position for an extended period of time. The term "orthostatic intolerance" does not imply a specific diagnosis but is better used to characterize a syndrome. Thus, it may be used to encompass OH of any etiology (whether symptomatic or asymptomatic), postural orthostatic tachycardia syndrome (POTS), and other less well-defined conditions in which symptoms are triggered by postural change.

12.2.2 Orthostatic Hypotension (OH)

OH has for some time been defined by consensus as a sustained reduction of systolic blood pressure of at least 20 mmHg or diastolic blood pressure of 10 mmHg within 3 min of standing or head-up tilt ($\geq 60°$) on a tilt table.[1,2] For the most part, this definition has stood the test of time. However, in patients with supine hypertension, a reduction in systolic blood pressure of at least 30 mmHg may be a more appropriate criterion.[2]

OH is a clinical sign that may or may not lead to symptoms. In the absence of symptoms, OH is not generally considered to be a clinically important observation, although it has been recently argued that it nonetheless has adverse prognostic implications.[7–9] Specifically, the presence of OH has been associated with subsequent susceptibility to falls in both hypertensive and normotensive older nursing home patients. Whether the same is also true in a free-living "younger" population is less certain; in the younger free-living patient a clinical diagnosis of symptomatic OH is best based upon both the demonstration of the blood pressure change and a concordant medical history indicating that symptoms (usually transient "grey-out," near-syncope, or syncope) are associated with movement to an upright posture or within a few moments after moving to the upright posture.

12.2.3 Postural Orthostatic Tachycardia Syndrome (POTS)

Postural orthostatic tachycardia syndrome (POTS) is a common form of orthostatic intolerance most often encountered in young persons.[4–6] POTS is conventionally defined by the presence of a "posturally triggered" sustained heart rate increment of ≥ 30 beats/min (>35 beats/min in teenagers) within 10 min of standing or head-up tilt. Most affected individuals will achieve quiet standing heart rates ≥ 120 beats/min for no apparent reason (Fig. 12.2). Associated symptoms often include palpitations,

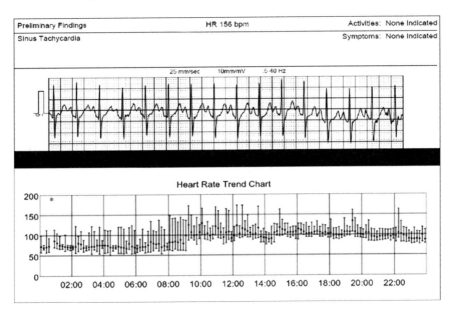

Fig. 12.2 ECG (*top panel*) and 24-h heart rate profile in an untreated 14-year-old male POTS patient. Note the persistent elevated heart rate throughout waking hours that subsides to some degree at night when the individual is resting seated or recumbent in bed. The ECG reveals sinus rhythm with heart rates often >150 beats/min for no apparent reason

weakness, exertional incapacity, inability to concentrate, and fatigue. The autonomic over-activity associated with POTS may be temporarily diminished by supine rest but often not completely; symptoms return with resumption of upright posture.

12.2.4 Dysautonomia

Although the term dysautonomia has had a specific meaning to neurologists (e.g., when used to describe "familial dysautonomia" [Riley-Day syndrome]), it has in recent years come to be used more broadly to characterize abnormal functioning of the autonomic nervous system (including transient forms such as those that occur in the neurally mediated faints).[10–12] This newer usage is unfortunate, inasmuch as the term "dysautonomia" has for a long time implied an underlying "structural" disturbance of the autonomic nervous system. The latter is not typically the case in neurally mediated faints. It would be better to reserve the term "dysautonomia" for drug-induced, disease-induced (e.g., diabetes), or familial autonomic dysfunction, and perhaps certain less well-understood but prolonged autonomic disturbances such as POTS. Transient disturbances of autonomic function such as those that occur in the neurally mediated faints should be excluded.

12.3 Physiology of Blood Pressure Control

An adequate blood pressure is essential to ensure an adequate supply of oxygen and nutrients to body organs, and particularly the brain since it has only limited energy reserves (see Chapter 2). Maintenance of blood pressure is determined by the combination of cardiac output and arterial vascular resistance. In this regard, venous vasculature tone and fluid volume status play a crucial role by contributing to preload (a major determinant of cardiac output).

The interaction among cardiac function and vascular tone with respect to cerebral blood flow is particularly important when subjects are upright, since gravitational force tends to reduce arterial and venous pressure. Vascular tone is affected by circulating hormones (e.g., angiotensin II and epinephrine), synaptic norepinephrine release, and by locally active hormones such as endothelin and nitric oxide.[13,14] Intravascular and extravascular fluid volumes are determined by various factors including the renin–angiotensin–aldosterone system and atrial natriuretic peptide. However, while these factors are important over relatively long time periods, none exhibit the speed and sensitivity of the baroreceptor reflex system; the latter controls blood pressure on a beat-to-beat basis. Afferents from the carotid sinus, heart, and major cardiopulmonary vessels relay information to the brain through the vagus and glossopharyngeal nerves. Within the brain stem, numerous regions interact to determine efferent sympathetic outflow to blood vessels and both sympathetic and parasympathetic (vagus) nerves to the heart.

12.4 Failure to Maintain Blood Pressure

Levels of blood pressure need to be adequately maintained not only during resting upright posture but also during various daily activities (e.g., physical exercise, emotional stress, and digestion). In health, the flexibility and responsiveness of the autonomic nervous system enables appropriate regional circulatory adjustments, thereby accounting for changing needs. However, in many individuals, especially in older and frail individuals or those encountering environmental extremes of altitude or temperature, the adjustments may be inadequate.

Inability to maintain blood pressure, especially when upright, may lead to reduced perfusion of organs and in particular to those organs (particularly the brain) that lie above the level of the heart. A reduction in cerebral perfusion may cause symptoms that vary from transient confusion and memory lapse to falls, temporary loss of vision and/or hearing, and ultimately loss of consciousness or syncope. Less often, if a regional vascular system is compromised (e.g., obstructive coronary artery disease), symptoms may arise due to disturbance of specific organ function (e.g., myocardial ischemia resulting in angina pectoris). On the other hand, in some individuals, it is the necessary but perhaps "hyperactive" autonomic nervous system response itself that causes symptoms (e.g., racing heart sensation in POTS patients).

Apart from postural change, certain other activities of daily life, such as physical exertion and exposure to hot crowded places, may also act to lower blood pressure. Thus, splanchnic vasodilatation during food ingestion and increased skeletal muscle blood flow during exercise can contribute to near-syncope and syncope, especially when an individual is upright. Recognition of these factors is important as they may account for certain presenting symptom scenarios (e.g., syncope or near-syncope when climbing stairs or walking up hill, so-called coat-hanger distribution of muscle pain thought to be due to inadequate blood flow to that region during modest exertion).

12.5 Clinical Conditions

12.5.1 Orthostatic Syncope and Near-syncope

As the name implies, orthostatic syncope occurs as a result of a transient excessive cerebral hypotension that may occur when susceptible individuals arise from a lying or a sitting to a standing position. Loss of consciousness is usually of gradual onset but may occur suddenly. Some patients may also manifest more non-specific complaints such as weakness, fatigue, cognitive slowing, leg buckling, visual blurring, headache, neck pain, orthostatic breathlessness, and chest pain.

Soon after standing, blood volume is redistributed with pooling of 0.5–1.0 L of blood from the upper part of the body to the lower extremities and splanchnic venous capacitance system. As a result, venous return to the heart falls and cardiac filling pressure are reduced. This results in diminished stroke volume and cardiac output and a lower blood pressure. In response, autonomic nervous system adjustments act to increase vascular tone, heart rate, and cardiac contractility. In addition, during active standing, contraction of skeletal muscle acts to mitigate pooling and augments venous return to the heart. The goal is to stabilize arterial pressure and organ blood flow.

Patients with OH exhibit inability to maintain arterial blood pressure adequately when in the upright posture (this may not occur every time, but often enough to cause lifestyle issues and potential for injury). A significant and persistent decrease in systemic pressure may occur leading to symptoms arising from transient retinal and/or cerebral ischemia, including visual disturbances ("grey out" or "blackout"), light-headedness, or "dizziness," postural instability, and/or loss of consciousness (i.e., orthostatic syncope). Additionally, symptoms may result from impaired perfusion of certain muscle groups (particularly those above heart level) causing symptoms such as pain in the neck region ("coat-hanger" distribution) and symptoms suggesting angina pectoris. Typically symptoms resolve on lying down. Susceptibility to OH may be aggravated by concomitant chronotropic incompetence (due to sinus node dysfunction and/or drug effects) in older subjects.

12.5.1.1 Presentation

Since orthostatic faints are those in which symptoms are associated with OH triggered by movement from a more gravitationally neutral position (e.g., supine position) to one in which gravitation tends to further diminish cerebral blood flow (e.g., upright posture), a careful medical history is usually diagnostic.[15–17] Two basic forms of OH (and consequently OH-induced syncope) are recognized (see also Chapter 7, Section 7.3):

Rapid forms. These forms occur rapidly upon "active" standing (not during tilt testing) and may be observed in young healthy individuals as well as in older patients.[17] In fact, many healthy individuals experience a minor form of "immediate hypotension" when they need to support themselves momentarily as they stand up. The cause is a transient mismatch between cardiac output (diminished as preload falls) and vascular tone (insufficient constriction). Essentially, in these instances, "immediate OH" causes a transient self-limited "grey-out" primarily due to inadequate retinal perfusion. On the other hand, immediate OH may not always be benign; frank syncope can occur, and even in the absence of syncope, instability and falls are a risk in more frail individuals.

Delayed form (including delayed OH followed by vasovagal syncope). In delayed OH, as the name implies, symptoms usually occur a few minutes after standing up.[1,15] Commonly, the patient has already walked some distance, then collapses. It is the delayed form that is detected when multiple standing blood pressure measures are taken over several minutes after movement to the upright posture (Fig. 12.3).

In both forms of orthostatic syncope, the underlying cause is failure of the vascular and autonomic nervous systems to respond to an increased gravitational stress. Lack of an appropriate response can be due to either extrinsic factors or autonomic failure (Table 12.1). Extrinsic factors include dehydration from prolonged exposure to hot environments, inadequate fluid intake or excessive use of diuretics, anti-hypertensive agents, beta-adrenergic blockers, or vasodilators. Similarly, concomitant conditions such as diabetes or alcohol abuse may cause neuropathies that predispose patients to orthostatic syncope. Less often the problem is the result of a primary autonomic failure with inadequate reflex adaptations to upright posture (e.g., multi-system atrophy or Parkinson's disease). Once again, chronotropic incompetence (a frequent comorbidity in older patients) may contribute to increased susceptibility.

The importance of considering autonomic dysfunction as a cause of orthostatic syncope has been emphasized by the findings of Low et al.,[18] who reviewed an experience in 155 patients referred for assessment of suspected orthostatic hypotension. Although a highly select population were referred to a neurology department, findings revealed that among the most severely affected symptomatic patients ($n = 90$, mean age 64 years), pure autonomic failure accounted for 33%, multi-system atrophy for 26%, and autonomic/diabetic neuropathy for 31%. Finally, secondary autonomic dysfunction due to neuropathies associated with chronic diseases (e.g., diabetes mellitus), or toxic agents (e.g., alcohol), or infections (e.g.,

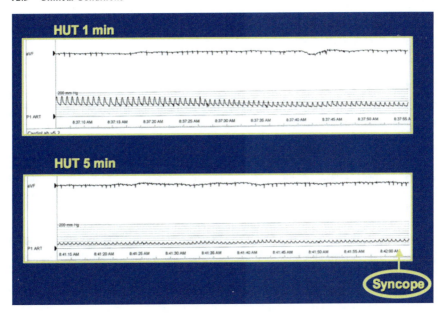

Fig. 12.3 ECG (*upper trace*) and arterial blood pressure (BP, *lower trace*) traces during delayed symptomatic OH provoked by head-up tilt. The BP recording reveals steady gradual fall in arterial pressure with onset of syncope when pressure reaches approximately 55/35 mmHg. The ECG reveals a relatively stable sinus rhythm without evidence of attempt at compensatory tachycardia. The absence of tachycardia suggests an element of chronotropic incompetence of uncertain etiology

Table 12.1   Neurogenic and non-neurogenic causes of inadequate blood pressure control

---

Non-neurogenic causes
- Impaired cardiac output
  - Diseases affecting ventricular myocardium (heart failure, hypertrophic cardiomyopathy)
  - Valvular heart disease (e.g., aortic stenosis)
  - Arrhythmias (tachyarrhythmias or bradyarrhythmias)
- Inadequate intravascular volume (e.g., acute blood loss, diminished intake)
- Vasodilatation (e.g., drug effects)

Neurogenic factors
- Neurally mediated (e.g., vasovagal syncope, carotid sinus hypersensitivity)
- Primary autonomic disease
- Secondary autonomic dysfunction (e.g., diabetes, alcohol abuse)

Guillain-Barre syndrome) are relatively common in medical practice and may also cause syncope in association with orthostatic hypotension.

Elderly institutionalized individuals are at particular risk for OH.[14,16,19,20] In elderly non-volume-depleted patients, in whom central or peripheral autonomic nervous system diseases have been excluded, the prevalence of OH is about 9% over the age of 80 and about 12% over the age of 85. It is a significant independent predictor of all-cause mortality.

12.5.1.2 Diagnosis

The medical history is the most important diagnostic tool for identifying orthostatic syncope. Apart from the association of symptoms with change of posture, other common historical features include the following[19–21]:

- OH is more common and more severe in the morning most likely due to high supine nocturnal blood pressure that causes a relative overnight "pressure diuresis" and results in intravascular volume depletion.
- Patients with autonomic failure and the elderly are susceptible to significant falls in blood pressure associated with meals. This is exacerbated by large meals, meals high in carbohydrate, and alcohol intake.
- Orthostatic blood pressure fall increases with age due to age-associated changes in baroreflex function, reduced cardiac and vascular compliance, and supine hypertension.

Orthostatic syncope is confirmed when documented OH is accompanied by symptoms that reproduce spontaneous events (i.e., syncope or near-syncope). For purposes of establishing the diagnosis of "orthostatic hypotension," arterial blood pressure should be measured when the patient adopts the standing position after 5 min of lying supine. As discussed earlier, OH is defined as a decline in systolic blood pressure of at least 20 mmHg and/or a diastolic fall of 10 mmHg within 3 min of standing (30 mmHg in hypertensive patients), regardless of whether or not symptoms occur.[1–3] Optimally, the blood pressure recording should be made with the patient's arm at heart level. If the patient does not tolerate standing for this period, the lowest systolic blood pressure during the upright position should be recorded. Measurements should be continued after 3 min of standing if blood pressure is still falling.

There are some patients with syncope in whom there is a history suggestive of impaired orthostatic blood pressure control but in whom measurements in upright position may be normal. In these patients, if the clinical history suggests the need, additional tests after major provocative stimuli (e.g., food ingestion, exercise) may be needed to unmask the abnormality. An alternative approach is the use of a 24-h or longer ambulatory blood pressure recording during daily living circumstances. These devices offer the potential to capture spontaneous events. However, the available technology is less than optimal and cumbersome for the patient to use.

Establishing the specific underlying "causative" diagnosis is valuable for OH patients. First, it is important to identify non-neurogenic potentially reversible causes of OH such as drug effects, volume depletion, or adrenal insufficiency (uncommon). Second, if there is evidence for a neurological cause, the patient should be appropriately informed of the nature of the problem and its prognosis.

12.5.2 *Postural Orthostatic Tachycardia Syndrome (POTS)*

POTS tends to occur principally in a relatively young population and is more preva-lent in women than men.[4-6] Orthostatic symptoms consist of racing heart (especially with change of posture or with minor physical activity), light-headedness, visual disturbances, palpitations, tremulousness, and weakness. Other symptoms include fatigue, hyperventilation, shortness of breath, anxiety, chest pain, nausea, cold or painful fingers, concentration difficulties, various gastrointestinal complaints, and headaches.

The etiology and pathophysiology of POTS is currently unknown but it is likely that as more is learned the causes will prove to be heterogeneous. Current inter-est in subtle inflammatory conditions or auto-antibodies, although reported in some patients,[22,23] has yet to pay convincing treatment dividends. In any event, the clini-cal final common pathway in most cases is a symptomatic hyper-adrenergic state. It is assumed that the autonomic hyperactivity is induced by a perceived need to main-tain cardiovascular stability. Targeting this apparently excessive adrenergic state is usually necessary in order to diminish symptoms but does not appear to alter the course of the disease.

The differential diagnosis of POTS includes many other conditions that cause seemingly unexplained sinus tachycardia, such as the syndrome of inappropri-ate sinus tachycardia, dehydration, anemia, inflammatory states, thyrotoxicosis, pheochromocytoma, and Addison's disease. Medications (e.g., vasodilators, diuret-ics, thyroid supplements, certain herbal agents, and ß-agonists) may also contribute.

12.5.2.1 Diagnosis

The onset of POTS is often recorded as being abrupt and closely associated with a recent viral or other illness, or surgery. While in many cases this historical con-nection may be largely circumstantial, it seems that an abrupt onset of symptoms is associated with a shorter ultimate disease course (but nonetheless many months to several years). On the other hand, the slower the onset, the longer the course of the illness. Reversal may take many years.

Apart from the usually distinctive medical history, physical examination may also reveal reduced pulse pressure, signs of poor peripheral perfusion (e.g., coldness of the hands and fingers) in addition to an expected excessive postural heart rate increment. Continued standing may lead to venous prominence, lower extremity edema, and cyanosis. A hyper-adrenergic state is present in some patients, with additional complaints of sweating, tremulousness, anxiety, and diminished ability to concentrate. Symptoms are often sufficiently severe to undermine work or school performance.

12.6 Treatment of Orthostatic Intolerance

Treatment strategies for prevention of orthostatic syncope and for amelioration of symptoms in patients with POTS and related orthostatic intolerance conditions are similar in many respects. The objective is to enhance appropriate neural and vascular responsiveness to upright postural stress and in essence normalize orthostatic tolerance as much as possible. The goal is to diminish risk of symptomatic OH in the former condition and reduce the tendency to autonomic hyperactivity in the latter.

12.6.1 General Measures

Initial treatment in patients with orthostatic intolerance should include advice and education about factors that can aggravate or provoke symptoms. In particular, in the case of orthostatic syncope the objective is to reduce both the risk and the severity of hypotension upon assuming the upright posture. Pertinent factors include avoiding:

- sudden head-up postural change (especially in the morning when OH susceptibility is usually greatest),
- standing still for a prolonged period of time, and
- straining during micturition and defecation.

Other important considerations are minimizing exposure to high environmental temperature (including hot baths, showers, and saunas or low humidity environments) that might lead to dehydration and vasodilatation, large meals, and severe exertion.

Iatrogenic factors are critically important in many orthostatic syncope patients. The patients are often older individuals who are being treated for a number of commonly occurring comorbidities such as hypertension, coronary artery disease, and benign prostatic hyperplasia. As a result, they may be prescribed drugs such as diuretics, vasodilators, beta-adrenergic blockers, and alpha-adrenergic blockers. Each of these can aggravate a predisposition to OH, and in some instances (e.g., excessive diuresis) may induce orthostatic symptoms. Concomitant sinus node dysfunction with chronotropic incompetence (sometimes drug-induced) may also exacerbate susceptibility.

Some patients with autonomic failure exhibit post-prandial hypotension. In these patients, symptoms typically begin about 30 min after food ingestion and can last, even while supine, for several hours. Carbohydrate load appears to be a particular problem. Alcohol can exert an additional effect by causing splanchnic vasodilatation. Consequently, advice should include the recommendation that affected patients eat smaller meals with reduced carbohydrate content and avoid alcohol.

Volume expansion can improve orthostatic tolerance markedly, with relatively small increases in arterial pressure.[24,25] It may only be necessary for treatment to shift mean arterial pressure from just below to just above the critical level of perfusion of the brain. To this end, patients with OH or POTS should be encouraged to increase dietary salt intake (about 6 to 8 g of salt per day, assuming no contraindications such as concomitant hypertension or heart failure) with liberal use of salt at mealtimes and by eating foods with a high salt content. The use of salt tablets is not advocated for typical OH patients as they tend to provoke an undesirable transfer of volume from the vascular system into the gastric/intestinal lumen.

Additionally, patients should drink 2–2.5 l of fluids every day, focusing when possible on electrolyte-containing beverages. Elderly patients may have a decreased sense of thirst and may need to be encouraged to increase fluid intake. This latter point is particularly important as many older individuals, apart from not taking in enough fluid, may also tend to avoid fluids to prevent urinary frequency or incontinence. In patients with supine hypertension, it may be necessary to "tolerate" higher than desired pressures so as to reduce OH-induced falls risk.

12.6.2 Non-pharmacological Treatment Strategies

For patients with orthostatic intolerance in whom, despite the general measures discussed above, symptoms persist, several non-pharmacological strategies may be helpful.

12.6.2.1 Head-up Sleeping at Night

Sleeping with the head somewhat elevated tends to increase extracellular fluid volume and improve orthostatic tolerance. Head-up sleeping may diminish renal filtration and increase angiotensin II production, thereby reducing risk of volume depletion in the morning. Additionally, some transfer of fluid to the dependent extravascular space in the lower extremities during the night, while initially undesirable, may increase tissue pressure and prevent further losses when the individual arises. Effective head-up tilt sleeping can be achieved by elevating the head of the bed about 20–25 cm. To avoid sliding down while sleeping, a hospital bed can be employed or more inexpensively, a hard pillow can be placed under the mattress at the level of the buttocks.

12.6.2.2 Physical Counter-maneuvers

Several physical maneuvers that reduce venous pooling have been described to abort or diminish OH symptoms. The techniques (Table 12.2) are simple and most patients (apart from the extremely frail) can be trained to apply them relatively effectively. There are two groups of physical maneuvers[26–30]:

- *Acute measures*: patients are advised to apply these physical maneuvers as soon as symptoms begin.
- *Longer term prevention*: those techniques are designed to improve longer-term orthostatic tolerance.

12.6.2.3 Lower Body Compression Techniques

Abdominal binders and graded lower extremity compression stockings (worn from the feet to the waist) may be helpful in severe cases of postural OH and POTS. Similarly, although more troublesome to apply, lower limb compression bandages may be applied but there is concern that they may obstruct venous flow if placed by

Table 12.2 Physical maneuvers to enhance orthostatic tolerance

Technique	Mechanism of benefit
Acute measures	
Leg crossing	Mechanical compression of the venous vascular beds in the legs, buttocks, and abdomen enhances venous return. Leg crossing can be performed casually without drawing attention to the patient's problem
Muscle tensing	Increases the beneficial effect of leg crossing. Patients may need to "casually" support themselves by leaning on a wall or a piece of furniture
Squatting	Increases venous return rapidly and produces an important increase in systolic and diastolic arterial blood pressure. Often used as an emergency maneuver to prevent loss of consciousness
Bending forward	Lowering the head between the knees is a rapid way to enhance cerebral perfusion by decreasing the hydrostatic column between the heart and the brain
Long-term prevention	
Standing training	Also known as "tilt training," this procedure requires that patients undertake progressively longer periods of quiet upright standing to build tolerance to upright posture. The value in OH is not proven, but the technique is advocated
Support hose and abdominal binders	Both are used to enhance venous return to the heart
Isometric exercise	This is designed to enhance effectiveness of lower body "muscle pump" capability

a non-expert.[31] "Bikers pants" may be easy to put on for many patients and can be comfortably worn under conventional clothing (see also Chapter 21).

12.6.2.4 Standing Training

Standing training (sometimes referred to as "tilt training") has been advocated to help improve vascular responsiveness to upright posture over a long period of time (see more detail in Chapter 21). This technique is controversial in terms of demonstrable benefit but is simple and may help some individuals. In essence, the affected patient is asked to stand absolutely still for progressively longer periods of time each day. Conceptually this "exercise" results in greater tolerance to upright position.

12.6.2.5 Isometric Exercise

Isometric exercise involving the lower extremities may also enhance vascular responsiveness over time. Additionally, muscle tensing (a form of isometric exercise) may be used acutely to ameliorate a hypotensive episode in progress and allow the affected individual to seek a safe position (i.e., seated or supine) before they collapse. See more detail in Chapter 21.

12.6.3 Pharmacological Treatment

Pharmacological approaches are widely used to enhance orthostatic tolerance, but supportive evidence of effectiveness is limited. In any event, when non-pharmacological treatments described above are inadequate, several drugs have been advocated. In most cases these are used in OH to prevent syncope or falls, but some have also been widely employed in POTS patients. The most important of these drugs are summarized below, but in each case the potential for aggravating supine hypertension must be considered.

12.6.3.1 Fludrocortisone

Fludrocortisone is a synthetic mineralocorticoid with minimal glucocorticoid effect. Given the apparent value of increased salt intake for enhancing orthostatic tolerance, fludrocortisone has for some time been used in patients with orthostatic symptoms.[32,33] It offers the potential to expand intravascular and extravascular body fluid, sensitize vascular receptors to pressor amines, and increase fluid content of vessel walls that makes them more resistant to stretching. In POTS, its role is to diminish autonomic hyper-activity. Treatment is usually begun with a dose of 0.1 mg once a day, and if necessary increased only very cautiously by 0.1 mg at 1–2 weeks intervals up to at most 0.3 mg daily (at the higher doses the risk of hypokalemia increases while the benefit is not necessarily substantially improved). The pressor action does not take effect immediately and may take some days to be manifest. Side effects are primarily accounted for by its expected pharmacological action, including mild dependent edema can be expected. However, hypokalemia is a serious concern that requires monitoring and often potassium repletion.

12.6.3.2 Midodrine

Midodrine is a pro-drug that is converted to its active metabolite desglymidodrine after absorption. It acts on α-adrenoreceptors to cause constriction of both arterial resistance and venous capacitance vessels, with the predominant effect being on the venous side. It does not tend to cross the blood–brain barrier and consequently it has little central stimulant effects. Midodrine may be of particular value in patients with severe postural hypotension and in those with peripheral neurological lesions, as in pure autonomic failure.[34] In POTS patients, by helping maintain arterial pressure, it is thought to reduce the apparent need for excessive autonomic activation.[35] Midodrine is administered in doses of 2.5–10 mg, three times daily. Supine hypertension is a potentially important but infrequent side effect. Scalp tingling is a very frequent effect as is increased urinary frequency.

12.6.3.3 Beta-Adrenergic Blockers and Acetylcholine (Ach) Esterase Inhibitors

These agents are used primarily in POTS patients to reduce heart rate increment and diminish symptoms.[36,37] In the case of beta-blockers, current recommendations are for use of low doses of non-selective agents (e.g., propranolol 20 mg twice daily). However, many older OH patients are taking beta-adrenergic blockers for treatment of other ailments such as ischemic heart disease, hypertension, and tremor. In these patients, the drugs may actually aggravate postural orthostatic symptoms. Ach-esterase inhibitors such as pyridostigmine may help diminish the sensation of rapid heart beat, but are not usually adequate as sole therapy.

12.6.3.4 Others Drugs

The following agents have been used in a limited fashion for symptomatic OH but are not usually recommended for treatment of POTS patients:

- Octreotide may benefit patients with post-prandial hypotension.
- Erythropoietin has been reported to help in patients with anemia.
- Yohimbine, a vasoconstrictor.
- Norepinephrine re-uptake blocker in selected cases (e.g., atomoxetine).

12.6.4 Other Methods

12.6.4.1 Pressor Response to Water Drinking

Ingestion of a substantial amount of water is an intervention that is reported to be effective in combating orthostatic intolerance in patients with autonomic failure.[25,38,39] After rapid drinking of about half a liter of water, an increase in blood pressure is apparent within several minutes. The maximum effect (20–30 mmHg increase of seated and standing systolic blood pressure) is reached after approximately 30 min and the effects are sustained for about 1 h. For patients with autonomic failure, water ingestion is also effective to combat post-prandial hypotension. Drinking of water also increases blood pressure substantially in healthy elderly, but not in healthy young subjects or patients with Parkinson's disease. The mechanisms underlying the rapid pressor response elicited by water drinking are debated. Sympathetic activation resulting in increased vasoconstrictor tone has been reported. Others have emphasized that the time course of the blood pressure response is unusually slow for sympathetic activation. These authors have suggested that minor elevations of intra- and extravascular fluid volume might be involved in patients with autonomic failure who are extremely sensitive to changes in fluid balance. The afferent signal that activates the sympathetic system through water drinking is not known.

12.6.4.2 Impedance Threshold Device (ITD)

Improvement in cardiac output and blood pressure can be achieved by enhancing venous return by use of an ITD (Fig. 12.4). This device, which the patient breaths through for 30–40 s before standing, provides some resistance to inspiratory effort

Fig. 12.4 The handheld impedance threshold device (Advanced Circulatory Systems, Roseville, MN, USA) provides a low level of resistance to inspiration, thereby further diminishing intra-thoracic pressure. The lower pressure facilitates venous return to the heart and enhances cardiac output. Preliminary studies suggest the possibility that the ITD may reduce susceptibility to OH[40]

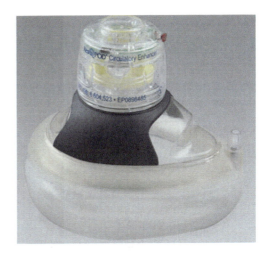

but not to expiration. Thus, the patient is forced to develop greater negative intra-thoracic pressure during inspiration than is usually the case. The greater negative pressure forces more venous blood to move from the periphery to the central circulation and thereby increases cardiac output. The ITD is available in Europe and North America (Advanced Circulatory Systems, Inc., Roseville, MN) and has been mainly used for improving circulatory support during cardiopulmonary resuscitation (CPR). Its value in orthostatic hypotension has only very recently been the subject of clinical study but appears to be promising.[40]

12.6.4.3   Cardiac Pacing

The use of cardiac pacing for OH is not advocated. The major physiological abnormality, inadequate venous return, is not addressed and consequently the likelihood of benefit (an unrelated conventional indication for pacing being absent) is at best remote.

12.7   Clinical Perspectives

Orthostatic intolerance syndromes are common and often very disabling. Of these syndromes, orthostatic hypotension (OH) is the most common; while OH may be asymptomatic in many individuals, it can also be the source of important clinical consequences. In this regard, whether drug-induced or the result of concomitant conditions such as Parkinsonism or other diseases associated with autonomic dysfunction, OH is a serious concern in older individuals in whom it may be responsible for triggering falls with considerable risk of injury. In younger persons, OH (particularly of the "immediate form") is usually no more than a nuisance; in the absence of severe underlying neurological disease, OH is much less often serious than it is in the elderly. On the other hand, postural orthostatic tachycardia syndrome (POTS), which tends to occur much more frequently in younger than in older individuals, may be very disabling for many years. Treatment of these and other less well-defined orthostatic intolerance syndromes is imperfect at best and in most cases focuses on symptom relief rather than cure (with the exception of eliminating offending drugs whenever possible). The overall strategy must address improving venous return to the heart in both OH and POTS and in POTS patients diminishing adrenergic hyperactivity. However, while the goals are clear and now widely accepted, they are often difficult to accomplish and the treatment approach must be adapted to each individual.

References

1. Schatz IJ, et al. Consensus statement on the definition of orthostatic hypotension, pure autonomic failure, and multiple system atrophy. Neurology. 46:1470 and *Clin Autonom Res.* 1996;6:125–126.
2. Wieling W, Schatz IJ. The consensus statement on the definition of orthostatic hypotension: a revisit after 13 years. *J Hypertens.* 2009;27:935–938.
3. Robertson D. The pathophysiology and diagnosis of orthostatic hypotension. *Clin Autonom Res.* 2008;18(Suppl 1):2–7.
4. Low PA, et al. Postural tachycardia syndrome (POTS). *J Cardiovasc Electrophysiol.* 2009;20:352–358.
5. Stewart JM. Chronic orthostatic intolerance and the postural tachycardia syndrome (POTS). *J Pediatr.* 2004;145:725–730.
6. Joyner MJ, Masuki S. POTS versus deconditioning: the same or different? *Clin Autonom Res.* 2008;18:300–307.
7. Davis BR, et al. The association of postural changes in systolic blood pressure and mortality in persons with hypertension. *Circulation.* 1987;75:340–346.
8. Masaki KH, et al. Orthostatic hypotension predicts mortality in elderly men: the Honolulu Heart Program. *Circulation.* 1998;98:2290–2295.
9. Federowski A. Orthostatic hypotension in genetically related hypertensive and normotensive subjects. *J Hypertens.* 2009;27:976–982.
10. Mathias CJ. Autonomic diseases – clinical features and laboratory evaluation. *J Neurol Neurosurg Psychiatr.* 2003;74:31–41.
11. Mathias CJ. Autonomic diseases – management. *J Neurol Neurosurg Psychiatr.* 2003;74:42–47.
12. Mathias CJ. Disorders of the autonomic nervous system. In: Bradley WG, et al. (eds) *Neurology in Clinical Practice* (2004). 3rd edn. Boston, MA: Butterworth-Heinemann; 2003:pp 2403–2440.
13. Mathias CJ. To stand on one's own legs. *Clin Med.* 2003;2:237–245.
14. Smit AAJ, et al. Topical review. Pathophysiological basis of orthostatic hypotension in autonomic failure. *J Physiol.* 1999;519:1–10.
15. Lahrmann H, et al. EFNS guidelines on the diagnosis and management of orthostatic hypotension. *Eur J Neurol.* 2006;13:930–936.
16. Freeman R. Neurogenic orthostatic hypotension. *N Engl J Med.* 2008;358:615–624.
17. Wieling W, et al. Initial hypotension: review of a forgotten condition. *Clin Sci.* 2007;112:157–165.
18. Low PA, et al. Prospective evaluation of clinical characteristics of orthostatic hypotension. *Mayo Clin Proc.* 1995;70:617–622.
21. Mathias CJ, et al. Observations on recurrent syncope and presyncope in 641 patients. *Lancet.* 2001;357:348–353.

19. Lipsitz LA. Orthostatic hypotension in the elderly. *N Engl J Med*. 1989;321:952–957.
20. Rutan GH, et al. Orthostatic hypotension in older adults. The Cardiovascular Health Study. *Hypertension*. 1992;9:508–519.
22. Stewart JM, et al. Defects in cutaneous angiotensin-converting enzyme 2 and angiotensin-(1–7) production in postural tachycardia syndrome. *Hypertension*. 2009;53:767–774.
23. Sandroni P, Low PA. Other autonomic neuropathies associated with ganglionic antibody. *Auton Neurosci*. 2009;146:13–17.
24. El-Sayed H, Hainsworth R. Relationship between plasma volume, carotid baroreceptor sensitivity and orthostatic tolerance. *Clin Sci*. 1995;88:463–470.
25. Wieling W, et al. Extracellular fluid volume expansion in patients with posturally related syncope. *Clin Autonom Res*. 2002;12:243–249.
26. Wieling W, et al. Physical manoeuvres that reduce postural hypotension in autonomic failure. *Clin Autonom Res*. 1993;3:57–65.
27. van Dijk N, et al. Hemodynamic effects of leg crossing and skeletal muscle tensing during free standing in patients with vasovagal syncope. *J Appl Physiol*. 2005;98: 584–590.
28. Krediet CT, et al. Management of vasovagal syncope: Controlling or aborting faints by leg crossing and muscle tensing. *Circulation*. 2002;106:1684–1689.
29. Brignole M, et al. Isometric arm counter-pressure maneuvers to abort impending vasovagal syncope. *J Am Coll Cardiol*. 2002;40:2053–2059.
30. Reybrouck T, et al. Long-term follow-up results of tilt training therapy in patients with recurrent neurocardiogenic syncope. *Pacing Clin Electrophysiol*. 2002;25:1441–1446.
31. Podoleanu C, et al. Lower limb and abdominal compression bandages prevent progressive orthostatic hypotension in elderly persons a randomized single-blind controlled study. *J Am Coll Cardiol*. 2006;48:1425–1432.
32. Hussain RM, et al. Fludrocortisone in the treatment of hypotensive disorders in the elderly. *Heart*. 1996;76:507–509.
33. Claydon VE, Hainsworth R. Salt supplementation improves orthostatic cerebral and peripheral vascular control in patients with syncope. *Hypertension*. 2004;43:809–813.
34. Low PA, et al. Efficacy of midodrine vs placebo in neurogenic orthostatic hypotension. A randomized, double-blind multicenter study. *J Am Med Assoc*. 1997;277:1046–1051.
35. Lai CC, et al. Outcomes in adolescents with postural orthostatic tachycardia syndrome treated with midodrine and beta-blockers. *Pacing Clin Electrophysiol*. 2009;32:234–238.
36. Raj SR, et al. Propranolol decreases tachycardia and improves symptoms in the postural tachycardia syndrome: less is more. *Circulation*. 2009;120:725–734.
37. Singer W, et al. Pyridostigmine treatment trial in neurogenic orthostatic hypotension. *Arch Neurol*. 2006;63:513–518.
38. Cariga P, Mathias CJ. Haemodynamics of the pressor effect of oral water in human sympathetic denervation due to autonomic failure. *Clin Sci*. 2001;101:313–319.
39. Young TM, Mathias CJ. The effects of water ingestion on orthostatic hypotension in two groups of chronic autonomic failure: Multiple system atrophy and pure autonomic failure. *J Neurol Neurosurg Psychiatry*. 2004;75:1737–1741.
40. Melby DP, et al. Increased impedance to inspiration ameliorates hemodynamic changes associated with movement to upright posture in orthostatic hypotension: A randomized pilot study. *Heart Rhythm*. 2007;4:128–135.

Chapter 13
Cardiac Syncope

Contents

Key points: Cardiac syncope

- The European Society of Cardiology Syncope Task Force guideline classifies "Cardiac syncope" as incorporating all of the causes of syncope that are primarily due to disturbances of cardiac or cardiovascular function.

M. Brignole, D.G. Benditt, *Syncope*, DOI 10.1007/978-0-85729-201-8_13,
© Springer-Verlag London Limited 2011

- Cardiac syncope may be the result of cardiac conduction system disease, primary cardiac rhythm disturbances, or cardiovascular structural abnormalities.
- Identifying whether syncope is of a "cardiac origin" is important from both prognostic and treatment perspectives.
- Findings obtainable during the initial clinical evaluation can be used to determine whether cardiac syncope is a high probability. These include, apart from the patient's personal and family medical history, findings on physical examination and results of 12-lead ECG and echocardiogram.
- Alone, the presence of underlying cardiac disease is not sufficient evidence to support a cardiac cause for syncope. Syncope of more innocent etiologies may be the cause, even in "cardiac" patients. Thus, further evaluation is necessary in most cases.
- Additional studies are selected as deemed appropriate by the suspected diagnosis.
- In some cases, evaluation will need to be carried out in hospital (or in a "syncope management unit"), while in many others it is reasonable to conduct studies in the outpatient environment.
- In all cases, the goal is to establish an etiologic diagnosis that can be relied upon to permit informing the patient and family of the expected prognosis, as well as leading to an effective treatment strategy. Nevertheless, in clinical practice the relation between observed abnormalities and syncope is often inferential despite a thorough series of diagnostic studies; this is understandable and inevitably one must proceed with treatment based on best judgment. In clinical trials, on the other hand, the diagnostic bar is set higher; a much stronger correspondence between symptoms and abnormal findings should be sought.

13.1 Introduction

"Cardiac syncope" comprises those causes of syncope that are primarily due to disturbances of cardiac or cardiovascular function.[1] Thus, cardiac conduction system disease, primary cardiac rhythm disturbances, and cardiovascular structural abnormalities are incorporated within this category (previously "cardiac arrhythmias" and "structural cardiac and cardiovascular disease" were considered as separate classes[2,3]). It is understood that despite the presence of one or other evident cardiac disease, the pathophysiology of "cardiac syncope" is often multifactorial (Table 13.1). For example, syncope occurring in conjunction with an acute myocardial infarction may be triggered by an arrhythmia, or transient fall of cardiac output on a structural basis, or both; however, neural reflex effects and inappropriate vascular responsiveness as well as volumne status likely contribute in many instances. Similarly, syncope occurring at the

Table 13.1 Multifactorial components contributing to "cardiac" syncope

Cardiac condition	Basic cause	Contributing factors
Acute MI	Arrhythmia, reduced CO	Neural reflex effects and inadequate vascular responsiveness, low volume status, drug effects
Dilated CM	Reduced CO	Inadequate vascular responsiveness, arrhythmia, dehydration, drugs
Aortic stenosis	Obstruction	Abnormal vascular responsiveness Hydration, arrhythmia
HCM	Obstruction	CO inadequate for exertion Abnormal vascular responsiveness Arrhythmia
QTS, Brugada	Arrhythmia	
Pulmonary hypertension	Low CO	Neural reflex effects
Acute dissection	Neural reflex	Cerebral vascular obstruction
Tachyarrhythmia onset	Reduced CO	Inadequate vascular responsiveness
Bradycardia onset	Reduced CO	Inappropriate vascular response

CM, cardiomyopathy; CO, cardiac output; HCM, hypertrophic cardiomyopathy; LQTS, long QT syndrome; MI, myocardial infarction.

onset of a tachyarrhythmia may be due in part to an abrupt fall in cardiac output, but once again the inability of vascular tone to compensate promptly (largely a responsibility of the autonomic nervous system) is often the key determinant of the severity of hypotension and hence the likelihood that a faint will occur. Finally, the mere presence of cardiac disease, while not to be overlooked, should not be immediately assumed to be the cause of syncope. These patients may also experience reflex faints, orthostatic syncope, or other causes of transient loss of consciousness.

This chapter reviews the prognostic importance of identifying "cardiac" causes for syncope and reviews the most frequent of these causes. In this regard, a number of specific conditions have already been addressed in other chapters in this volume and, inasmuch as they are covered in less depth here, the reader is referred to those chapters.

13.2 Prognosis

In syncope patients, the presence and the severity of coexisting structural heart disease are the most important predictors of mortality risk. Thus, among individuals with cardiac syncope (i.e., primary cardiac arrhythmia, an ischemic episode, or severe valvular heart disease), the 1-year mortality is high (ranging between 18 and 33%) compared to that for patients with either non-cardiac (including "vasovagal") causes of syncope (0–12%) or unexplained syncope. Differences in the risk of death are even more striking when considering "sudden cardiac death" events; the 1-year incidence of sudden death is approximately 24% in patients with a cardiac cause of syncope versus about 3% in the other two groups.[4,5]

In general, while patients with cardiac syncope have higher mortality rates compared with those of non-cardiac or unknown causes, the bulk of evidence does not suggest that cardiac syncope patients actually exhibit a higher mortality when

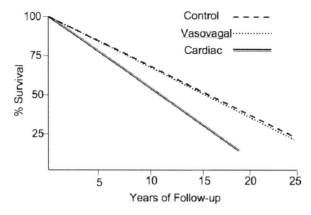

Fig. 13.1 Comparison of prognosis in patients with presumed cardiac syncope versus vasovagal syncope and no-syncope control subjects modified after Framingham study published data[4]

compared with matched controls having similar degrees of heart disease[6-9] (Fig. 13.1). There are, however, some important exceptions to this rule. The association of syncope with aortic stenosis has been long recognized as having an increased mortality risk (average survival without valve replacement of 2 years). Similarly, in hypertrophic cardiomyopathy, the combination of young age and syncope at diagnosis, severe dyspnea, and a family history of sudden death are predictors of increased sudden death risk. The mortality risk associated with syncope in the setting of one of the channelopathies (e.g., Brugada syndrome, long QT syndrome), or in the presence of arrhythmogenic right ventricular dysplasia (ARVD), may fall into this exception as well, although the literature varies in this regard. Finally, Olshansky et al.[10] in reviewing the SCD-HeFT (Sudden Cardiac Death in Heart Failure Trial) data indicated that the presence of syncope was an independent predictor of ICD shocks in that population. Similarly in one large prospective observational trial[11] of long QT syndrome (LQTS), comprising >800 patients, syncope was associated with a fivefold increased risk of cardiac arrest or sudden death, but it was not a sensitive indicator of death risk. A similar observation has been made in some studies of patients with the ECG Brugada pattern who have a history of syncope, but not in all such studies[12-15] (see Chapter 15).

Failing to distinguish the additional risks associated with recurrent syncope from the risks accompanying any underlying comorbidity (especially, heart disease) is a common error. The result is that physicians may overlook the need to address syncope risk directly as they focus on the treatment of the underlying heart disease (or occasionally vice versa). For instance, ICD therapy is often recommended in patients with syncope and left ventricular ejection fraction (LVEF) <30%. Clearly, an ICD may well be indicated, but it would be indicated even in the absence of syncope. On the other hand, while the ICD may prevent sudden death, it takes time to detect an arrhythmia and initiate treatment; consequently, it may not protect the patient from injury due to recurrent syncope (even if the syncope is due to ventricular tachyarrhythmias). Further assessment of the patient is needed.

13.3 Identifying a "Cardiac Origin"

It is well known now that identifying whether syncope is of a "cardiac origin" is crucial from a prognostic perspective as well as being essential for targeting therapy. In this regard, the single piece of information of greatest importance is whether or not the fainter has a history of heart disease[16] or a family history of cardiac conditions known to be genetically transmitted. The presence of such conditions substantially raises the likelihood of a cardiac origin for the faint. Second in importance is characterizing the circumstances associated with syncope. Syncope in the supine position or during physical exertion (not afterward) tends to favor cardiac syncope. Beyond these key points, the description of premonitory or post-event symptoms is not sufficiently reliable to clearly differentiate cardiac syncope from more benign reflex faints.[16,17]

In terms of the fainter's overall medical history, it is important to inquire regarding evidence of known structural heart disease, such as prior myocardial infarction, valvular heart disease, congenital conditions, or previous cardiac surgery. Drug treatment, particularly vasodilators, beta-adrenergic blockers, antiarrhythmic drugs, and QT prolonging agents, any of which may trigger syncope, should be documented (Table 13.2). Additionally determine whether there has been any recent dosing change and whether any new agents have been added that might produce an undesirable drug interaction.

In regard to the family history, initial evaluation should query whether there is a family history of sudden death or certain known genetically transmitted conditions such as long/short QT syndromes, Brugada syndrome, arrhythmogenic ventricular cardiomyopathy, infiltrative disease (e.g., amyloid), or hypertrophic cardiomyopathy. Additionally, since even some "benign" faints seem to have familial connections, it is important to ascertain if there might be a familial predisposition to syncope.

Abnormal findings during physical examination only infrequently provide direct evidence of a basis for syncope, but any of the following observations increase the likelihood of a cardiac origin:

Table 13.2 Common "cardiac" medications predisposing to syncope

- Antihypertensives
- Beta-adrenergic blockers
- Calcium channel blockers
- Nitroglycerin-based antianginal drugs
- Antidepressant agents
- Antiarrhythmics
- Diuretics and
- QT prolonging agents including:
  - commonly used antibiotics, and
  - psychoactive agents

- differences in blood pressure/pulse in upper extremities suggesting subclavian steal, or aortic dissection,
- evidence of heart failure (e.g., elevated jugular venous pulse, peripheral edema),
- pathologic cardiac murmurs and/or vascular bruits, including signs of pulmonary embolism/hypertension (loud pulmonic component of the second heart sound),
- peripheral pulse findings suggestive of severe aortic stenosis or hypertrophic obstructive cardiomyopathy,
- findings suggesting pericardial disease (e.g., paradoxical pulse, Kussmaul's sign).

The 12-lead ECG and echocardiogram are considered basic laboratory tests that should be readily available to physicians undertaking the initial evaluation of the syncope patient.[1] Both tests are usually indicated if a cardiac origin for syncope is suspected. In this regard, the 12-lead ECG only rarely (about 5%) identifies a specific cause of syncope (e.g., an arrhythmia that persists such as complete heart block). However, 12-lead ECG findings such as Q waves and/or "acute" ST segment changes, left ventricular hypertrophy, a prolonged QT interval, or ventricular pre-excitation may suggest the presence of organic heart disease and thereby provide a basis for proceeding with further directed testing. Similar limitations apply to the echocardiogram. However, echocardiography is of particular value when the status of underlying cardiac disease is unclear based on history or prior studies. In essence, the echocardiogram is usually essential for assessing left ventricular function and the severity of valvular abnormalities (e.g., severe aortic stenosis), intra-cardiac tumors, or pulmonary hypertension.

In summary, multiple findings readily obtainable during the initial clinical evaluation can be used to determine whether cardiac syncope is a high probability. Given the prognostic importance of this determination, Del Rosso et al.[18] calculated a risk score (the EGSYS score); using derivation ($n = 260$) and validation ($n = 256$) cohorts (mean age 63 years), the authors assigned positive (or negative) points to the presence (absence) of selected clinical observations. A score ≥ 3 identified cardiac syncope with a sensitivity of approximately 95% and a specificity of about 65%. The prognostic importance of the score was evident in an approximate 2-year follow-up, with the score ≥ 3 population having a mortality of about 20% versus only 2–3% in the <3 group. However, the mean age of the Del Rosso et al.[18] cohort limits the application of this risk assessment approach to older individuals. The findings in younger individuals require further assessment. For instance, Colivicchi et al.[19] assessed syncope risk in over 7,500 young athletes (mostly male) who had pre-participation evaluation. During 6 years of follow-up, syncope was reported in 6.2%, with six athletes having syncope during exertion (four were normal, one had right ventricular outflow tract tachycardia, and one had hypertrophic cardiomyopathy). This latter study suggests that most syncope in younger patients is of the reflex type and that exertional syncope is rare in these individuals but not necessarily associated with an adverse outcome in the absence of structural heart disease.

13.4 Cardiac Conduction System Disease and Arrhythmias

13.4.1 Sinus Node Dysfunction (SND)

SND comprises several types of rhythm disturbances, including sinus or junctional bradycardia, sinus pauses, and episodes of primary atrial arrhythmias, tachyarrhythmia (most commonly paroxysmal atrial fibrillation or other primary atrial tachycardias) often (but not always) with a relatively slow ventricular response.[20] Syncope can be caused by severe bradycardia (e.g., sustained severe bradycardia, sinus pauses, or sinus arrest) or may be associated with tachycardia. In the latter case, the faint may occur at the beginning of the paroxysm of atrial fibrillation (before blood vessels have had a chance to constrict adequately). Alternatively, it is not uncommon for syncope to be due to a long asystolic pause occurring at the end of an episode of atrial fibrillation (before the sinus pacemaker has an opportunity to resume at a relatively normal rate). In patients with syncope of unknown origin, SND can be suspected in the presence of severe sinus bradycardia (heart rates persistently <40–50 beats/min), long asystolic pauses (>3–5 s) due to sinus arrest, or episodes of sinoatrial block[20] (Fig. 13.2).

Electrophysiological testing (EPS) for the diagnosis of SND as a cause of syncope is of limited value[20,21] (see also Chapter 7). The tests used to evaluate the function of sinus node [sinus node recovery time (SNRT) and sinoatrial conduction time (SACT)] exhibit adequate specificity, but they are relatively insensitive and may miss many affected individuals. Furthermore, with the possible exception of a very prolonged corrected sinus node recovery time (CSNRT),[22,23] testing does not provide sufficient evidence whether SND was the cause of syncope or whether it was tachycardia or bradycardia component; more information must be sought. Recently, there has been interest in assessing the presence of SND by adenosine provocation. For instance, Fragakis et al.[24] observed that the pause induced by adenosine was comparable to the post-pacing recovery times recorded in SND patients.

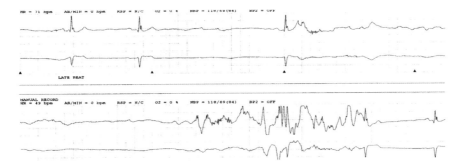

Fig. 13.2 Prolonged asystolic pause during telemetry monitoring, suggesting a basis for syncope. Artifact in *lower trace* may have been generated by a fall or possibly by jerky muscular motion associated with cerebral hypoperfusion

The diagnosis of SND as the cause of syncope is best established when a clear correlation of symptoms with arrhythmia (usually a bradycardic event) is documented. Ambulatory ECG "event" recorders or implanted loop recorders (ILRs) have the best chance of making the diagnosis by virtue of their long recording periods.

In patients with SND and syncope due to bradyarrhythmia, pacemaker implantation improves symptoms. In these patients, physiologic pacing (atrial or dual chamber) is generally considered to be superior to single-chamber ventricular (VVI or VVIR) pacing, especially if the patient is likely to be pacing frequently. Further, since many of these patients also exhibit inappropriate chronotropic response (i.e., so-called chronotropic incompetence), the use of rate-adaptive pacing is recommended.[20]

In patients with paroxysmal atrial tachycardias associated with SND, antiarrhythmic drug therapy or even mapping and transcatheter ablation may be advocated. In such cases, however, if drugs are chosen, unsuspected susceptibility to bradycardia may be provoked by drug administration. Once again, assuming alternative drugs or ablation is not available, pacing may be a necessary element of therapy.

13.4.2 Atrioventricular Conduction Disorders

Bradycardia due to intermittent AV block is among the more important causes of syncope.[25–29] The presence of Mobitz II type second-degree AV block, third-degree AV block, or alternating left and right bundle branch block in an individual who presents with syncope is generally considered to be sufficiently diagnostic of the probable cause that no further testing is needed. In the absence of these ECG findings, there are other suggestive observations the recognition of which may help direct further assessment but alone they are inferential only and further evidence is needed. Such observations include the following:

- bifascicular block (left bundle branch block or right bundle branch block associated with left anterior or left posterior fascicular block);
- other intraventricular conduction abnormalities with a QRS duration >120 ms; or
- documented Mobitz I second-degree AV block, in older (>70 years) individuals.

Electrophysiological study (EPS) may be useful to help confirm the severity of conduction system disease in cases where a direct correlation with transient AV block cannot be readily obtained (see also Chapter 7). In those cases, the assessment of the His–Purkinje system during EPS should include the measurement of baseline HV interval, effects of incremental atrial pacing and, if baseline study is inconclusive, pharmacologic provocation with ajmaline, procainamide, or disopyramide to further stress the integrity of the intracardiac conduction system. In addition, EPS should assess inducibility of ventricular arrhythmias. The latter is particularly important in patients with structural heart disease (e.g., prior myocardial infarction, cardiomyopathy, and ventricular hypertrophy).

EPS findings that are generally considered sufficiently diagnostic in terms of suggesting a basis for syncope include[1] the following:

- HV interval >100 ms,
- presence of 2nd or 3rd degree infra-His AV block with progressively rapid atrial pacing,
- high-degree AV block after intravenous administration of ajmaline, disopyramide, or procainamide, and
- induction of sustained monomorphic ventricular tachycardia (VT) at a rate deemed fast enough to account for hypotension in an upright patient.

The presence of an abnormal EPS finding cannot be accepted as definitive evidence that the cause of syncope has been established; the diagnosis remains inferential. Thus, in clinical trials, a higher diagnostic bar would be preferred. Specifically direct correlation of symptoms and ECG findings (e.g., ILR findings during a spontaneous syncope). However, in clinical practice, the findings obtained at EPS are deemed reasonable to act upon.

The absence of abnormal EPS findings in these patients does not exclude an arrhythmia as a possible etiology of syncope, and implantation of an ILR (if not already done) is justified. Findings from the ISSUE trial strongly suggest that prolonged recording periods (often 5–10 months) may be needed to document a correlation between arrhythmia (often paroxysmal AV block) and syncope.[30,31]

Paroxysmal AV block is a particularly important and often overlooked cause of "syncope of unknown origin" in older patients (especially women) in whom there may not be overt ECG evidence to suggest a cardiac conduction system disorder. Establishing the diagnosis may be difficult and an ILR may be essential to confirm clinical suspicions. Findings can be considered diagnostic when a correlation between syncope and AV block is obtained.

Congenital AV block is a special case of conduction system disease that may be associated with syncope. Patients with congenital AV block may remain asymptomatic for a long period of time. Consequently, congenital AV block was, until recently, considered to be a relatively benign condition. However, detailed follow-up studies have demonstrated that such patients, especially if they have suffered syncope, have an increased mortality, and while numbers of paced patients were small, it seemed as though cardiac pacing may have been protective.[32,33] Consequently, it is now believed that these individuals are best advised to undergo pacemaker implantation at an earlier age than was previously thought appropriate, probably by early adulthood. Rarer conditions such as mesothelioma of the AV node may mimic congenital complete heart block; these also have a risk for sudden death. However, making an antemortem diagnosis is uncommon.

13.4.3 Supraventricular Tachyarrhythmias

13.4.3.1 Atrial Fibrillation/Flutter

Of the supraventricular tachycardias, paroxysmal atrial fibrillation (PAF) is probably the most frequent cause of near-syncope and syncope. In part, this may be due to the fact that these arrhythmias are very common, and they tend to occur in older more fragile individuals who also exhibit evidence of sinus node dysfunction. In these cases, as noted earlier, syncope most often occurs at the beginning of the tachycardia episode before the vascular constriction has had a chance to compensate. However, syncope may also occur when the episode terminates if a long asystolic pause occurs before a regular heart rhythm resumes.

Patients with atrial flutter have many of the same risks for syncope as do those with atrial fibrillation, except that atrial flutter is much less likely to be paroxysmal. However, two important considerations are important in patients with atrial flutter:

- Exertion in patients with atrial flutter can lead to very rapid ventricular rates (e.g., 1:1 AV conduction). At rapid rates, hypotension may ensue.
- Use of class membrane-active antiarrhythmic agents without concomitant pharmacologic AV nodal blockade may slow the flutter cycle length, reduce the degree of physiologic block offered by the AV node, and result in even greater propensity to 1:1 AV conduction. The result may be a sufficiently fast ventricular rate to cause severe hemodynamic compromise and syncope.

13.4.3.2 Paroxysmal Supraventricular Tachycardia

Although the paroxysmal supraventricular tachycardias (PSVTs) are among the most frequently encountered cardiac arrhythmias, they are relatively uncommon causes of syncope[34]; the latter may be in part due to the tendency for PSVT to occur in otherwise healthy younger individuals. Nevertheless, PSVT is important to consider as most forms of this arrhythmia are easily treated (including cure by transcatheter ablation techniques).

Syncope in patients with PSVT is multifactorial. Symptomatic hypotension is not solely due to a rapid heart rate. The affected individual being in an upright posture and/or the absence of a prompt vasoconstrictor response at the onset of an arrhythmia episode will exacerbate the degree of hypotension and increase the chance of syncope. Susceptibility to syncope may also be increased by dehydration, vasodilator drugs, and underlying SND. The last of these (SND), although much less frequent in PSVT patients than in PAF patients, predisposes to long post-tachycardia pauses and consequent transient hypotension at termination of the tachycardia.

In those patients in whom PSVT is the suspected cause of syncope, electrophysiological study (EPS) is indicated. The induction of PSVT, especially if it provokes hypotension or reproduces clinical symptoms (this may not happen with the patient lying supine in the laboratory), can be considered diagnostic. More often than not, hypotension and symptom reproduction is achieved only if tachycardia is induced with the patient in an upright posture such as on a tilt table. In any case, if tachycardia with a rapid rate consistent with the potential for hypotension is observed, transcatheter ablation (typically using radiofrequency or cryoablation methodology) is the treatment of choice.

Patients with evidence of pre-excitation on baseline ECG (e.g., WPW syndrome) have additional clinical risks that may contribute to syncope (or even sudden death on rare occasion). In these patients, apart from PSVT (i.e., paroxysmal tachycardias using an accessory AV connection as part of their reentrant circuit), possible susceptibility to episodes of atrial fibrillation with very fast ventricular response (due to conduction over the accessory connection) can not only cause hypotension and syncope but may also induce ventricular fibrillation leading to sudden death. In these patients, transcatheter ablation of the accessory connection is clearly the treatment of choice.

13.4.4 *Ventricular Tachycardias*

13.4.4.1 Ischemic Heart Disease and Dilated Cardiomyopathy (CM)

Ventricular tachyarrhythmias (VTs) are a major cause for concern in patients with ischemic disease or dilated CM, and have been reported to be responsible for syncope in up to 20% of patients referred for EPS assessment of syncope.[1,34] Again, as with the supraventricular tachycardias, posture at the time of arrhythmia onset, tachycardia rate, status of left ventricular function, and the promptness of peripheral vasoconstriction determine whether syncope occurs. Establishing the correct diagnosis requires a level of suspicion based on the risk factors discussed above,

The mere presence of frequent ventricular ectopy is insufficient to establish a connection between syncope and VT. Even the presence of couplets and/or asymptomatic non-sustained VT may not be considered to be definitive. In fact, non-sustained (VT) is a common finding during ambulatory ECG monitoring, especially in patients with known or suspected ischemic heart disease or cardiomyopathy. Consequently, such a finding during the assessment of a syncope patient may not be very helpful in the absence of documented concomitant symptoms. On the other hand, while syncope may need further evaluation, non-sustained VT in the presence of severely diminished left ventricular function (i.e., ejection fractions <35%) predicts a high mortality rate and implantable cardioverter defibrillators (ICDs) may be warranted to protect against sudden death (MADIT); however, an ICD cannot be counted upon to prevent syncope.[7] ICDs require a period of time to detect the tachyarrhythmia and initiate therapy, whether it be antitachycardia pacing or a defibrillation shock (a shock requires charging capacitors, reconfirming the arrhythmia, and discharging the shock). Loss of consciousness may have already developed by the time therapy is delivered. In fact, loss of consciousness may be a desirable feature for patients who are going to be subject to an ICD shock.

Apart from patients with ischemic heart disease and dilated cardiomyopathies, a number of special forms of VT may cause syncope. These are important to identify as the prognostic implications for the affected individual and family members may be important, and treatment choices may be quite different.

13.4.4.2 Arrhythmogenic Right Ventricular Dysplasia/Cardiomyopathy (ARVC)

ARVC is a hereditary disease in which right ventricular myocardium is replaced to varying degrees by fatty infiltration. In some cases the left ventricle is affected as well, but rarely as a solitary finding. Recent thought suggests that ARVC may be better considered a problem of intercellular communication.[35,36] The clinical picture ranges from asymptomatic patients to symptoms secondary to ventricular tachyarrhythmias (VTs) or right ventricular failure. The outcome may vary from palpitations to syncopal episodes, or even sudden death. Of patients referred for evaluation to tertiary care centers, about one-third have a history of syncope, and while of only borderline significance, Corrado et al.[36] identified syncope as one of the important risk factors associated with sudden death (Table 13.3). Syncope related to exercise should bring this diagnosis to mind, especially in individuals without evident underlying structural heart disease.[37] ARVC should be suspected in patients with syncope of unknown origin in whom there is a family history of premature sudden death or unexplained syncope, and ventricular premature beats of left bundle branch block morphology, suggesting a right ventricular site of origin, or who exhibit certain ECG abnormalities[37,38]: epsilon waves (analogous to "late" potentials in ischemic heart disease), found mainly in ECG lead V1; and/or inverted T waves in right precordial leads in the absence of right bundle branch block. However, it must be pointed out that no test is per se diagnostic and a combination of diagnostic tests is needed to evaluate the presence of right ventricular structural, functional, and electrical abnormalities. Electrocardiogram, echocardiography, right ventricular angiography, signal-averaged ECG, and Holter monitoring provide optimal clinical evaluation of patients suspected of ARVC (13.4).

The optimum treatment strategy for patients with ARVC and syncope has not been fully established. Drug therapy is not well proven, and ablation success may be hard to predict by virtue of the potential for many regions of the heart to be affected. Consequently, in those patients with syncope in whom VT is either documented

Table 13.3 Clinical characteristics associated with appropriate ICD intervention[36]

Risk factor	p	OR[a]	95% CI
Age/5 years	0.007	0.77	0.57–0.96
LVEF	0.037	0.94	0.89–0.95
Cardiac arrest	<0.001	79	6.8–90.6
VT with hypotension	0.015	14	1.7–21.1
Unexplained syncope	0.07	7.5	0.84–1.81

[a]OR per 5 year interval.

Table 13.4 Clinical and laboratory features in arrhythmogenic right ventricular dysplasia/ cardiomyopathy (ARVD/CM) patients from Marcus et al.[38]

• Age at symptom onset	36±15 years
• Age at diagnosis	38±13 years
• Gender(M/F) $n = 108$	62/46
• Family history	21%
• Symptoms (%)	
– Palpitations	56%
– Dizziness	27%
– Syncope	21%
– Chest pain	14%
• Abnormal ECG (negative T waves in precordial leads)	57%
• Late potentials (2/3 criteria on signal averaging ECG)	51%
• >1,000 PVC on Holter monitoring	52%
• Induction of sustained VT on EPS	49%
• RV dilatation and/or wall motion abnormalities (echocardiogram)	66%
• RV dilatation and/or wall motion abnormalities (angiography)	56%
• RV dilatation and/or wall motion abnormalities (MRI)	36%

during a spontaneous recording or induced at EPS, an ICD is recommended (once again recognizing the caveat discussed earlier regarding the limitation of ICDs for syncope prevention).

13.4.4.3 Outflow Tract Tachycardias

Idiopathic right ventricular outflow tract (RVOT) tachycardia is the most frequent type of idiopathic VT[39,40]; it can be present at any age, but it is most frequently detected between the 2nd and 4th decade of life and appears to be due to cyclic AMP-mediated "triggered activity." Patients may be asymptomatic or they can experience palpitations, dizziness, or on occasion syncope. Most often this tachycardia has a benign course from a mortality perspective, but it may have a very negative impact on patient lifestyle. The baseline ECG in (RVOT) patients is usually normal. Some patients have frequent premature ventricular beats with the same morphology as the recorded tachycardia (i.e., a QRS which appears to have a left bundle branch block appearance but relatively narrow, with a vertical or rightward frontal axis). Tachycardia in these patients can manifest as episodes of non-sustained VT, repetitive monomorphic VT interrupted by short periods of sinus rhythm or episodes of paroxysmal sustained VT. As the morphology of this tachycardia can be similar to tachycardia observed in the prognostically more worrisome ARVC patients, it is important that ARVC be excluded.

Idiopathic left ventricular outflow tract (LVOT) tachycardia is less common than but analogous to RVOT tachycardia. It exhibits subtle variations in QRS morphology during tachycardia, consisting mainly of the presence of an R wave in V1 and V2 leads. It has been shown, by intracavitary mapping techniques, that the QRS morphology of the VT may not only suggest LVOT but assist in defining the site of origin even more precisely.

Treatment of both RVOT and LVOT tachycardias is indicated in symptomatic patients with palpitations or syncope. Beta-blockers have been considered as the first-choice drug for the treatment of these patients. Other antiarrhythmic drugs may also be tried. However, drug therapy is often associated with troublesome side effects, and since most of these patients are diagnosed at a relatively young age, transcatheter ablation is often preferable. Ablation has a reported success rate of approximately 85%.

13.4.4.4 Idiopathic Left Fascicular Tachycardia

Idiopathic LV fascicular tachycardia is a relatively common tachycardia and is most frequently seen in otherwise healthy patients between the 2nd and 4th decade of life; it predominates in males. The mechanism of tachycardia seems to be a re-entry in the left distal fascicular system (usually the posterior fascicle). During EPS, the arrhythmia can usually be induced and stopped by programmed ventricular stimulation. Usually, fascicular VT can be easily terminated by verapamil infusion (although long-term oral verapamil is not generally effective for prevention of recurrences). The most frequent form of presentation is as paroxysmal VT, with a QRS pattern of right bundle branch block and left axis deviation. Occasionally, similar right bundle branch block but with right axis deviation can be seen, suggesting that re-entry arises from the left anterior fascicle. Clinically, these patients may be asymptomatic, but when they have symptoms, they usually experience palpitations, dizziness, or syncope. As in RVOT tachycardia, the prognosis in left fascicular tachycardia is generally benign, but symptomatic patients require treatment, and transcatheter ablation has been highly effective.

13.4.4.5 Long QT Syndromes (Primary, Secondary)

The long QT syndromes may be a primary disorder or secondary to other factors, most commonly various drugs (Table 13.5).[11,41–47] The primary long QT syndromes comprise a group of disorders, generally considered to be genetically transmitted in nature and characterized by a prolongation of ventricular repolarization (i.e., long QT interval). It is also understood that there are some affected patients who have normal baseline QT interval durations but who are predisposed to QT interval prolongation and "torsade de pointes" VT when exposed to QT prolonging drugs or certain metabolic disturbances (e.g., hypokalemia). The clinical manifestations may be syncope, but sudden death is a major concern. In the most common form of long QT syndrome, syncope episodes are triggered by adrenergic stimulus, such as exercise or stressful situations. However, other forms of long QT syndrome may result in torsades being apparently triggered either by, or at least in the setting of bradycardia.

In patients with syncope of unknown origin, the presence of primary long QT syndrome must be suspected when there are abnormalities of repolarization, or family history of long QT syndrome, syncope, or sudden death. As a rule, these patients should be advised to avoid vigorous exercise. They should also not be exposed to drugs that can further prolong QT interval. For patients with a first syncopal

Table 13.5 Drugs commonly associated with QT interval prolongation[a]

Antiarrhythmic agents
Class IA
  Quinidine
  Procainamide
  Disopyramide
Class III
  Sotalol
  Ibutilide
  N-Acetylprocainamide (NAPA)
  Dofetilide
  Amiodarone, dronedarone (relatively low risk)

Antianginal agents
Ranolazine[b]
Bepridil (removed from market in USA)

Psychoactive/antidepression agents
Phenothiazines
Thioridazine
Amitriptyline
Imipramine
Resperidone[b]
Lithium
Methadone

Anti-infective, antibiotics
Clarithromycin
Erythromycin
Pentamidine
Fluconazole
Ciprofloxacin, levofloxacin[b]
Pentamidine

Non-sedating antihistamines
Terfenadine (removed from market in USA)
Astemizole

Miscellaneous
Cisapride (removed from market in USA)
Droperidol
Vardenafil[b]
Octreotide[b]

---

[a]Only the more commonly used agents are listed here.
[b]Drug is considered a "possible" risk only.

episode and no other risk factors, treatment with beta-blockers is considered as a first-line treatment. When bradycardia-triggered syncope is implicated, the use of beta-blockers is questionable while it can be argued that the use of implanted cardiac pacemakers is justified. In patients that have other risk factors in addition to syncope (see above) or those who have syncope recurrences in spite of beta-blockers, implantation of an ICD is indicated. A strong family history of sudden death is probably a strong indicator for an ICD (see also Chapter 15).

Secondary forms of long QT syndrome may be the result of drug effects, electrolyte disturbances, or a combination of these. Drug-induced long QT syndrome is by far the most frequently encountered of these conditions, and new drugs capable of inducing the problem are being identified each year. Given the substantial public health hazard associated with drug-induced long QT, physicians must be very attentive to the risk (Table 13.5). Internet sites such as www.torsades.org are helpful in terms of maintaining relatively up-to-date lists of drugs associated with triggering torsades.

Eliminating the offending agent is the key to treatment of drug-induced torsades. In an emergent situation (i.e., recurrent torsades), infusion of magnesium sulfate, restoration of normal electrolyte status, and prevention of bradycardia are important therapeutic steps.

13.4.4.6 Brugada Syndrome

Brugada syndrome is a hereditary disease characterized by an ECG pattern of right bundle branch block and coved ST segment elevation in V1–V3.[12–15,48] However, the ECG findings do not always reveal the characteristic pattern. In those patients with suspected Brugada syndrome who have an apparently normal ECG, intravenous administration of a class I antiarrhythmic drug (e.g., ajmaline, procainamide) can provoke the typical QRS-ST segment changes, thereby confirming the diagnosis.

These individuals are at risk of developing syncope (and sudden death) due to episodes of polymorphous ventricular tachycardia. Although the risk of sudden death in asymptomatic patients with Brugada syndrome is uncertain, those patients who have had syncope or an aborted sudden death are generally considered to be at increased risk. Currently, sudden death prevention requires an ICD, but syncope may still occur (see also Chapter 15).

13.4.4.7 Short QT Syndrome

Short QT syndrome appears to be a very rare inherited condition described to date in only a few families. Characteristically, the corrected QT interval is shorter than 320 ms. Clinical manifestations include syncope, palpitations, paroxysmal atrial fibrillation, and sudden death. ICD therapy is again considered the treatment of choice for sudden death prevention. However, it has been suggested that it may be beneficial to try and prolong the QT interval and reduce ventricular arrhythmia risk; it may also be helpful to diminish syncope risk, since as has been emphasized earlier, ICD therapy alone may not be effective for syncope prevention.

13.5 Structural Cardiopulmonary Diseases

A variety of structural cardiac, vascular, or pulmonary disease may be associated with syncope (Table 13.6). However, most often the relationship of structural cardiopulmonary abnormalities to syncope is indirect (i.e., operating through

Table 13.6 Principal structural cardiac and pulmonary disease conditions associated with syncope

Condition	Mechanism(s) excluding arrhythmia
Acute MI or ischemia	Reflex, reduced CO, VT
Chronic ischemic heart disease	VT, AV block
Aortic stenosis	Reflex
Atrial myxoma	Transient blood flow obstruction
Acute aortic dissection	Reflex
Pulmonary embolism	Reflex
Primary pulmonary hypertension	Reflex
Pericardial disease	Inflow obstruction, reduced CO
Dilated cardiomyopathy	VT
ARVD	VT
HOCM	Outflow obstruction, VT

Abbreviations: AV, atrioventricular; ARVD, arrhythmogenic RV, dysplasia/cardiomyopathy; CO, cardiac output; HOCM, hypertrophic obstructive cardiomyopathy; MI, myocardial infarction; reflex, neural reflex vasodepressor/bradycardia; VT, ventricular tachycardia.

susceptibility to tachy- or bradyarrhythmias, or hypotension of other cause [e.g., acute myocardial infarction, acute aortic dissection]). Additionally, in many cases a reflex mechanism contributes to the faint (e.g., syncope associated with acute myocardial ischemia, severe aortic stenosis, or pulmonary hypertension). On the other hand, whether structural disease is a "direct" or an "indirect" participant, the associated mortality risk must be taken seriously. Careful consideration needs to be given to hospitalizing these patients for prompt evaluation.

In patients in whom structural cardiovascular or cardiopulmonary disease is the cause of syncope, treatment is best directed toward ameliorating the specific structural lesion or its consequences. Thus, in syncope associated with myocardial ischemia, pharmacologic therapy and/or revascularization is clearly the appropriate strategy in most cases. Similarly, when syncope is closely associated with surgically addressable lesions (e.g., valvular aortic stenosis, atrial myxoma, congenital cardiac anomaly), a direct corrective approach is often feasible. On the other hand, when syncope is caused by certain difficult to treat conditions such as primary pulmonary hypertension or restrictive cardiomyopathy, it is often impossible to ameliorate the underlying problem adequately. Even modifying outflow gradients in HCM is not readily achieved surgically. In the latter condition, the effectiveness of standard pharmacological therapies remains uncertain, and despite ongoing controversy, cardiac pacing techniques continue to be employed (often as an ICD) in individuals who have experienced syncope or who have a worrisome family history.

13.5.1 *Myocardial Ischemia, Pulmonary Embolism, and Pericardial Tamponade*

In terms of syncope directly attributable to structural disease, the most common is that which occurs in conjunction with acute myocardial ischemia or infarction. Other relatively common acute conditions associated with syncope include pulmonary embolism and pericardial tamponade. The basis of syncope in these conditions is multifactorial, including both the hemodynamic impact of the specific lesion and neurally mediated reflex effects leading to inappropriate bradycardia and peripheral vascular dilatation. The latter is especially important in the setting of acute ischemic events. One of the most commonly observed examples is the atropine-responsive bradycardia and hypotension often associated with inferior wall myocardial infarction.

13.5.2 Outflow Tract Obstruction

Syncope is of considerable concern when it is associated with conditions in which there is fixed or dynamic obstruction to left ventricular outflow (e.g., *aortic stenosis, hypertrophic obstructive cardiomyopathy, prosthetic valve malfunction*). In such cases, symptoms are often provoked by physical exertion but may also develop if an otherwise benign arrhythmia should occur (e.g., atrial fibrillation). The basis for the faint is in part inadequate blood flow due to the mechanical obstruction. However, and especially in the case of valvular aortic stenosis, neurally mediated reflex disturbance of vascular control is an important contributor to hypotension.

Hypertrophic cardiomyopathy (HCM, i.e., non-dilated left ventricle with increased wall thickness [typically ≥ 15 mm] with no other cause) warrants particular attention among the structural diseases associated with syncope as it

- is a relatively common condition,
- tends to affect young persons (particularly those taking part in vigorous, often competitive, physical activity),
- is readily diagnosed by physical examination and echocardiography,
- has been associated with substantial sudden death risk, of which syncope is a recognized risk factor.

In HCM, with or without left ventricle outflow obstruction, reflex mechanisms may play a role in triggering syncope. However, in the obstructive form of HCM, the occurrence of atrial tachyarrhythmias (particularly atrial fibrillation) or ventricular tachycardia (even at relatively modest rates) may diminish cardiac output sufficiently to cause transient loss of consciousness. Syncope is a recognized risk factor for sudden death in HCM, particularly in younger individuals who have experienced syncope relatively recently prior to their condition being diagnosed.[49,50] The reader is referred to Chapter 15 for more detail.

13.5.3 Other Cardiopulmonary Conditions That May Cause Syncope

A number of less common causes of syncope associated with cardiopulmonary disease may need to be considered depending on clinical circumstances. The mechanism of the faint is once again multifactorial, with hemodynamic, arrhythmic, and neurally mediated origins in need of evaluation. These conditions include the following:

- vascular steal syndromes (particularly "subclavian steal")
- pacemaker/ICD malfunction
- acute aortic dissection
- left ventricular inflow obstruction in patients with mitral stenosis or atrial myxoma
- right ventricular outflow obstruction and
- right-to-left shunting secondary to pulmonic stenosis or pulmonary hypertension.

Subclavian steal syndrome, albeit very uncommon, is the most important of the vascular steal conditions and may occur on a congenital or acquired basis. Low pressure within the subclavian artery due to a stenosis near its origin causes retrograde flow to occur in the ipsilateral vertebral artery. The result is a diminution of cerebral blood flow due to "steal" from the Circle of Willis. Syncope is typically associated with ipsilateral upper extremity exercise. Direct corrective angioplasty or surgery is usually feasible and effective. Other forms of vascular steal, particularly within the cranium, are recognized as potential causes of syncope but are virtually impossible to diagnose.

Intermittent failure to pace due to lead fracture, device failure or battery depletion, or a loose setscrew may cause syncope in a pacemaker-dependent individual. Similarly, an ICD may trigger syncope by failing to pace appropriately or by introducing burst pacing inappropriately. However, acute device failures are rare. The device should be interrogated as the true cause of the faint may in fact prove to be a tachyarrhythmia; these events are often recorded by the device diagnostics.

Acute dissection of the aorta is a relatively frequent occurrence; syncope has been reported to be a presenting feature in 5–20% of patients. For example, in one recent multicenter report comprising 728 patients with acute aortic dissection, syncope was reported in 19%.[51] Further, those patients presenting with syncope appeared to have an increased in-hospital mortality (34 versus 23% without syncope), as well as greater propensity for cardiac tamponade, stroke, and other neurological deficits.[51]

13.6 Diagnostic Strategies

13.6.1 Evaluation In or Out of Hospital?

The evaluation of patients with suspected cardiac syncope entails both a thorough evaluation of the underlying lesion(s) and determination of the role (if any) played by the structural disease in triggering the faint. Among the first steps is ascertaining whether it is safe to assess the patient as an outpatient (day patient) or if in-hospital evaluation is needed.[1] This issue has been discussed earlier in this volume, but here we provide a brief summary of important considerations (Table 13.7).

Table 13.7 Recommendations regarding inpatient versus outpatient evaluation (based on ESC syncope task force guidelines[1])

Hospital admission strongly recommended for diagnosis
- Suspected or known significant heart disease
- ECG abnormalities suggestive of arrhythmic syncope
- Syncope during exercise
- Syncope in supine position
- Syncope causing severe injury
- Family history of sudden death

Hospital admission recommended for treatment
- Cardiac arrhythmias
- Syncope due to cardiac ischemia
- Syncope secondary to structural cardiac or cardiopulmonary diseases
- Cardioinhibitory neurally mediated syncope when a pacemaker implantation is planned (usually older patients >60 years)

Usually not admitted
- Patients without heart disease but sudden onset of palpitations shortly before syncope
- History suggests neurally mediated reflex or orthostatic syncope
- Very frequent recurrent episodes (suggesting psychogenic pseudosyncope)
- Patients with minimal or mild heart disease when there is a high suspicion for cardiac syncope

---

13.6.1.1 In-hospital Recommended

Several markers identify syncope patients who should be considered for in-hospital evaluation. Syncope associated with an acute myocardial ischemia or infarction, and/or hemodynamically concerning underlying structural heart disease is thought to have the highest immediate mortality risk. At similar high risk are syncope patients with certain ECG abnormalities, including high-grade AV block, preexcitation syndromes (e.g., Wolff–Parkinson–White syndrome), arrhythmogenic RV cardiomyopathy (ARVD/C), long QT syndrome (LQTS), Brugada syndrome, and short QT syndrome. Patients with syncope during exercise (i.e., collapse during "full flight") should also be evaluated in hospital. As discussed earlier, some of these latter patients may have unrecognized myocardial ischemia and exercise-induced AV block, while others may be susceptible to catecholamine-triggered tachyarrhythmias (e.g., idiopathic ventricular tachycardia/fibrillation, HCM). An additional troublesome prognostic marker is a family history of premature sudden death. This history may be indicative of not only ischemic heart disease but also any of a variety of familial conditions which may first present as syncope (e.g., LQTS, Brugada syndrome, familial cardiomyopathies, and arrhythmogenic RV cardiomyopathy). See also Chapter 6.

13.6.1.2 Hospitalization Can Be Avoided

For patients with isolated or rare syncope episodes in whom there is no evidence of structural heart disease and who have a normal baseline ECG, the immediate risk of a life-threatening cardiac syncope is low and outpatient care is often appropriate.

Similarly, even in patients with known structural heart disease, the history may favor a neurally mediated reflex or orthostatic origin for the faint. In such cases, given a sufficiently safe supportive home environment, outpatient valuation is reasonable. Nevertheless, syncope recurrences can occur, and cautionary advice regarding driving, occupation, and avocation should be provided until such time as one is confident that the susceptibility to fainting has been suppressed.

13.6.2 Specific Testing

Apart from identifying the nature and severity of any underlying cardiopulmonary disease in a patient with syncope, the cause of the faint needs special consideration. As has already been emphasized, the same disease may induce syncope by different mechanisms. Consequently, the mere presence of structural disease does not necessarily provide a diagnosis that can be relied upon to prevent future syncope events. Furthermore, non-invasive risk assessment, while arguably of value to assess sudden death risk in patients with structural heart disease, does not address the cause of syncope.

In those cases in whom structural cardiopulmonary disease is known to be present and its severity is not thought to be critical, then only the mechanism of the syncope has to be determined. This aspect is facilitated if an arrhythmia has already been documented during or immediately after the syncope episode, or if the patient has a clear-cut evidence of channelopathy on ECG, or if the medical history strongly supports a neurally mediated reflex mechanism. In the absence of such findings, ambulatory ECG monitoring (typically an ILR or a Mobile Cardiac Outpatient Telemetry [MCOT] system) is generally the first step.[1,52-54] Short duration ECG monitoring (e.g., 24–48 h Holter monitors) is usually insufficient due to the low probability that a spontaneous event will occur during the recording period. EPS with or without autonomic studies (i.e., head-up tilt, carotid massage, and response to cough and Valsalva) may also prove to be needed (see later).

In cases where the presence of cardiopulmonary disease is known, but the severity has not been characterized, referral for selected non-invasive (e.g., echocardiogram, exercise testing, and radionuclide imaging) and possibly invasive (e.g., angiography and hemodynamic measurements) evaluation is recommended. Thereafter the strategy for evaluation depends on the nature of the disease process. If severe, in-hospital monitoring and/or EPS/autonomic assessment may be elected. If not severe, then outpatient ambulatory monitoring as discussed above is appropriate.

EPS has not proven to be as effective for assessment of syncope patients as was initially hoped, but it may be helpful in selected circumstances, particularly in individuals with underlying structural heart disease.[34,55-61] For example, in a review by Camm and Lau,[34] testing was clearly more successful in patients with structural cardiac disease (71%) than in patients without (36%). Further, the addition of isoproterenol infusion during EPS is reported to increase diagnostic sensitivity,[59] again primarily in patients with structural heart disease. Nevertheless, it is evident that care must be taken in interpreting findings of electrophysiological testing in syncope patients. Fujimura et al.[57] were the first to demonstrate the need for caution; their study summarized outcomes of EPS testing in syncope patients in whom bradyarrhythmias were known to be the cause of syncope. Among 21 syncope patients with known symptomatic AV block or sinus pauses, EPS testing correctly identified only 3 of 8 patients with documented sinus pauses (sensitivity 37%) and 2 of 13 patients with documented AV block (sensitivity 15%). On the other hand, the induction of reentry supraventricular or ventricular tachycardia in a syncope patient is highly likely to be significant. These arrhythmias are rarely inconsequential bystanders; however, in order to demonstrate their hemodynamic significance in an individual patient, it may be necessary to initiate the arrhythmia with the patient in an appropriately secured upright tilt position.

The combination of tilt-table testing and invasive EPS testing has been evaluated in syncope patients, but the reports are few, date from the pre-ILR era in which a true "gold standard" was not available to confirm findings, and were not controlled. By way of example, Sra et al.[56] reported results of EPS in conjunction with head-up tilt testing in 86 consecutive patients referred for evaluation of unexplained syncope. EPS was abnormal in 29 (34%) of patients, with the majority of these (21 patients) exhibiting inducible sustained monomorphic VT. Among the remaining patients, head-up tilt testing proved positive in 34 (40%) cases, while 23 patients (26%) remained undiagnosed. In general, patients exhibiting positive EPS findings were older, more frequently male, and exhibited lower left ventricular ejection fractions (LVEFs) and higher frequency of evident heart disease than was the case in patients with positive head-up tilt tests or patients in whom no diagnosis was determined.

In a further evaluation of the combined use of EPS and head-up tilt testing in assessment of syncope, Fitzpatrick et al.[62] analyzed findings in 322 syncope patients. Conventional EPS provided a basis for syncope in 229 of 322 cases (71%), with 93 patients having a normal study. Among the patients with abnormal EPS findings, AV conduction disease was diagnosed in 34%, sinus node dysfunction in 21%, CSS in 10%, and an inducible sustained tachyarrhythmia in 6%. In the 93 patients with normal EPS studies, tilt-table testing was undertaken in 71 cases and resulted in syncope consistent with a vasovagal faint, in 53/71 (75%) of this subset.

13.7 Treatment

13.7.1 Addressing Underlying Structural Disease as the Treatment of Syncope

The treatment of syncope in the setting of structural cardiopulmonary disease is dependent on the nature and severity of the underlying structural abnormalities, and the apparent mechanism(s) (i.e., arrhythmia and hemodynamic abnormality) of the faint. In an emergency situation, the underlying structural disturbance must be treated first (e.g., acute myocardial infarction and severe aortic stenosis). Referral to a facility experienced in and capable of dealing with the acute problem is essential.

In non-emergency circumstances, evaluation of the structural disease and optimal corrective approach if needed can be undertaken on an elective basis (e.g., aortic valve replacement in the case of severe aortic stenosis).

Among patients seen acutely for evaluation of syncope, acute myocardial infarction (AMI) is an uncommon but important cause of the faint. McDermott et al.[63] found only a 3% incidence of AMI among 1,474 patients seen in the ED for syncope or near-syncope. In any case, it is clear that when syncope is the principal feature of AMI presentation, the priority is treatment of the acute ischemic syndrome including revascularization as appropriate. Exceptions would be patients presenting with high-grade or complete AV block, or recurrent ventricular tachyarrhythmias.

When syncope is closely associated with surgically addressable lesions (e.g., valvular aortic stenosis, atrial myxoma, congenital cardiac anomaly, and implanted device malfunction), a direct corrective approach is often feasible. In HCM, there are no convincing data on the effect of reducing outflow gradient for prevention relief of syncope relapses. Nevertheless, it would seem reasonable to consider such a step using medications and/or pacing, and on occasion of surgical intervention.

13.7.2 Addressing Underlying Structural Disease Is Not Feasible or Adequate

When syncope is caused by certain difficult-to-treat conditions such as in many instances of severe left ventricular dysfunction, primary pulmonary hypertension, or restrictive cardiomyopathy, it is often impossible to ameliorate the underlying problem adequately. In such cases it is reasonable to turn attention to determining the cause of syncope (e.g., ventricular tachycardia in dilated cardiomyopathy) and focusing on its treatment (e.g., antiarrhythmic drugs and ICD). In addition, it should be emphasized that for patients with structural cardiopulmonary disease, additional factors could participate in the triggering of a syncope event. For instance, electrolyte disturbances, increasing heart failure, dehydration (over-diuresis) or worsening oxygenation may all aggravate susceptibility to arrhythmia initiation, leading to syncope. Hypokalemia occurring as a side effect of diuretic therapy is one of the most common scenarios to keep in mind. It is of course of crucial importance to recognize these triggering factors as their reversal can eliminate the symptoms.

13.8 Clinical Perspectives

The most recent update of the European Society of Cardiology Syncope Task Force guideline classifies "cardiac syncope" as incorporating all of the causes of syncope that are primarily due to disturbances of cardiac or cardiovascular function. Consequently, cardiac syncope may be the result of cardiac conduction system disease, primary cardiac rhythm disturbances, or cardiovascular structural abnormalities.

Identifying whether syncope is of a "cardiac origin" is important from both prognostic and treatment perspectives. In this regard, a medical history indicating that the fainter is known to have heart disease him- or herself or a family history of certain genetically transmitted cardiac conditions is an important clue to the possibility of a cardiac etiology of syncope. In effect, the presence of these conditions substantially raises the likelihood of a cardiac origin, but nonetheless further evaluation remains necessary in most cases. Multiple findings readily obtainable during the initial clinical evaluation can be used to determine whether cardiac syncope is a high probability. These include, apart from the patient's personal and family medical history, findings on physical examination and results of 12-lead ECG and echocardiogram. Thereafter, additional studies are selected as deemed appropriate by the suspected diagnosis. In some cases, evaluation will need to be carried out in hospital (or in a "syncope management unit"), while in many others it is reasonable to conduct studies in the outpatient environment. In all cases, the goal is to establish an etiologic diagnosis that can be relied upon to permit informing the patient and family of the expected prognosis, as well as leading to an effective treatment strategy.

References

1. Moya A, et al. Guidelines for the diagnosis and management of syncope (version 2009). *Eur Heart J*. 2009;30:2631–2671.
2. Brignole M, et al. Guidelines on management (diagnosis and treatment) of syncope. *Europace*. 2004;6:467–537.
3. Jhanjee R, et al. *Syncope*. Mosby: Disease-a-Month; 2009:527–586.
4. Soteriades ES, et al. Incidence and prognosis of syncope. *N Engl J Med*. 2002;347:878–885.
5. Savage DD, et al. Epidemiologic features of isolated syncope: The Framingham Study. *Stroke*. 1985;16:626–629.
6. Pires LA, et al. Comparison of event rates and survival in patients with unexplained syncope without documented ventricular tachyarrhythmias versus patients with documented sustained ventricular tachyarrhythmias both treated with implantable cardioverter-defibrillators. *Am J Cardiol*. 2000;85:725–728.
7. Olshansky B, et al. Clinical significance of syncope in the electrophysiologic study versus electrocardiographic monitoring (ESVEM) trial. The ESVEM Investigators. *Am Heart J*. 1999;137:878–886.
8. Steinberg JS, et al. Follow-up of patients with unexplained syncope and inducible ventricular tachyarrhythmias: analysis of the AVID registry and an AVID substudy. Antiarrhythmics versus implantable defibrillators. *J Cardiovasc Electrophysiol*. 2001;12:996–1001.
9. Knight BP, et al. Outcome of patients with nonischemic dilated cardiomyopathy and unexplained syncope treated with an implantable defibrillator. *J Am Coll Cardiol*. 1999;33:1964–1970.
10. Olshansky B, et al. Syncope predicts the outcome of cardiomyopathy patients: Analysis of the SCD-HeFT study. *J Am Coll Cardiol*. 2008;51:1277–1282.
11. Sauer A, et al. Long QT Syndrome in Adults. *J Am Coll Cardiol*. 2007;49:329–337.
12. Sacher F, et al. Outcome after implantation of a cardioverter-defibrillator in patients with Brugada syndrome. A Multicenter Study. *Circulation*. 2006;114:2317–2324.
13. Sarkozy A, et al. Long-term follow-up of primary prophylactic implantable cardioverter-defibrillator therapy in Brugada syndrome. *Eur Heart J*. 2007;28:334–344.

14. Paparella G, et al. Brugada syndrome: The prognostic dilemma and value of syncope. *Minerva Med.* 2009;100:307–319.
15. Paul M, et al. Role of programmed ventricular stimulation in patients with Brugada syndrome: A meta-analysis of worldwide published data. *Eur Heart J.* 2007;28:2126–2133.
16. Alboni P, et al. The diagnostic value of history in patients with syncope with or without heart disease. *J Am Coll Cardiol.* 2001;37:1921–1928.
17. Del Rosso A, et al. Relation of clinical presentation of syncope to the age of patients. *Am J Cardiol.* 2005;96:1431–1435.
18. Del Rosso A, et al. Clinical predictors of cardiac syncope at initial evaluation in patients referred urgently to a general hospital: the EGSYS score. *Heart.* 2008;94:1620–1626.
19. Colivicchi F, et al. Epidemiology and prognostic implications of syncope in young competing athletes. *Eur Heart J.* 2004;25:1749–1753.
20. Benditt DG, et al. Sinus node dysfunction. In: Willerson JT, Cohn JN, eds. *Cardiovascular Medicine.* 3rd edn. Edinburgh: Churchill Livingstone; 2006:1925–1935.
21. Benditt DG, et al. Indications for electrophysiologic testing in the diagnosis and assessment of sinus node dysfunction. *Circulation.* 1987;75(Suppl III):93–99.
22. Raj S. Highlights in clinical autonomic neurosciences. Orthostatic tachycardia and orthostatic hypotension. *Autonom Neurosci Basic and Clin.* 2010;154:1–2.
23. Gann D, et al. Electrophysiologic evaluation of elderly patients with sinus bradycardia: a long-term follow-up study. *Ann Intern Med.* 1979;90:24–29.
24. Fragakis N, et al. The value of adenosine test in the diagnosis of sick sinus syndrome: susceptibility of sinus and atrioventricular node to adenosine in patients with sick sinus syndrome and unexplained syncope. *Europace.* 2007;9:559–562.
25. Flammang D, et al. The adenosine triphosphate (ATP) test for evaluation of syncope of unknown origin. *J Cardiovasc Electrophysiol.* 2005;16:1388–1389.
26. Perennes A, et al. Epidemiology, clinical features, and follow-up of patients with syncope and a positive adenosine triphosphate test result. *J Am Coll Cardiol.* 2006;47:594–597.
27. Brignole M, et al. Lack of correlation between the responses to tilt testing and adenosine triphosphate test and the mechanism of spontaneous neurally mediated syncope. *Eur Heart J.* 2006;27:2232–2239.
28. Menozzi C, et al. Mechanism of syncope in patients with heart disease and negative electrophysiologic test. *Circulation.* 2002;105:2741–2745.
29. Brignole M, et al. Investigators. Mechanism of syncope in patients with bundle branch block and negative electrophysiological test. *Circulation.* 2001;104:2045–2050.
30. Brignole M, et al. Indications for the use of diagnostic implantable and external ECG loop recorders. Task Force members. *Europace.* 2009;11:671–687.
31. Brignole M, et al. Improved arrhythmia detection in implantable loop recorders. *J Cardiovasc Electrophysiol.* 2008;19:928–934.
32. Villain E. Indications for pacing in patients with congenital heart disease. *Pacing Clin Electrophysiol.* 2008;31(Suppl 1):S17–S20.
33. Michaelsson M, et al. A natural history of congenital atrio-ventricular block. *Pacing Clin Electrophysiol.* 1997;20:2098–2101.
34. Camm AJ, Lau CP. Syncope of undetermined origin: diagnosis and management. *Prog Cardiol.* 1988;1:139–156.
35. Maron BJ, et al. Contemporary definitions and classification of the cardiomyopathies. *Circulation.* 2006;113:1807–1816.
36. Corrado D, et al. Implantable cardioverter-defibrillator therapy for prevention of sudden death in patients with arrhythmogenic right ventricular cardiomyopathy/dysplasia. *Circulation.* 2003;108:3084–3091.
37. Maron BJ, et al. Recommendations for physical activity and recreational sports participation for young patients with genetic cardiovascular diseases. *Circulation.* 2004;109:2807–2816.
38. Marcus FI, et al. Arrhythmogenic right ventricular cardiomyopathy/dysplasia clinical presentation and diagnostic evaluation: results from the North American Multidisciplinary Study. *Heart Rhythm.* 2009;6:984–992.

39. Farzaneh-Far A, Lerman BB. Idiopathic ventricular outflow tract tachycardia. *Heart*. 2005;91:136–138.

40. Chun KR, et al. Left ventricular outflow tract tachycardia including ventricular tachycardia from the aortic cusps and epicardial ventricular tachycardia. *Herz*. 2007;32:226–232.

41. Jackman WM, et al. The long QT syndromes: a critical review, new clinical observations and a unifying hypothesis. *Prog Cardiovasc Dis*. 1988;31:115–172.

42. Moss AJ, et al. The long QT syndrome: prospective longitudinal study of 328 families. *Circulation*. 1991;84:1136–1144.

43. Schwartz PJ, et al. Stress and sudden death: the case of the long QT syndrome. *Circulation*. 1991;83(Suppl II):71–80.

44. Moss AJ, et al. ECG T-wave patterns in genetically distinct forms of the hereditary long QT syndrome. *Circulation*. 1995;92:2929–2934.

45. Zareba W, Cygankiewicz I. Long QT syndrome and short QT syndrome. *Prog Cardiovasc Dis*. 2008;51:264–278.

46. Johnson JN, Ackerman MJ. QTc: How long is too long? *Br J Sports Med*. 2009;43:657–662.

47. Colman N, et al. Value of history-taking in syncope patients: In whom to suspect long QT syndrome?. *Europace*. 2009;11:937–943.

48. Antzelevitch C, et al. Brugada syndrome: report of the second consensus conference. *Circulation*. 2005;111:659–670.

49. Spirito P, et al. Implantable cardioverter defibrillators and prevention of sudden death in hypertrophic cardiomyopathy. *J Am Med Assoc*. 2007;298:405–412.

50. Spirito P, et al. Syncope and risk of sudden death in hypertrophic cardiomyopathy. *Circulation*. 2009;119:1703–1710.

51. Nallamothu BK, et al. Syncope in acute aortic dissection: Diagnostic, prognostic and clinical implications. *Am J Med*. 2002;113:468–471.

52. Krahn AD, et al. Randomized assessment of syncope trial: conventional diagnostic testing versus a prolonged monitoring strategy. *Circulation*. 2001;104:46–51.

53. Krahn AD, et al. Cost implications of testing strategy in patients with syncope. Randomized assessment of syncope trial. *J Am Coll Cardiol*. 2003;42:495–501.

54. Brignole M, et al. Early application of an implantable loop recorder allows a mechanism-based effective therapy in patients with recurrent suspected neurally-mediated syncope. *Eur Heart J*. 2006;27:1085–1092.

55. Morady F, et al. Long-term follow-up of patients with recurrent unexplained syncope evaluated by electrophysiologic testing. *J Am Coll Cardiol*. 1983;2:1053–1059.

56. Sra JS, et al. Unexplained syncope evaluated by electrophysiologic studies and head-up tilt testing. *Ann Intern Med*. 1991;114:1013–1019.

57. Fujimura O, et al. The diagnostic sensitivity of electrophysiologic testing in patients with syncope caused by bradycardia. *N Engl J Med*. 1989;321:1703–1707.

58. Brembilla-Perrot B, et al. Are the results of electrophysiological study different in patients with a pre-excitation syndrome, with and without syncope? *Europace*. 2008;10:175–180.

59. Brembilla-Perrot B, et al. Increased sensitivity of electrophysiological study by isoproterenol infusion in unexplained syncope. *Int J Cardiol*. 2006;106:82–87.

60. Chen LY, et al. Score indices for predicting electrophysiologic outcomes in patients with unexplained syncope. *J Interv Card Electrophysiol*. 2005 Nov;14:99–105.

61. Brilakis ES, et al. Programmed ventricular stimulation in patients with idiopathic dilated cardiomyopathy and syncope receiving implantable cardioverter-defibrillators: A case series and a systematic review of the literature. *Int J Cardiol*. 2005;98:395–401.

62. Fitzpatrick A, et al. The incidence of malignant vasovagal syndrome in patients with recurrent syncope. *Eur Heart J*. 1991;12:389–394.

63. McDermott D, et al. Acute myocardial infarction in patients with syncope. *Can J Emerg Med*. 2009;11:156–160.

Chapter 14
Conditions that Mimic Syncope

Contents

Key points: Conditions that mimic syncope

- "Syncope" consists of a relatively brief, self-limited period of transient loss of consciousness (T-LOC) caused by a temporary period of global cerebral hypoperfusion; in most cases the final common pathway is transient systemic hypotension.
- There are other non-syncope conditions that may cause T-LOC without inducing cerebral hypoperfusion (e.g., epilepsy, concussion, and metabolic/endocrine disorders). These conditions have a different pathophysiology and require a different treatment strategy than does true syncope.
- Distinguishing epileptic seizures from syncope is often a difficult challenge when patients come to medical attention after a "blackout" or "collapse." Therefore, despite apparent clinical differences between

---

M. Brignole, D.G. Benditt, *Syncope*, DOI 10.1007/978-0-85729-201-8_14,
© Springer-Verlag London Limited 2011

seizure and syncope, a patient who presents with apparent or real T-LOC
often triggers a costly but misdirected cascade of testing (e.g., MRIs and
EEGs).

- The characteristics of the skeletal muscle motor activity during generalized epilepsy may help an experienced observer distinguish seizure from
syncope. However, for the non-expert, the often subtle differences may be
nearly impossible to appreciate with a high level of confidence.
- There are yet other conditions that mimic syncope (e.g., pseudosyncope, pseudoseizures) but in which true loss of consciousness does not
occur ("syncope mimics"). The key historical finding favoring a diagnosis of "pseudosyncope" or "pseudoseizures" is a very high frequency of
"attacks"; the patient may report that many episodes occur each day or
each week. Injury may occur but is uncommon.
- For "syncope mimics," the event rate is much greater, and symptoms are
reported to be recurrent over a longer duration of time than is usually
observed even in patients with extreme susceptibility to "true" syncope.
- The "syncope mimics" often occur in the setting of certain psychiatric conditions, and their recognition is the crucial first step in directing affected
individuals toward proper care.

14.1 Introduction

Consciousness is a complex physiologic state that is difficult to account for scientif-
ically but is nonetheless widely understood in intuitive terms. From an operational
perspective, the loss of consciousness (i.e., unconsciousness) that most physicians
concern themselves with (e.g., in the context of syncope and related disorders)
relates to loss of alertness. As discussed by van Dijk et al.,[1] this concept of
unconsciousness is restricted to a disturbance of the "arousal" part of consciousness that resides either in the brainstem or in the integrity of a very large part
of the cerebral cortex. Loss of consciousness in this context is always associated
with inability to control posture and consequently the affected individual falls or
slumps over.

Real or seemingly real transient loss of consciousness (T-LOC) is among the
most common reasons that patients to present for urgent medical assessment. Many
conditions may cause a period of real T-LOC; "syncope" is but one of the conditions
that cause real T-LOC. As has been emphasized in previous chapters, syncope is a
syndrome that consists of self-limited and spontaneously terminating period of loss
of consciousness that is caused by a temporary period of global cerebral hypoperfusion (most often due to systemic hypotension).[2] Typically, syncope episodes are
relatively rapid in onset and brief in duration (usually 1–2 min at most). Epilepsy
and concussion are two other important examples of conditions that cause T-LOC;

however, in these last two conditions, despite the fact that T-LOC is real, the loss of consciousness is not due to cerebral hypoperfusion. Consequently neither epilepsy nor concussion is to be considered syncope; they are best classified as "non-syncope T-LOC." Further, there are a number of other conditions that might also appear to be syncope but in which consciousness is not really lost. These latter conditions, which are often termed "syncope mimics" (although they might reasonably also be termed "T-LOC mimics"), are important to recognize in order for affected patients to be appropriately diagnosed and receive proper therapy.

It is the goal of this chapter to review the most frequently encountered conditions that by virtue of their presentation may seem to be "syncope," but which in fact are really something else (i.e., "syncope mimics").

14.2 Syncope Mimics and Pseudosyncope

As alluded to above, there are two broad groups of conditions that may present with real or apparent T-LOC but that should not be considered as true "syncope" (Table 14.1):

- *"Non-syncope T-LOC"* – conditions that cause true T-LOC, but without cerebral hypoperfusion (i.e., the mechanism differs from true syncope). Epilepsy, concussion, and metabolic/endocrine disorders comprise this group.
- *Syncope/T-LOC mimic* – conditions in which T-LOC is reported, but after detailed evaluation it is determined that consciousness was never really lost. Most of these patients are ultimately determined to have psychiatric conditions (e.g., conversion disorders). The terms "pseudosyncope" or "pseudoseizure" be appropriate to many of these cases.

14.3 Non-syncope T-LOC

This category of so-called non-syncope T-LOC mainly comprises three circumstances in which unconsciousness actually occurs: (1) epilepsy, (2) concussion, and (3) metabolic and endocrine disturbances.

Table 14.1 Seemingly real syncope not due to cerebral hypoperfusion

Non-syncope T-LOC	Syncope/T-LOC mimic
• Epilepsy	• Somatization disorders:
• Trauma/concussion	– Pseudosyncope
• Metabolic/endocrine conditions	– Pseudoseizure
– Hypoglycemia	• Cataplexy
– Hypercapnia	• Hyperventilation
– Hyponatremia	• TIAs
– Acute intoxication (e.g., alcohol)	• "Drop attacks"

14.3.1 Epilepsy

The international classification of epilepsy is based on the concept of spreading abnormal neuronal activity (Table 14.2): the two main categories are partial seizures, beginning locally in a part of the cortex, and generalized seizures. Generalized epileptic seizures disrupt the function of the entire cerebral cortex and are therefore most likely to resemble syncope. Conversely, during complex partial seizures, patients may carry out seemingly complicated but purposeless tasks but do not respond or respond only vaguely when addressed; they do not lose postural tone and consequently the spells are less likely to be mistaken for syncope. These latter states are best considered as "altered" or "impaired" consciousness but not "loss of consciousness."[1]

Although epilepsy may be responsible for T-LOC, its pathophysiology differs importantly from that of syncope. Seizures occur due to an electrical disturbance of the brain resulting in abnormal functioning of neural networks; as a rule, nutrient supply to the brain is intact and cerebral perfusion is not an issue (i.e., therefore not "true" syncope).

Distinguishing epileptic seizures from syncope is a challenge often faced by frontline physicians when patients come to medical attention after a "blackout" or "collapse." Therefore, despite apparent clinical differences between seizure and syncope, a patient who presents with apparent or real T-LOC often triggers a costly but misdirected cascade of testing (e.g., magnetic resonance imaging or computed tomography of the head [MR or CT] and electroencephalography [EEGs]) designed to exclude a "seizure." In reality, epilepsy is much less common than syncope and a careful history taking can usually distinguish one from the other. It is far better to wait and make a carefully considered diagnosis (i.e., syncope versus seizure) than to label a patient prematurely with "epilepsy." The latter misdiagnosis is difficult to reverse at a later date.

Table 14.2 Abbreviated classification of epilepsy. Forms of epilepsy relevant to the differential diagnosis of syncope are noted by an asterisk (*)

1 *Partial seizures (seizures beginning locally)*
- Simple partial seizures (consciousness not impaired)
- Attacks may be motor, sensory, psychic, or autonomic in nature
- Complex partial seizures (with impairment of consciousness)
- Partial seizures with secondary generalization

2 *Generalized seizures (bilaterally symmetric and without local onset)*
- Absence seizures
- Myoclonic seizures
- Clonic seizures*
- Tonic seizures*
- Tonic–clonic seizures*
- Atonic seizures*

3 *Unclassified epileptic seizures* (term is used when there are inadequate or incomplete data to use the other two groups)

Table 14.3 Historical Features seizures versus syncope

Fall	
Keeling over, stiff	Tonic phase epilepsy, rarely syncope
Flaccid collapse	Syncope (all forms)
Movements[a]	
Beginning before the fall	Epilepsy
Beginning after the fall	Epilepsy, syncope
Symmetric, synchronous	Epilepsy
Asymmetric, asynchronous	Syncope, may be epilepsy
Beginning at the onset of unconsciousness	Epilepsy
Beginning after the onset of unconsciousness	Syncope
Lasting less than about 15 s	Syncope more likely than epilepsy
Lasting for 30 s to min	Epilepsy
Restricted to one limb or one side	Epilepsy
Other aspects	
Automatisms (chewing, smacking, blinking)	Epilepsy
Cyanotic face	Epilepsy
Eyes open	Epilepsy as likely as syncope
Tongue bitten	Epilepsy
Head consistently turned to one side	Epilepsy
Incontinence	Epilepsy as likely as syncope

[a]The word "clonic" is in everyday use restricted to epilepsy, while the word "myoclonus" is used for the movements in syncope as well as for certain types of epilepsy and to describe postanoxic movements.

Certain important distinguishing features may be helpful in terms of differentiating epilepsy from syncope (Table 14.3). Specifically,

(i) in epilepsy, the clinical picture is dominated by abnormal movements and complex behavior patterns, whereas syncope is principally characterized by loss of consciousness and postural tone often leading to a fall and occasionally some brief "jerky" movements; temporal lobe seizures are the form of epilepsy that may be most easily mistaken for syncope since they may either mimic or cause neurally mediated reflex bradycardia and hypotension;

(ii) epileptic seizures do not depend on posture, whereas syncope occurs primarily when the affected individual is in an upright position (arrhythmic causes of syncope are a possible exception as they may occur in supine patients);

(iii) epilepsy is often preceded by an aura or strange sensations, while "true syncope" if preceded by any warning at all, the warning symptoms are most often nausea (or less specific abdominal complaint), sweating, and palpitations;

(iv) after an epileptic seizure, the patient will typically be confused or may have a focal weakness (also known as Todd's paralysis), whereas after a syncope episode, the patient tends to recover mental and physical faculties promptly, although in the case of vasovagal faints, they may feel fatigued;

(v) some epileptic disorders affect the "content" aspect of consciousness. The best examples are "absence" seizures in children and complex partial seizures in adults. During such attacks the affected individual may blink and stare, or exhibit "automatisms" such as chewing or lip movements.

The characteristics of the skeletal muscle motor activity during generalized epilepsy may help an experienced observer distinguish seizure from syncope. However for the non-expert, the often subtle differences may be nearly impossible to appreciate with a high level of confidence.[3] In any case, the so-called tonic–clonic movements of a typical generalized epileptic spell refer to a succession of stiffness and movements synchronized over the body. As summarized by van Dijk,[1] "during the tonic phase the patient may utter a cry and may keel over like a falling log. Thereafter massive synchronous jerking movements occur. These gradually decrease in frequency and severity. This scenario lasts for a period of varying length, but usually only about a minute". "Atonic" seizures may also occur but are very rare and almost exclusively occur in children with other health issues such as learning disability. In these cases, there is no muscle jerking but control over postural muscles is lost, and the affected individual falls to the floor. The event is often brief (just enough to cause a fall), and it may be unclear whether consciousness was lost; these attacks can resemble syncope.

Stiffness and jerking movements (so-called myoclonic jerky movements) may occur in syncope and they are readily misinterpreted by eye witnesses who often report that the patient had a "fit" or "seizure." These types of movements have been observed in up to 12% of fainting blood donors.[4,5] However, in contrast to the tonic–clonic movements of an epileptic seizure, the jerky movements accompanying syncope tend to be less exaggerated and are not as synchronous in various parts of the body. The difference from the much more massive and synchronous clonic movements of a true seizure can be used to diagnostic advantage if reported accurately by a keen observer.

Additional features may help to determine whether the observed jerky movements are due to syncope or epilepsy. In syncope, onset of the movements tends to follow the fall, whereas the reverse often occurs in epilepsy. In fact, if the jerks start before consciousness is lost, and/or the jerks are unilateral at any moment during the attack, epilepsy is more likely than syncope.

Most epileptic attacks are unassociated with evident triggers ("reflex" epilepsy is an exception), whereas most forms of syncope can be attributed to certain triggering events (e.g., situational neural reflex faints; vasovagal faints in warm-crowded environments or after prolonged upright posture, or triggered by pain or fear; orthostatic faints associated with change of posture). Syncope due to cardiac arrhythmia is the principal confounder as it may occur under almost any circumstance (but most often with the patient upright).

"Reflex epilepsy" is often triggered by specific stimuli. The most common type is visually induced epilepsy; repeated visual stimuli may provoke an attack. Most triggers that are known to elicit reflex epilepsy do not trigger any type of syncope; therefore they should not cause diagnostic confusion. An important but very rare exception is auditory stimuli that not only may cause epilepsy but also can cause syncope in certain forms of long QT syndrome.

14.3.2 Concussion

Trauma leading to concussion and loss of consciousness may be mistaken for syncope in some circumstances, especially if the traumatic event is unwitnessed. Further, the mere occurrence of trauma does not absolutely exclude the possibility of syncope as the primary trigger; head injury may for instance, be secondary to the patient having fallen after a true syncope. Generally, however, the distinction is readily made and a diagnosis of concussion causing T-LOC is established.

14.3.3 Metabolic and Endocrine Conditions Mimicking Syncope

Diabetic coma, hypoglycemia, and *hypercapnia* are the metabolic and endocrine disturbances that are the most important conditions in this class. Very severe *hyponatremia* may also cause T-LOC, although this is quite rare. In any case, while these conditions may resemble syncope initially, they seldom reverse on their own without therapeutic interventions. Further, none of these conditions is associated with cerebral hypoperfusion. In the case of hypoglycemia, loss of consciousness is due to inadequate cerebral nutrition, whereas T-LOC due to hyperventilation and hyponatremia is the result of electrolyte or acid/base derangements. A careful medical history and straightforward laboratory evaluation should permit distinguishing these conditions from syncope.

Intoxications may also reasonably be considered in this category (e.g., alcohol). Generally, however, intoxications are readily diagnosed and not often misinterpreted as syncope.

14.4 Syncope/T-LOC Mimic

14.4.1 Somatization Disorders ("Pseudosyncope," "Pseudoseizures")

Although the term "psychogenic syncope" has been used in the past, "psychogenic pseudosyncope" or simply "pseudosyncope" are the preferred terms, since true "syncope" does not occur in this condition. "Pseudosyncope" is a relatively common clinical problem faced by cardiologists and internists, but one that can be a challenge to confirm. Ultimately, it is determined to be associated with one or more psychiatric disorders (particularly, conversion disorders, factitious disorders, and malingering) (Table 14.4). While these "psychogenic" pseudosyncope attacks mimic syncope, there is another type that mimics epilepsy and has been termed (primarily by neurologists and psychiatrists) "pseudoseizures" (Table 14.5).

Pseudoseizures are reported to be closely associated with the same group of psychiatric conditions as pseudosyncope and perhaps can be considered to be linked through "hypochondriasis." In fact, a study of psychiatric disorders in pseudoseizure patients found psychopathology in 89% of affected adults. A history of physical

Table 14.4 Psychiatric conditions associated with pseudosyncope/pseudoseizures

- Conversion disorder: unexplained somatic symptoms occur at a time when psychologic factors are also apparent
- Factitious disorder: patients intentionally pretend to be ill in order to assume the sick role
- Malingering: patients pretend illness to gain some advantage, such as avoiding some task or duty

Table 14.5 Diagnostic examination clues in pseudosyncope/pseudoseizure (derived from van Dijk[1])

- The state of pseudo-unconsciousness lasts too long to be confused with syncope (i.e., the differential diagnosis is coma rather than syncope)
- There are no gross abnormalities during a neurologic examination, except for a lack of responsiveness
- Patients may lie relaxed with their eyes shut (usually an unconscious person has eyes open)
- Muscle tone differs from that of unconscious subjects resulting in a non-flaccid posture of the limbs
- Tendency to sudden and active closure of the eyes when opened passively by the examiner
- If a lifted limb is let go, it may hesitate shortly in midair before it starts to fall
- If the patient's hand is held above the face and let go, it will not drop onto the face
- There may be reflexive gaze movements or the eyes may be turned upward, downward, or consistently away from the observer
- These patients often exhibit impressive ability to suppress any response to pain (i.e., painful stimuli have little diagnostic value)
- Ice-water irrigation of the ears produces an eye deviation in comatose subjects but an active nystagmus in awake ones

and/or sexual abuse was present in 84%. Consequently, more likely than not, there is no real difference between the pseudosyncope and pseudoseizures apart from whether the patient presents with what appears to be a faint (and is therefore referred to a cardiologist or an internist and diagnosed as "pseudosyncope") or alternatively presents with muscle activity that is more suggestive of a seizure (and is therefore seen by neurology or psychiatry and categorized as "pseudoseizure"). In both cases the individual is manifesting a conversion reaction. On the other hand, just as pseudosyncope patients may have true syncope on occasion, patients with pseudoseizures may at times have true epileptic seizures; Kanner et al.,[6] in summarizing the literature, reports that in 5–40% of patients, both epilepsy and pseudoseizures coexist.

Among epileptologists, "pseudoseizures" are sometimes labeled as "nonepileptic attack disorder" (NEAD) since they mimic epilepsy. van Dijk[1] argues that this is not a desirable terminology "as it states what it is not (epilepsy) instead of what it is (psychogenic). Taken literally, syncope falls under the NEAD heading, which is about as useful as labeling epilepsy as a non-syncopal attack disorder."

The key historical finding favoring a diagnosis of "pseudosyncope" is a very high frequency of "attacks"; the patient may report that many episodes occur each day or each week. The event rate is much greater, and symptoms are reported to be recurrent over a longer duration of time, than is usually observed even in patients with extreme susceptibility to "true" syncope.

As the name implies, true T-LOC does not occur in pseudosyncope/pseudoseizure cases, but the history from the patient and witnesses suggests that it had. Consequently, it may be useful to try and reproduce symptoms by head-up tilt testing. When witnessed in the clinical autonomic or tilt-table laboratory, pseudosyncope is unassociated with any changes in heart rate or blood pressure. The patient may, however, seem agitated and unusual muscle movements (not tonic–clonic activity) may be observed. The latter may lead one to use the descriptor "pseudoseizure." In any event, the apparent T-LOC event occurs despite an essentially normal blood pressure, and absence of any evidence of hyperventilation. Further, our laboratory often combines tilt testing with simultaneous video EEG recording to exclude a seizure disturbance. Often, however, the diagnosis is one of exclusion after other causes of presumed T-LOC have, usually at great expense, been excluded.

Diagnostic findings that may help to identify pseudosyncope/pseudoseizures are listed in Table 14.5. However, as has been appropriately cautioned by van Dijk,[1] the findings should not be used to embarrass patients; they are more productively used as a means of establishing communication and allowing the problem to be addressed. Often, simply establishing the true diagnosis has been proven therapeutic.

Pseudosyncope rarely results in serious injury. However, these patients may in fact have occasional "true" faints as well. Indeed, it may have been initial true syncope episodes that instigated the apparent subsequent susceptibility to "pseudosyncope." Further, in psychiatric conditions that may be associated with pseudosyncope, it should be kept in mind that many prescribed medications (e.g., phenothiazines, tricyclics and newer antidepressants, and monoamine oxidase inhibitors) may increase the risk of "true" syncope by increasing susceptibility to orthostatic hypotension or by prolonging QT interval on the ECG and predisposing to torsade de pointes.

"Pseudoseizures," like pseudosyncope, tend to have a high event rate, higher than one would expect of true epilepsy. Injury is also rare. Further, compared to epilepsy patients, pseudoseizure patients exhibit higher rates of depression and personality disorders. Psychiatric disturbance is reported in >50% of pseudoseizure patients. There is also reported correlation with post-traumatic stress disorder and high rates of sexual and physical abuse[7] (Table 14.6). Pre-adult sexual abuse and physical abuse were reported in one study to have occurred in 58% and 67% of pseudoseizure patients, respectively. The percentages were even more dramatic in women (69% and 56%, respectively)[7] (Table 14.6). The authors point out that the traumatic life events were often "remote in time (i.e., child abuse or rape)" and that the onset may be related in some to inadvertent re-visiting of the trauma (e.g., seeing the perpetrator many years later or a new traumatic event [e.g., motor vehicle accident] that in some fashion resembles trauma of an earlier time in life).[7] Video EEG monitoring, while the subject of some difference of opinion, appears to be the most effective diagnostic tool for confirming the diagnosis. In our laboratory this

Table 14.6 Abuse and trauma in pseudoseizure patients (from Bowman and Markand[7])

Event	All subjects (%)	Women (%)	Men (%)
Sexual abuse			
Any	67	80	20
Pre-adult	58	69	20
Physical abuse			
Any	67	77	30
Pre-adult	51	63	10
Spouse physical abuse	42	51	10
Any adult abuse/trauma	60	69	30

procedure is often carried out in conjunction with the neurology service during a tilt-table provocative test.

14.4.2 Cataplexy

Cataplexy occurs principally in the context of the disease narcolepsy and refers to loss of muscle tone in conjunction with certain emotions, particularly laughter. Consequently, when faced with laughter-related attacks, physicians should inquire of symptoms suggesting coexisting narcolepsy (e.g., excessive daytime sleepiness).

In terms of the clinical presentation, as described by van Dijk,[1] patients suddenly slump to the ground with complete or partial paralysis. Partial paralysis may present as dropping of the jaw and sagging or nodding of the head. Attacks may develop slowly enough to allow the patient to break the fall before he or she hits the floor. Complete attacks look like syncope in that the patient is unable to respond at all, although he or she is completely conscious and aware of what is going on.

Although emotions such as laughter often accompany onset of cataplexy, other emotions such as fear and anxiety, which are often triggers for reflex faints, are not often triggers for cataplexy. Further, consciousness is not really lost. However, the presence of consciousness can be confirmed only later by virtue of the fact that the affected individual has "recall" of the event. On the other hand, the physician must be alert to the possibility that the "recall" may in fact have been the result of the patient having been told of what happened by bystanders.

14.4.3 Hyperventilation

"Hyperventilation" (i.e., breathing in excess of metabolic needs) results in hypocapnia. Hypocapnia is known to constrict cerebral vessels and reduce cerebral blood flow. As such, hyperventilation might in very rare circumstances diminish cerebral perfusion sufficiently to cause syncope or at least to increase susceptibility to syncope of other origin. However, if syncope does occur, it is an infrequent consequence of hyperventilation.[8] Peri-oral numbness, light-headedness, and peripheral paresthesias (tingling fingers or toes) are much more common manifestations. The term "hyperventilation syndrome" is used when hyperventilation and its associated symptoms are seemingly triggered by stress.

14.4.4 Transient Ischemic Attacks

As a rule, carotid artery transient ischemic attacks (TIAs) do not cause T-LOC. Most such TIAs affect the downstream territory of one arterial vessel and consequently may cause specific transient neurologic disturbances, but not unconsciousness. Loss of consciousness would require substantial loss of brain stem function or of a very large portion of the cerebral cortex; while possible, this is not believed to be very common.

14.4.4.1 Vertebrobasilar TIAs

Vertebrobasilar TIAs may be expected to cause T-LOC more often than do carotid TIAs, but loss of consciousness would not be the sole symptom. Other concomitant posterior circulation symptoms (e.g., vertigo) should be sought and if present would tend to support a vertebrobasilar TIA.

14.4.4.2 Drop Attacks

The term "drop attack" is often used colloquially to describe various "faints" or "falls." However, the term is best reserved for a syndrome in which the patient experiences an abrupt fall with no apparent warning. The episode is a very short-lasting event in which a patient suddenly falls without any warning and without apparent loss of consciousness.[2,9] Commonly, the affected individual remembers the fall, so if there were any loss of consciousness, it would have to be extremely brief. Drop attacks tend to occur in middle-aged individuals, more often in women than men. Patients may bruise their knees or legs but otherwise rebound quickly without other injury. There are no other characteristic features. There is no known effective therapy. The basis for "drop attacks" is unknown, although in some cases there may be inner ear abnormalities with very transient disturbances of balance.[10,11] In this same context, "drop attacks" have been used to describe falling in patients with Ménière's disease. However, the descriptor "drop attacks" has also been attached to the collapse in "astatic" or "atonic" epileptic seizures, but these attacks last longer and are associated with EEG abnormalities; consequently, these latter collapses differ from the preferred usage of the term provided earlier. In brief, prior to diagnosiing a classical "drop attack", it is essential that every effort be made to be assured that T-LOC did not occur.

14.5 Clinical Perspectives

As discussed in other chapters, many conditions may be responsible for initiating a syncope event; in most cases the final common pathway is temporary systemic hypotension. On the other hand, there are many other non-syncope conditions that cause T-LOC without inducing cerebral hypoperfusion (e.g., epilepsy and concussion). These conditions have a different pathophysiology and require a different treatment strategy than does true syncope. Furthermore, there are yet other conditions that mimic syncope (e.g., pseudosyncope and pseudoseizures) but in which true loss of consciousness does not occur. These latter conditions often occur in the setting of a variety of psychiatric conditions, and their recognition is the crucial first step in directing affected individuals toward proper care.

References

1. van Dijk JG. Conditions that mimic syncope. In: Benditt DG, et al. eds. *The Evaluation and Treatment of Syncope: A Handbook of Clinical Practice*. 2nd edn. Oxford, UK: Blackwell Publishing; 2006:pp 242–258.
2. Moya A, et al. Guidelines for the diagnosis and management of syncope (version 2009). *Eur Heart J*. 2009;30:2631–2671.
3. Lin JT, et al. Convulsive syncope in blood donors. *Ann Neurol*. 1982;11:525–528.
4. Galena HJ. Complications occurring from diagnostic venipuncture. *J Fam Pract*. 1992;34:582–584.
5. Lempert T, et al. Syncope: a videometric analysis of 56 episodes of transient cerebral hypoxia. *Ann Neurol*. 1994;36:233–237.
6. Kanner AM, et al. Psychiatric and neurologic predictors of psychogenic pseudoseizure outcome. *Neurology*. 1999;53:933–938.
7. Bowman ES, Markand ON. Psychodynamics and psychiatric diagnoses of pseudoseizure subjects. *Am J Psychiatry*. 1996;153:57–63.
8. Hornsveld HK, et al. Double-blind placebo-controlled study of the hyperventilation provocation test and the validity of the hyperventilation syndrome. *Lancet*. 1996;348:154–158.
9. Meissner I, et al. The natural history of drop attacks. *Neurology*. 1986;36:1029–1034.
10. Ishiyama G, et al. Drop attacks and vertigo secondary to a non-Meniere otologic cause. *Arch Neurol*. 2003;60:71–75.
11. Ozeki H, et al. Vestibular drop attack secondary to Meniere's disease results from unstable otolithic function. *Acta Otolaryngol*. 2008;128:887–891.

Chapter 15
Unexplained Syncope in Patients with High Risk of Sudden Cardiac Death

Contents

Key points: Reduction of sudden death

- Patients with unexplained syncope and ischemic or non-ischemic cardiomyopathy are at a greater risk of death than are those without syncope. Syncope is more an expression of severity of the underlying disease rather than a surrogate of an undocumented ventricular tachyarrhythmia. Consequently, the benefit of ICD therapy may be lower than expected.
- Unexplained syncope is a major risk factor for sudden death in hypertrophic cardiomyopathy particularly if the syncope is of recent onset (<6 months) and occurs in young patients. However, the fact that most patients who experience a syncopal episode do not die suddenly emphasizes the need for an individual risk assessment that takes into account the presence of the several other risk factors that have been shown to be associated with sudden death.

M. Brignole, D.G. Benditt, *Syncope*, DOI 10.1007/978-0-85729-201-8_15,
© Springer-Verlag London Limited 2011

- Unexplained syncope is frequent in patients with arrhythmogenic right ventricular cardiomyopathy. The combination of syncope and ventricular tachycardia, but not syncope alone, identifies patients at higher risk of sudden death.
- Common presentations of the long QT syndrome are palpitations, presyncope, syncope, and cardiac arrest. The most powerful predictor of risk is the QT duration. Patients with recurrent unexplained syncope despite adherence to an adequate beta-blocking regimen are at high risk and an ICD implantation is warranted.
- In patients with Brugada syndrome, the strongest predictor of ventricular tachyarrhythmias is a history of previous cardiac arrest; syncope is much less powerful than cardiac arrest, but patients with syncope are at higher risk than are asymptomatic individuals. The usefulness of ICD in patients with syncope is controversial and is undoubtedly more questionable than in cardiac arrest survivors. A better stratification of the risk of arrhythmic events in Brugada syndrome is needed.
- In patients with catecholaminergic polymorphic ventricular tachycardia, unexplained syncope does not seem to carry an additive risk of sudden death.

15.1 Introduction

In patients at high risk of sudden cardiac death (SCD), a disease-specific treatment is essential in order to reduce risk of death and of life-threatening events, even if the exact mechanism of syncope is still unknown or uncertain at the end of a complete workup. In these patients the goal of treatment is primarily the reduction of mortality risk.

It is important to bear in mind, however, that even if an effective specific treatment of the underlying disease is found, patients may remain at risk of syncope recurrence. For example, ICD-treated patients may remain at risk for fainting because only the SCD risk is being addressed and not the cause of syncope. An analysis of the SCD-HeFT[1] has shown that ICD did not protect patients against syncope recurrence compared with those treated with amiodarone or placebo. This implies the need for precise identification of the mechanism of syncope and specific treatment as far as possible.

15.2 Ischemic and Non-ischemic Cardiomyopathies

There are two different clinical settings:

- syncope in patients with pre-existing established indications for an ICD, and
- syncope in patients without pre-existing established indication for an ICD.

15.2.1 *Pre-existing Established Indications for ICD Therapy*

The management of these patients is the same in patients with and without syncope. The risk of death in patients with acute or chronic coronary artery disease and depressed ejection fraction (EF) is increased. This necessitates evaluation of ischemia and, if indicated, revascularization. However, arrhythmia evaluation, including electrophysiological study with premature ventricular stimulation, may still be needed, especially in the syncope subset, because, when present, the substrate for malignant ventricular arrhythmia may not be completely eliminated by revascularization alone. Consequently, patients with heart failure and an established ICD indication by current guidelines should receive an ICD before and independently of the evaluation of the mechanism of syncope. This group includes, for example, patients with ischemic or dilated cardiomyopathy and depressed EF (ranging from <30 to <40% and NYHA class $\geq$ II according to current guidelines).[2–5] A prospective sub-study from the Antiarrhythmics Versus Implantable Defibrillators (AVID) trial[6] showed that patients affected by syncopal ventricular tachycardia derived important survival benefit from ICDs. A survival benefit from the device is also suggested by small retrospective studies of patients with syncope and inducible ventricular tachyarrhythmias at electrophysiological study (EPS).[7]

The situation of patients with unexplained syncope and undocumented arrhythmias is different. Patients with syncope and heart failure carry a high risk of death regardless of the cause of syncope.[8] In a retrospective analysis,[9] 60 of 491 patients with NYHA class III–IV heart failure and mean left ventricular EF of 20% had syncope. The 1-year rate of sudden death was 45% in patients with syncope regardless of cause versus 12% in patients without syncope ($p < 0.00001$). A recent analysis of the Sudden Cardiac Death in Heart Failure Trial (SCD-HeFT)[1] has shed new light regarding the use of ICDs in such patients. When comparing patients receiving amiodarone or placebo to those receiving ICD, while syncope was associated with a greater risk for all-cause and cardiovascular death, the ICD group had the same, if not greater, risk for death compared to the amiodarone or placebo group. Syncope predicted appropriate ICD shocks (hazard ratio 2.91, $p = 0.001$). Despite the fact that the ICD population with syncope received more ICD shocks than did the patient group that did not have syncope, they did not benefit in the sense that they still had a risk of death as great as or even greater than the amiodarone and placebo arm of the study. Recurrent syncope occurred at the same rate, independent of the treatment arm. This highlights the fact that heart failure patients are sick and may develop hemodynamic problems that could explain syncope (they are also often taking many drugs that predispose to greater syncope risk [e.g., vasodilators, diuretics]). In brief, heart failure patients with syncope may be at a greater risk of death compared to those without syncope.

15.2.2 *No Pre-existing Established Indications for ICD*

In patients with preserved systolic function not meeting the criteria for ICD implantation, syncope requires careful assessment of the risk of life-threatening arrhythmia and SCD. In other words, the occurrence of unexplained syncope is considered per se a risk factor. Even if the evaluation was negative, the possibility that syncope might have been caused by an undocumented ventricular arrhythmia cannot be absolutely ruled out. Nevertheless, the prognostic value of syncope as well as the efficacy of an empirical ICD implantation is largely unknown. This is not surprising in light of the study of Alboni et al.[10] in which many patients with suspected or diagnosed heart disease thought to be the cause of syncope were ultimately found not to have a cardiac cause for syncope. About half of them had neurally mediated reflex syncope despite the fact that they had an underlying cardiac diagnosis. In a small study,[11] an implantable loop recorder (ILR) was applied in 35 patients with overt heart disease deemed to be at risk of ventricular arrhythmia; these were patients with previous myocardial infarction or cardiomyopathy with moderately depressed EF or non-sustained ventricular tachycardia in whom an electrophysiological study was unremarkable. During follow-up of 3–15 months, no patient died, and the mechanism of recurrent syncope was heterogeneous; both arrhythmias and no arrhythmias were documented in association with syncope. Ventricular tachyarrhythmia was observed in only one case. The findings were not very much different from those observed in the patients without structural heart disease. A strategy of prolonged ILR monitoring has been shown to be safe in patients with mild-to-moderate structural heart disease (see Chapter 8). Thus, if the patient does not meet the criteria for an ICD and does not appear to be particularly at high risk of sudden death, long-term monitoring with an external or an implantable device would be an appropriate next diagnostic step.

In conclusion, at the two ends of the spectrum, we find on one side the group of syncope patients with preserved systolic function and negative EPS that do not warrant aggressive treatment with an ICD and on the other, those with congestive heart failure and severely depressed EF who warrant an ICD despite the fact that it will not provide protection against syncope. In this latter group, it was found that mortality was higher in patients with syncope compared with those without.[1]

15.3 Hypertrophic Cardiomyopathy

Many studies have examined the relation between syncope and outcomes in hypertrophic cardiomyopathy (HCM). Although the findings vary, the relative increased risk of sudden cardiac death (SCD) for syncope alone is on average twofold. Unexplained syncope is a major risk factor for SCD in hypertrophic cardiomyopathy particularly if it has occurred in close temporal proximity (<6 months) to the evaluation (relative risk >5).[12] Conversely, older (>40 years) patients with remote episodes of syncope (>5 years before evaluation) and patients with typical history of vasovagal syncope have low risk of SCD[12] (Table 15.1). However, the fact that most patients who experience a syncopal episode do not die suddenly emphasizes the need for individualized risk assessment.[13] Indeed, in addition to self-terminating ventricular tachyarrhythmia, many other mechanisms can cause

Table 15.1 Major risk factors for sudden death in hypertrophic cardiomyopathy

Prior cardiac arrest
Young age (<40 years)
Recent onset unexplained syncope
Family history of premature sudden cardiac death
Left ventricular wall thickness >30 mm
Abnormal blood pressure response to exercise
Non-sustained spontaneous ventricular tachycardia

Table 15.2 Causes of syncope in hypertrophic cardiomyopathy

- Arrhythmia:
  - Paroxysmal atrial fibrillation/supraventricular tachycardia
  - Complete heart block/sinus node dysfunction
  - Sustained ventricular tachycardia
- Primary hemodynamic mechanism:
  - Left ventricular outflow tract obstruction
  - Abnormal vascular control mechanisms (due to abnormal left ventricular mechanoreceptor behavior) leading to episodes of hypotension
  - Hypotension due to impaired filling when preload is reduced in the setting of diastolic dysfunction
- Non-cardiac:
  - Reflex syncope unrelated to the underlying disease
  - Others

syncope in hypertrophic cardiomyopathy, including supraventricular tachycardia, severe outflow tract obstruction, bradyarrhythmia, decreased blood pressure in response to exercise, and reflex syncope (Table 15.2). If a treatable mechanism for the syncopal episode is identified, it should, if possible, be remedied. For example, if an atrial arrhythmia or bradycardia is the cause, drug therapy, ablation, or a pacemaker may be appropriate. Similarly, patients with syncope caused by moderate-to-severe left ventricular outflow tract obstruction should receive pharmacological therapy followed, if symptoms persist, by invasive strategies to reduce the outflow gradient. In the minority of patients in whom abnormal vascular responses are the major mechanism, options are more limited. ICD therapy should be reserved for those HCM patients in whom a treatable (or avoidable) cause of syncope cannot be elucidated after extensive clinical evaluation. The decision to implant an ICD should take into account the age of the patient and the presence of other clinical risk factors. A consensus document on hypertrophic cardiomyopathy from the American College of Cardiology and European Society of Cardiology[14] categorized the following as "major" known risk factors for SCD in HCM (see also further details below and Table 15.1):

- prior cardiac arrest, spontaneous sustained VT, spontaneous non-sustained VT,
- family history of SCD, syncope,
- LV thickness ≥30 mm, and
- an abnormal hypotensive blood pressure response to exercise.

It is also important to consider the risks of intervention, ensuring that patients have sufficient time and access to appropriate resources in order to make informed decisions. The following algorithm for risk stratification is recommended for individual patients[15,16]:

(i) Patients with a prior cardiac arrest or spontaneous sustained VT are at high risk and should be advised to have prophylactic therapy with an ICD.

(ii) In the absence of an arrhythmia history summarized in (i), risk is probably best assessed on the basis of the total number of the following risk factors:

   (a) a history of at least one sudden death in a relative before the age of 45 years;
   (b) maximum wall thickness >30 mm;
   (c) abnormal systolic blood pressure response during maximal upright exercise in patients <40 years of age (defined as failure to increase by >25 mmHg or a fall from peak values during continued exercise of >15 mmHg);
   (d) non-sustained VT during 48-h ambulatory ECG monitoring;
   (e) a resting peak instantaneous LV outflow tract gradient of >30 mmHg.

Patients with no risk factors can be reassured. Those with two or more risk factors are at high risk and should be considered for prophylactic therapy with an ICD. Those with a single risk factor are at intermediate risk and no clear recommendation can be provided other than follow-up to periodically (e.g., annual review) reassess for possible appearance of other risk factors that would cause the patient to be moved to a "higher risk" group.

15.4 Arrhythmogenic Right Ventricular Cardiomyopathy/Dysplasia

Arrhythmogenic right ventricular cardiomyopathy (ARVC) patients present between the second and fifth decades of life either with symptoms of palpitations and syncope associated with ventricular tachycardia or with SCD. Electrocardiogram, echocardiography, right ventricular angiography, signal-averaged ECG, and Holter monitoring provide the essential tools for clinical evaluation of patients suspected of ARVC.[17] A combination of diagnostic tests is needed to evaluate the presence of right ventricular structural, functional, and electrical abnormalities (see Chapter 13). Syncope occurs in about one-third of ARVC patients referred to tertiary centers. In one report[18] comprising 130 patients (mean age at the onset of symptoms of 32 ± 14 years), followed-up for a mean of 8 years, the annual mortality rate was of 2.3%. The causes of death were progressive heart failure and SCD. All patients who died had a history of ventricular tachycardia. Multivariate analysis showed that history of syncope, chest pain, new ventricular tachycardia, recurrence of ventricular tachycardia, QRS dispersion, clinical signs of right ventricular failure, and left ventricular dysfunction were independently associated with cardiovascular mortality. The combined presence of one of these risk factors and ventricular tachycardia identifies high-risk subjects for cardiovascular mortality, whereas patients without ventricular tachycardia displayed the best prognosis.

When ICD is being considered for primary prevention, it should be kept in mind that predictive markers of SCD in patients with ARVC have not yet been defined in large prospective studies focusing on survival. As a consequence there is not yet clear consensus on the specific risk factors that identify those patients with ARVD/C in whom the probability of SCD is sufficiently high to warrant an ICD for primary prevention.[19] In a multicenter study[20] conducted on 132 patients in order to evaluate the impact of ICD for prevention of SCD, the patients with unexplained syncope had a rate of appropriate ICD intervention of around 15% per year, a figure which was similar to that of patients with cardiac arrest or ventricular tachycardia with hemodynamic compromise.

15.5   Primary Electrical Diseases

Unexplained syncope is regarded as an ominous finding in patients with inherited cardiac ion channel abnormalities, the so-called channelopathies. An ICD should be carefully considered in the absence of another competing syncope diagnosis or when ventricular tachyarrhythmia cannot be excluded as a cause of syncope. Nevertheless, the mechanism of syncope may be heterogeneous, being caused by life-threatening arrhythmias in some but being of a more benign origin, i.e., reflex, in many others. Therefore, in these settings, it seems that syncope does not necessarily carry a high risk of major life-threatening cardiac events and has a much lower sensitivity in that regard than does a history of documented prior cardiac arrest. However, differentiating between benign and malignant forms is usually very difficult in the setting of an inherited disease based on conventional investigations. Consequently, while there is a rationale for more precise diagnosis (i.e., ILR documentation) of the mechanism of syncope before embarking on ICD therapy, existing data are insufficient to make confident recommendations.[21]

15.5.1 Long QT Syndrome

Common presentations of the long QT syndrome (Fig. 15.1) are palpitations, presyncope, syncope, and cardiac arrest. In addition, asymptomatic persons may be identified because the diagnosis is established or suspected in a family member. Syncope in patients with the long QT syndrome is generally attributed to the form of polymorphic ventricular tachycardia called torsade de pointes. Death is usually due to ventricular fibrillation. This is a disease in which clinical concerns are primarily in the young, and syncope and sudden death appear to be unusual in patients older than 40 years of age. Genetic testing is progressing rapidly in the long QT syndromes, and only a brief incomplete update can be provided here.

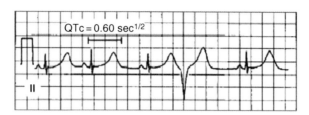

Fig. 15.1 ECG tracing from a patient with LQT1, the most frequent form of the long QT syndrome. LQT1 is associated with a broad T wave without a shortening of the QT interval due to exercise (not shown in the figure)

Mutations in three genes, each encoding a cardiac ion channel that is important for ventricular repolarization, account for the vast majority of cases; these three genetic subtypes are termed LQT1, LQT2, and LQT3. In LQT1, syncope or sudden death is triggered by emotional or physical stress; diving and swimming are LQT1-specific triggers. QT interval prolongation may be especially notable during or after exercise or epinephrine challenge. In LQT2, syncope or sudden death can occur with stress or at rest and the triggering of events by sudden loud noises, such as that produced by an alarm clock, is virtually diagnostic of this form.[22,23]

The most powerful predictor of risk is the QTc duration; patients at particularly high risk are those with a QTc interval >500 ms in carriers with LQT1 and LQT2 forms. The mainstay of therapy for the long QT syndrome has been beta-adrenergic blockade. Long-acting preparations such as nadolol and atenolol are usually used, and the efficacy of beta-blockade is assessed by blunting of the exercise heart rate (e.g., by >20%); beta-blockers do not substantially shorten the QT interval. Extensive observational data have shown superior survival among symptomatic LQT1 and LQT2 patients who received beta-blockers as compared with those who did not. The role of beta-blockers in LQT3 is less clear. The major cardiology and electrophysiology societies in the USA and Europe have jointly issued guidelines for the care of patients who are at risk for sudden death from cardiac causes[3,5,21] (Table 15.3).

The use of ICDs is widely considered, especially those with LQT2 and LQT3 and female gender, in patients at high risk for sudden death based on family history or documented arrhythmia, including those with symptoms before the age of 18, those with very long QTc intervals (e.g., >500 ms), and those with recurrent syncope thought to be due to arrhythmias despite adherence to an adequate beta-blocking regimen.

15.5.2 Brugada Syndrome

Spontaneous Brugada type I pattern ECGs (Fig. 15.2) and a history of syncope have been reported as adverse prognostic indicators. The strongest predictor of ventricular tachyarrhythmias is a history of previous cardiac arrest; again, syncope is a much less powerful predictor of prognosis than is prior cardiac arrest, but patients with syncope are at higher risk than are asymptomatic individuals (Fig. 15.3).

Table 15.3 American and European joint guidelines for management of long QT syndrome

Recommendation	Level of evidence	Comment
No participation in competitive sports	I	Includes patients with the diagnosis established by means of genetic testing only
Beta-blockers	I	For patients who have QTc-interval prolongation (>460 ms in women and >440 ms in men)
	IIa	For patients with a normal QTc interval
ICD	I	For survivors of cardiac arrest
	IIa	For patients with *syncope* while receiving beta-blockers
	IIb	For primary prevention in patients with characteristics that suggest high risk; these include LQT2, LQT3, and QTc interval >500 ms

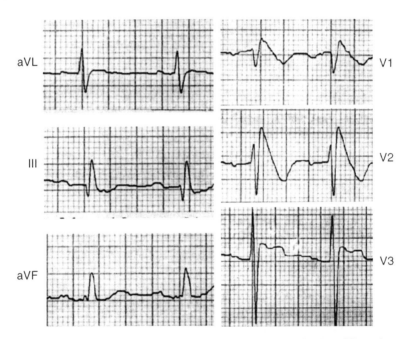

Fig. 15.2 Brugada syndrome is characterized by coved-type ST elevation (type I Brugada pattern ECG described in the consensus report on Brugada syndrome[24] in the right precordial leads), which represents abnormal repolarization in the right ventricle

In general, Brugada syndrome patients with a spontaneous type 1 ECG pattern have a worse outcome than do those with a type 2 or drug-induced pattern. Inducibility of ventricular tachyarrhythmia by means of ventricular premature stimulation is unable to predict the outcome.[24,25] Recently fragmented QRSs have been

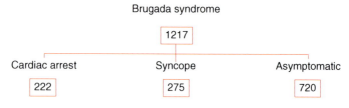

Brugada syndrome

Follow-up (34 mos): ventricular arrhythmias

	Odds ratio	P value
Cardiac arrest *versus* Asymptomatic	14.4	0.001
Cardiac arrest *versus* Syncope	3.1	0.003
Syncope *versus* Asymptomatic	4.7	0.002

Fig. 15.3 Risk stratification of patients with Brugada syndrome in a meta-analysis of published data[25]

shown to be a marker for the substrate for spontaneous VF in Brugada patients and predict patients at high risk of syncope.[26] Indeed, among patients with a history of syncope or ventricular fibrillation, only 6% of those without fragmented QRSs experienced ventricular fibrillation during follow-up, but 58% of patients with fragmented QRSs had recurrent ventricular fibrillation. The usefulness of ICD in patients with syncope is controversial and more questionable than is the case for cardiac arrest survivors. In a large multicenter study[27] comprising 220 patients with Brugada syndrome and ICD, of whom 18 (8%) had a history of cardiac arrest and 88 (40%) had a history of syncope, the rates of appropriate ICD shocks were 22 and 10%, respectively, during a mean follow-up period of 38 ± 27 months. ICD discharge in syncope patients was similar to that of asymptomatic patients; inappropriate shocks occurred in 28% and 20% respectively. In a recent study that evaluated the outcome of 59 Brugada patients treated with ICD,[28] none of the 31 patients with syncope received an appropriate ICD shock during a mean of 39% months follow-up; appropriate device therapy was limited to cardiac arrest survivors. The overall complication rate of ICD therapy was 32% (27% inappropriate shocks). In the largest series of Brugada syndrome patients thus far-which included 1029 patients- cardiac arrhythmic event rate per year was 7.7% in patients with aborted sudden death, 1.9% in patients with syncope, and 0.5% in asymptomatic patients.[29]

15.5.3 Catecholaminergic Polymorphic Ventricular Tachycardia

Catecholaminergic polymorphic ventricular tachycardia is a familial arrhythmogenic disorder characterized by polymorphic ventricular tachyarrhythmias induced by physical or emotional stress without any detectable morphological abnormalities of the heart. Syncope is a frequent manifestation of the disease. In an analysis of 101 patients followed up for 8 years,[30] fatal or near-fatal event rates occurred in 32% and 13%, respectively. In most of the patients (92%), a fatal or near-fatal event occurred at between 13 and 26 years of age. In the multivariable analyses, absence of therapy with any beta-blockers, younger age at the time of the diagnosis, and history of cardiac arrest were independent predictors for fatal or near-fatal events. No difference was observed in the cardiac or fatal or near-fatal event rate between the patients with and without a prior syncopal event. Prescription of beta-adrenergic blockers was associated with lower event rates but did not provide sufficient prevention of arrhythmias. Beta-blockers should be prescribed in every patient regardless of any prior syncopal events. ICD should be considered for patients intolerant of beta-blockers and those with documented ventricular tachyarrhythmias.

15.5.4 Short QT Syndrome

The electrocardiogram is characterized by a short QT interval (typically <320 ms), virtual absence of the ST segment, and tall, peaked, narrow-based T waves.[31] The available data in the literature on patients with syncope and short QT syndrome are too limited to permit any recommendation.

15.6 Clinical Perspectives: The Role of ICD

In patients with severe structural heart disease and in those with primary electrical disease, the goal of treatment is primarily reduction of mortality risk. A history of syncope in general increases the risk of sudden death in patients who are already at high risk. When disease-specific treatments are not possible or ineffective, ICD therapy should be considered as the most powerful protection against sudden death caused by ventricular tachycardia/fibrillation, even though syncope may still be a risk (due to the time it takes for an ICD to determine that an arrhythmia is present and to charge the capacitors in preparation for delivering a shock).

Two situations need to be clearly differentiated. In patients in whom syncope was documented to have been caused by ventricular tachyarrhythmias, ICD is very effective in reducing sudden and total mortality. On the other hand, in cases of undocumented syncope, in which a causal relationship with ventricular tachyarrhythmia is only suspected but not proven, the efficacy of ICD therapy is much less evident. The likely explanation for the latter is the multifactorial nature of syncope. Many other mechanisms other than a ventricular tachyarrhythmia are responsible for episodes of loss of consciousness:

- different arrhythmias (for example, atrial fibrillation or other atrial tachycardias or bradyarrhythmias),
- hemodynamic compromise due to the underlying disease,
- abnormal vascular control mechanisms leading to reflex hypotension, etc.

For these reasons, syncope per se is in general a moderate risk factor and only the combination of syncope with other risk factors is helpful to identify the patients at highest risk. Not surprisingly then, evidence of benefit of ICD therapy is much less convincing in those instances in which the cause of the faint is undocumented than in the case of documented ventricular arrhythmias. Furthermore, it is important to keep in mind that ICD insertion is unlike an "insurance policy" to be adopted for all patients; many patients may not benefit from device therapy while still being exposed to procedural and device-related complications. The risk of complication is particularly high in young patients with primary electrical disease who have a potential long life expectancy. The most frequent and severe complications are inappropriate shocks, lead failure, and site infections; together these complications

Table 15.4 Indications for ICD in patients with unexplained syncope and a high risk of SCD (modified from Recommendations of the 2009 ESC Task Force on Syncope)

Clinical situation	Class[a]	Level[b]	Comments
• In patients with ischemic and non-ischemic cardiomyopathy with severely depressed LVEF or HF, ICD therapy is indicated according to current guidelines for ICD-cardiac resynchronization therapy implantation	I	A	
• In hypertrophic cardiomyopathy, ICD therapy should be considered in patients at high risk (see text)	IIa	C	In non-high risk, consider ILR
• In right ventricular cardiomyopathy, ICD therapy should be considered in patients at high risk (see text)	IIa	C	In non-high risk, consider ILR
• In Brugada syndrome, ICD therapy should be considered in patients at high risk with spontaneous type I ECG	IIa	B	In non-high risk, consider ILR
• In long QT syndrome, ICD therapy, in conjunction with beta-blockers, should be considered in patients at risk	IIa	B	In non-high risk, consider ILR
• In patients with ischemic and cardiomyopathy without severely depressed LVEF or HF and negative programmed electrical stimulation, ICD therapy may be considered in high-risk patients	IIb	C	Consider ILR to help define the nature of unexplained syncope
• In patients with non-ischemic cardiomyopathy without severely depressed LVEF or HF, ICD therapy may be considered in high-risk patients	IIb	C	Consider ILR to help define the nature of unexplained syncope

HF, heart failure; ECG, electrocardiogram; ICD, implantable cardioverter defibrillator; ILR, implantable cardioverter defibrillator; LVEF, left ventricular ejection fraction; SCD, sudden cardiac death.
[a]Class of recommendation.
[b]Level of evidence.

occur in up to 30% of cases. A reappraisal of the benefits and potential hazards of ICD therapy will enable physicians to a have a more mutually informed and balanced dialogue with their patients.[32] The current indications proposed by the ESC guidelines (Table 15.4) and AHA/ACC guidelines should act as a reference guide for recommendations offered to individual patients.

The development of better risk stratification tools to identify who should (and should not) get an ICD is clearly a research priority. However, there is no doubt that optimal risk stratification requires documentation of the cause of syncope. Every effort should be undertaken to determine whether there is a causal relationship between syncope and life-threatening arrhythmias, especially in patients with primary electrical disease; these are the individuals who have the most uncertain risk/benefit ratio from ICD therapy. To this end, a strategy of aggressive utilization of powerful ambulatory ECG monitoring technology, particularly implantable loop recorders, is strongly advocated by the current ESC guidelines (Table 15.4).

References

1. Olshansky B, et al. Syncope predicts the outcome of cardiomyopathy patients: Analysis of the SCD-HeFT study. *J Am Coll Cardiol.* 2008;51:1277–1282.
2. Vardas PE, et al. Guidelines for cardiac pacing and cardiac resynchronization therapy. *Eur Heart J.* 2007;28:2256–2295.
3. Goldberger JJ, et al. Scientific statement on noninvasive risk stratification techniques for identifying patients at risk for sudden cardiac death. *Circulation.* 2008;118:1497–1518.
4. Epstein AE, et al. ACC/AHA/HRS 2008 guidelines for device-based therapy of cardiac rhythm abnormalities. *J Am Coll Cardiol.* 2008;51:e1–e62.
5. Zipes DP, et al. ACC/AHA/ESC 2006 guidelines for management of patients with ventricular arrhythmias and the prevention of sudden cardiac death. *Europace.* 2006;8:746–837.
6. Steinberg JS, et al. Follow-up of patients with unexplained syncope and inducible ventricular tachyarrhythmias: analysis of the AVID registry and AVID substudy. Antiarrhythmics Versus Implantable Defibrillators. *J Cardiovasc Electrophysiol.* 2001;12:996–1001.
7. Andrews NP, et al. Implantable defibrillator event rates in patients with unexplained syncope and inducible sustained ventricular tachyarrhythmias: a comparison with patients known to have sustained ventricular tachycardia. *J Am Coll Cardiol.* 1999;34:2023–2030.
8. Brembilla-Perrot B, et al. Differences in mechanism and outcomes of syncope patients with coronary artery disease or idiopathic left ventricular dysfunction as assessed by electrophysiologic testing. *J Am Coll Cardiol.* 2004;44:594–601.
9. Middlekauff HR, et al. Syncope in advanced heart failure: high risk of sudden death regardless of origin of syncope. *J Am Coll Cardiol.* 1993;21:110–116.
10. Alboni P, et al. Diagnostic value of history in patients with syncope with or without heart disease. *J Am Coll Cardiol.* 2001;37:1921–1928.
11. Menozzi C, et al. Mechanism of syncope in patients with heart disease and negative electrophysiologic test. *Circulation.* 2002;105:2741–2745.
12. Spirito P, et al. Syncope and risk of sudden death in hypertrophic cardiomyopathy. *Circulation.* 2009;119:1703–1710.
13. Elliott P, McKenna W. The science of uncertainty and the art of probability: syncope and its consequences in hypertrophic cardiomyopathy. *Circulation.* 2009;119:1697–1699.
14. Maron BJ, et al. American College of Cardiology/European Society of Cardiology clinical expert consensus document on hypertrophic cardiomyopathy. *J Am Coll Cardiol.* 2003;42:1687–1713.

15. Frenneaux MP. Assessing the risk of sudden cardiac death in a patient with hypertrophic cardiomyopathy. *Heart*. 2004;90:570–575.
16. Williams L, Frenneaux M. Syncope in hypertrophic cardiomyopathy: mechanisms and consequences for treatment. *Europace*. 2007;9:817–822.
17. Marcus FI, et al. Arrhythmogenic right ventricular cardiomyopathy/dysplasia clinical presentation and diagnostic evaluation: results from the North American Multidisciplinary Study. *Heart Rhythm*. 2009;6:984–992.
18. Hulot JS, et al. Natural history and risk stratification of arrhythmogenic right ventricular dysplasia/cardiomyopathy. *Circulation*. 2004;110:1879–1884.
19. Dalal D, et al. Arrhythmogenic right ventricular dysplasia: a United States experience. *Circulation*. 2005;112:3823–3832.
20. Corrado D, et al. Implantable cardioverter-defibrillator therapy for prevention of sudden death in patients with arrhythmogenic right ventricular cardiomyopathy/dysplasia. *Circulation*. 2003;108:3084–3091.
21. Moya A, et al. Guidelines for the diagnosis and management of syncope (version 2009). *Eur Heart J*. 2009;30:2631–2671.
22. Goldenberg J, Moss A. Long QT syndrome. *J Am Coll Cardiol*. 2008;51:2291–2300.
23. Roden DM. Clinical practice. Long-QT syndrome. *N Engl J Med*. 2008;358:169–176.
24. Antzelevitch C, et al. Brugada syndrome: report of the second consensus conference. *Circulation*. 2005;111:659–670.
25. Paul M, et al. Role of programmed ventricular stimulation in patients with Brugada syndrome: a meta-analysis of worldwide published data. *Eur Heart J*. 2007;28:2126–2133.
26. Morita H, et al. Fragmented QRS as a marker of conduction abnormality and a predictor of prognosis of Brugada syndrome. *Circulation*. 2008;118:1697–1704.
27. Sacher F, et al. Outcome after implantation of a cardioverter-defibrillator in patients with Brugada syndrome: a multicenter study. *Circulation*. 2006;114:2317–2324.
28. Rosso R, et al. Outcome after implantation of cardioverter defibrillator [corrected] in patients with Brugada syndrome: a multicenter Israeli study (ISRABRU). *Isr Med Assoc J*. 2008;10:435–439.
29. Probst V, et al. Long-term prognosis of patients diagnosed with Brugada syndrome. Results from the FINGER Brugada Syndrome Registry. *Circulation*. 2010;121:635–643.
30. Hayashi M, et al. Incidence and risk factors of arrhythmic events in catecholaminergic polymorphic ventricular tachycardia. *Circulation*. 2009;119:2426–2434.
31. Gaita F, et al. Short QT syndrome: A familial cause of sudden death. *Circulation*. 2003;108:965–970.
32. Brignole M. Are complications of implantable defibrillators under-estimated and benefits over-estimated?. *Europace*. 2009;11:1129–1133.

Section II
Syncope Management in Clinical Practice: How to Do It

Chapter 16
How to: Role of Questionnaires and Risk Stratification at the Initial Evaluation in the Clinic and in the Emergency Department

Contents

This chapter describes two case studies as an educational guide for training in utilization of specific questionnaires and risk score tables for the evaluation of syncope.

16.1 Case Study #1. An 82-Year-Old Female Is in the Emergency Room with Head Trauma After a Transient Loss of Consciousness Episode: How Do I Evaluate and Triage This Patient?

16.1.1 Initial Evaluation

History taking:

– *Present illness*. The patient reports that she had a sudden onset of transient loss of consciousness (T-LOC) while walking to the store. The event was not triggered by any known circumstance and was not preceded by any prodrome. When she recovered, she found herself in an ambulance. She sustained a small laceration

M. Brignole, D.G. Benditt, *Syncope*, DOI 10.1007/978-0-85729-201-8_16,
© Springer-Verlag London Limited 2011

above the right eyebrow. No witness was present but the patient thinks that she passed out for few seconds. The patient had no previous episodes of loss of consciousness.

−*Past illnesses*. She had an uncomplicated myocardial infarction 15 years ago and diabetes mellitus treated by diet.
−*Medications*. Aspirin and atenolol 50 mg.

Physical exam:

−No apparent distress, alert and oriented to time, place, and person.
−*Vitals*. Afebrile, BP 142/65 HR 68 bpm supine and 138/60, 72 bpm standing, respectively, respiratory rate 16 with oxygen saturation 94% on room air.
−*Cardiovascular*. Regular rhythm, no abnormal heart sounds.
−*Neurological*. Non-focal, no gait disturbance.
−*Skin*. Ecchymosis and 1-cm wound above the right eyebrow.
−Remainder of the examination is unremarkable.

Standard 12-lead ECG:

−Sinus rhythm at 70 bpm, Q waves in inferior leads, no changes when compared to prior tracing.

CBC and blood chemistry:

−Hemoglobin 12 g/dL, hematocrit 37%, the rest of the panel was within normal limits.

Results from the initial evaluation. Syncopal spell likely, uncertain etiology, cardiac likely due to history of structural heart disease. Please refer to Section 5.1 (Fig. 5.1) on how to differentiate syncope from other forms of T-LOC and to Section 5.3 (Table 5.3) for the clinical features which suggest a cardiac cause.

16.1.2 Triage and Subsequent Evaluation

There are three main questions to answer for an evidence-based management of the patient.

16.1.2.1 *Question 1* – Do I Have to Admit This Patient? (i.e., Risk Stratification)

To answer this question we can utilize several validated risk scores shown in Table 16.1[1–5] (see also Chapter 6).

Table 16.1 Validated risk score useful for management of patients with syncope

Study	Risk factors	Score	Outcome	Risk score	Case #1	Case #2
San Francisco Rule[1]	– Abnormal ECG – Congestive heart failure – Shortness of breath – Hematocrit <30% – Systolic blood pressure <90 mmHg	No risk= 0 item Risk = ≥1 item	Serious events at 7 days		*Score 0* (no risk factor)	*Score 0* (no risk factor)
Rose rule[2]	– BNP concentration ≥300 pg/mL – Positive fecal occult blood – Hemoglobin ≤90 g/l – Oxygen saturation ≤94% – Q wave on ECG – Syncope during chest pain – Bradycardia <50 bpm	No risk= 0 item Risk = ≥1 item	Serious events at 1 month		*Score 1* (Q wave)	*Score 0* (no risk factor)
Martin et al.[3]	– Abnormal ECG* – History of ventricular arrhythmia – History of congestive heart failure – Age >45 years	0–4 (1 point each item)	1-Year severe arrhythmias or arrhythmic death	0: 0% 1: 5% 2: 16% 3–4: 27%	*Score 2* (abn ECG and age >45)	*Score 2* (abn ECG and age >45)
OESIL score[4]	– Abnormal ECG* – History of cardiovascular disease – Lack of prodrome – Age >65 years	0–4 (1 point each item)	1-Year total mortality	0: 0% 1: 0.6% 2: 14% 3: 29% 4: 53%	*Score 4* (all factors)	*Score 2–3* (abn ECG/age)

Table 16.1 (continued)

Study	Risk factors	Score	Outcome	Risk score	Case #1	Case #2
EGSYS score[5]	– Palpitations before syncope (+4) – Abnormal ECG and/or heart disease (+3) – Syncope during effort (+3) – Syncope while supine (+2) – Autonomic activation (−1) – Predisposing and/or precipitating factors (−1)	Sum of + and − points	2-Year total mortality	<3: 2% ≥3: 21%	*Score 3* (abn ECG/SHD)	*Score 2* (abn ECG/ predisposing)
			Cardiac syncope probability	<3: 2% 3: 13% 4: 33% >4: 77%	*Score 3*	*Score 2*

Instruction for use:

Abnormal ECG is defined in different ways in these reports:

– In San Francisco Rule it is defined as "new changes or non-sinus rhythm."
– In the ROSE study it is defined as "Q wave (not in lead III).
– In OESIL it is defined as "rhythm abnormalities, conduction disorders, hypertrophy, old myocardial infarction, possible acute ischemia and AV block."
– In EGSYS it is defined as "sinus bradycardia, atrioventricular block greater than first degree, bundle branch block, acute or old myocardial infarction, supraventricular or ventricular tachycardia, left or right ventricular hypertrophy, ventricular preexcitation, long QT and Brugada pattern."

Serious events during the follow-up are defined in different ways:

– In San Francisco Rule they are defined as "death, myocardial infarction, arrhythmia, pulmonary embolism, stroke, subarachnoid hemorrhage, significant hemorrhage, or any condition causing a return ED visit and hospitalization for a related event."
– In the Rose study, serious adverse event within 1 month of emergency department evaluation were defined as death, acute myocardial infarction, life-threatening arrhythmia, decision to implant a pacemaker or a cardiac defibrillator within 1 month of index collapse, pulmonary embolus, cerebrovascular accident, hemorrhage requiring a blood transfusion, acute surgical procedure or endoscopic intervention.
– In the Martin study, the outcome was defined as "severe arrhythmia (sustained ventricular tachycardia, symptomatic supraventricular tachycardia, pauses >3 s, AV block, pacemaker malfunction), or 1-year arrhythmic mortality."

Autonomic activation in EGSYS score: syncope preceded or followed by nausea/vomiting, abdominal pain, feeling of cold or sweating.
Precipitating and/or predisposing factors in EGSYS score:

– warm-crowded place, and/or prolonged orthostasis; or
– in relationship with emotional distress (fear, pain, instrumentation).

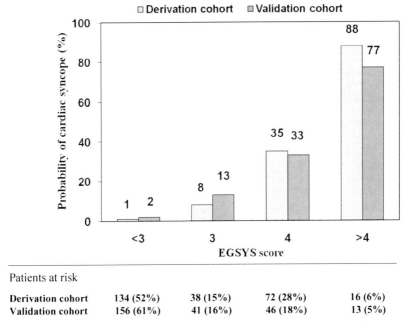

Patients at risk

Derivation cohort	134 (52%)	38 (15%)	72 (28%)	16 (6%)
Validation cohort	156 (61%)	41 (16%)	46 (18%)	13 (5%)

Fig. 16.1 Probability of cardiac syncope in the derivation cohort and in the validation cohort of the EGSYS score

Based on the risk score, the risk assessment of this patient indicates the following:

- *San Francisco Rule (SFR).*[1] Low short-term risk at 7 days of life-threatening conditions and death.
- *Rose rule.*[2] High short-term risk at 1 month of life-threatening conditions and death.
- *Martin.*[3] 16% risk of life-threatening arrhythmias or arrhythmic death at 1 year.
- *OESIL.*[4] 53% total mortality at 1 year.
- *EGSYS.*[5] 21% total mortality at 2 years and 13% probability of cardiac syncope (Fig. 16.1).

Answer to question 1. In summary, the risk stratification of the patient indicates a low short-term risk of serious events with one instrument and high short-term risk with another and considerable risk at 1–2 years. The probability of cardiac syncope is low but not negligible.

- According to the guidelines of the American College of Emergency Physician,[6] patients with any of the high-risk factors listed in Table 16.2 should be admitted. In our patient, structural heart disease (old myocardial infarction) and older age are indications for admission.

Table 16.2 Factors that lead to high-risk stratification requiring hospitalization according to a clinical policy statement of the American College of Emergency Physicians

---

- Old age and associated comorbidities[a]
- Abnormal ECG (defined as acute ischemia, dysrhythmias, or significant conduction abnormalities)
- Hematocrit <30%
- History or presence of heart failure, coronary artery disease, or structural heart disease

---

[a]Different studies use different ages as threshold for decision making. Age is likely a continuous variable.

- According to ESC guidelines,[7] previous myocardial infarction is a criterion for early intensive evaluation that can be performed with or without hospitalization (this latter possibility is also consistent with patient's SFR risk score) (see Chapter 6, Tables 6.2 and 6.3). However, in this particular case, the hospitalization can probably be avoided provided that the patient receives immediate ECG monitoring (external loop recorder) and is scheduled for an early outpatient evaluation (see below). Additional considerations include the patient's safety at home. Does she live alone? Is there risk of falls on stairs? Is there any concern that she may have sustained a more severe head injury?

16.1.2.2 *Question 2 –* **Which Test Should Be Performed Next? (i.e., Identifying the Mechanism of Syncope)**

Some features of the initial evaluation suggest a possible cardiac cause of syncope in this patient. Among those relevant for this patient and listed in Chapter 5, Tables 5.3 and 5.6 are absence of prodrome and old myocardial infarction. Moreover, the EGSYS score[5] indicates a probability of 13% of cardiac syncope; this is a relatively low probability but the possibility must nonetheless be ruled out.

Answer to question 2. Owing to the presence of structural heart disease, both AHA/ACCF document[8] and ESC/HRS guidelines[7] recommend further cardiac testing as initial step in evaluation based on the "cardiac syncope likely" algorithm (Fig. 16.2):

– *Echocardiogram.* If LVEF<30%, ICD may be indicated, but this neither provides a diagnosis nor necessarily prevents T-LOC recurrences.

    A stress test and thereafter likely an electrophysiological study (EPS) will be the next reasonable steps. In this case, the indications for EPS could be perhaps reconsidered given a low probability of a diagnostic finding (no history of arrhythmia or palpitations and preserved stable systolic function).

– *Stress test.* Ischemia workup and intervention if possible.

– *Electrophysiological study (EPS).* If negative, AHA/ACCF[8] did not recommend further investigation, while ESC guidelines[7] recommend reappraisal with investigating of possible reflex mechanism (carotid sinus message and tilt testing).

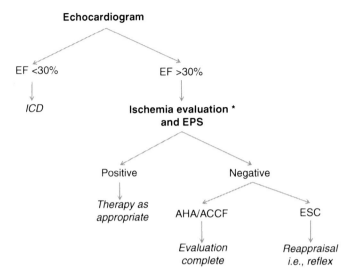

Fig. 16.2 Algorithm for cardiac likely syncope (*includes stress test and angiography if applicable)

16.1.2.3   *Question 3* – Is Head Imaging Justified as Part of the Initial Evaluation to Rule Out Possibility of Intracranial Hemorrhage?

As a consequence of T-LOC, the patient sustained minor head trauma and experienced a brief period of amnesia without abnormal neurological findings.

"Concussion" refers to a condition in which there is more often than not an immediate and transient loss of consciousness usually accompanied by a *brief period of amnesia* after a blow to the head.[9-11] The clinical status of the momentary sensation of being "starstruck," or dazed, after head injury without a brief period of loss of consciousness is uncertain, but it is generally considered the mildest form of concussion. Owing to the absence of witnesses in our patient's case, concussion cannot be excluded with certainty. The fact that apparently the patient did not have any prodrome could be explained by retrograde amnesia caused by the concussion.

Evidence that the injury was minor, including a normal neurologic examination and absence of post-concussion symptoms, does not ensure the absence of an intracranial lesion. Cranial computed tomography (CT) without contrast enhancement is adequate to detect important intracranial bleeding; magnetic resonance imaging is not necessary. To refine the criteria for CT scanning, several clinical decision rules have been developed. Two of these rules – the New Orleans Criteria[12] and the Canadian CT Head Rule[13] (Table 16.3) – have been validated prospectively. The presence of at least one criterion from the New Orleans Criteria or the Canadian CT Head Rule is considered an indication for a cranial CT scan. The patient did not show short-term memory deficits, convulsion, headache, and vomiting which are findings suggesting intracranial damage. Nevertheless patients older than 65 years are by virtue of age alone at a small additional risk of intracranial

Table 16.3 The New Orleans and Canadian Clinical Decision Rules for CT after concussion[a]

New Orleans Criteria[12] – *Glasgow Coma Scale score of 15*
– Headache
– Vomiting
– Age >60 years
– Drug or alcohol intoxication
– Persistent anterograde amnesia (deficits in short-term memory)
– Evidence of traumatic soft tissue or bone injury above clavicles
– Seizure

Canadian CT Head Rule[13] – *Glasgow Coma Scale score of 13–15 for patients 16 years and older*

High risk of neurosurgical intervention:
– Glasgow Coma Scale score <15 within 2 h after injury
– Suspected open or depressed skull fracture
– Any sign of basal skull fracture
– Two or more episodes of vomiting
– Age >65 years

Moderate risk of brain injury detected by CT:
– Retrograde amnesia for ≥30 min
– Dangerous mechanism[b]

---

[a]The presence of at least one criterion from the New Orleans Criteria or the Canadian CT Head Rule is considered an indication for a cranial CT scan. A score on the Glasgow Coma Scale of 15 signifies a fully alert and oriented patient.
[b]Refers to a motor vehicle that strikes a pedestrian, ejection from a motor vehicle, or a fall from an elevation of about 1 m or five or more stairs.

damage. According to NICE criteria,[10] amnesia and age drive the management in this case. Indeed, in the presence of age ≥65 years and retrograde amnesia for events more than 30 min before impact, it is acceptable to admit a patient for overnight observation and delay the CT scan until the next morning. Adult patients who have sustained a head injury and present with any one of the risk factors reported in Table 16.4 should have CT scanning of the head. The present case is borderline. Thus, weak evidence exists in favor of non-contrast brain CT scan in addition to a period of careful clinical observation.

16.2 Case Study #2. A 69-Year-Old Man Is Referred by His Primary Care Physician to a Syncope Unit for Recurrent Episodes of Transient Loss of Consciousness Syncope: How Do I Evaluate Him?

16.2.1 Initial Evaluation

History taking:

  –*Present illness*. The patient reports that he had three episodes of transient loss of consciousness (T-LOC) in the last year. Two of them occurred while

Table 16.4 NICE clinical guideline for CT scan after a head trauma

---

Criteria for immediate request for CT scan of the head (adults):
- GCS less than 13 on initial assessment in the emergency department
- GCS less than 15 at 2 h after the injury on assessment in the emergency department
- Suspected open or depressed skull fracture
- Any sign of basal skull fracture (hemotympanum, "panda" eyes, cerebrospinal fluid leakage from the ear or nose, Battle's sign)
- Post-traumatic seizure
- Focal neurological deficit
- More than one episode of vomiting
- Amnesia for events more than 30 min before impact

Criteria for immediate request for CT scan of the head provided patient has experienced some loss of consciousness or amnesia since the injury (adults):
- Age 65 years or older
- Coagulopathy (history of bleeding, clotting disorder, current treatment with warfarin)
- Dangerous mechanism of injury (a pedestrian or a cyclist struck by a motor vehicle, an occupant ejected from a motor vehicle or a fall from a height of greater than 1 m or five stairs)

GCS = Glasgow Coma Score.

standing; prodromes were short ("feeling about to faint") so that he was unable to prevent a fall; the loss of consciousness was brief and recovery rapid and complete. The most recent episode, similar to previous ones, occurred while driving his car; he could just stop the car before fainting. He had had other episodes of syncope 3 years ago and further two episodes during the previous 10 years (total six episodes during his life) and sporadic presyncopal episodes. Most of the episodes occurred during prolonged standing or shortly after a meal. Only once did he suffer minor injury as a consequence of T-LOC. As a consequence of the previous syncopal episodes, he underwent cardiac assessment: ECG showed a right BBB and normal axis; echocardiogram and Holter were normal. He had been having sporadic episodes of atypical chest pain over the past 10 years; a stress test last year was negative.

–*Past illnesses.* Hypertension and hyperlipidemia.
–*Medications.* ACE inhibitor for hypertension.

Physical exam:

- No apparent distress, alert, and oriented to time, place, and person.
- *Vitals.* Afebrile, BP 155/95 (HR 74) supine and 140/100 (HR72) standing, RR 18 with oxygen saturation 98% on room air.
- *Cardiovascular.* Regular rhythm, no added sounds.
- *Neurological.* Non-focal, no gait disturbance.
- Remainder of the exam is unremarkable.

Standard 12-lead ECG:

- Sinus rhythm at 78 bpm, right BBB(RBBB), no changes when compared to old tracing.

Table 16.5 Factors predicting arrhythmic (ECG-documented AV block or ventricular tachycardia) versus reflex syncope (from Calkins et al.[14])

Predictive factors	Sensitivity (%)	Specificity (%)
Age >54	94	81
Male sex	85	69
Warmings of <5 s	81	66
≤2 syncopes during life	77	88

Table 16.6 Variables associated with syncope due to primary arrhythmia (ECG documented by means of implanted loop recorders) (from Sud et al.[15])

Risk factors	Multiple logistic regression	
	Odds ratio (95% CI)	*p* value
Syncope without warnings	4.10 (1–17)	0.05
Structural heart disease	4.9 (1.1–22)	0.04
Normal ECG	0.16 (0.04–0.67)	0.01

Interpretation of the findings of the initial evaluation. Please refer to Section 5.1 (Fig. 5.1) regarding how to differentiate syncope from other forms of T-LOC and to Section 5.3 (Table 5.3) for the clinical features which suggest the cause of syncope. In particular, in this case the presence of right bundle branch block (RBBB) is weakly suggestive of a possible cardiac cause, whereas the long history of syncope > 3 years, some of them during prolonged standing or shortly after a meal, suggests a reflex cause. Prodromes were present but too short to permit the patient to avoid the faint. Absence of prodromes suggests a cardiac cause; in one study,[14] 81% of patients with syncope due to documented AV block or ventricular tachycardia had absence of prodromes or very brief prodromes (estimated at lasting <5 s), whereas only 34% of patients with reflex syncope had this feature (Table 16.5). In another study,[15] syncope without prodromes increased by approximately fourfold the probability of a primary arrhythmia (Table 16.6). In the present case the brevity of prodromes suggests an arrhythmic cause. Thus, the initial evaluation indicates that the T-LOC was indeed syncope but remained of uncertain etiology (reflex or primary arrhythmic).

16.2.2 Subsequent Evaluation

There are three main questions to answer for an evidence-based management of this patient.

16.2.2.1 *Question 1* – What Is the Prognosis of This Patient? (i.e., Risk Stratification)

With regard to the prognosis associated with syncope, two important elements should be considered:

Table 16.7 Prognosis of patients with uncertain diagnosis and low risk >40 years according to the number of syncopes during the previous 2 years

Number of syncopes during last 2 years	Risk of recurrence of syncope after the index episode		
	Actuarial risk 1 year (%)	Actuarial risk 2 years (%)	Estimated risk 4 years[a] (%)
1–2	23	27	37
3	29	36	49
4–6	43	51	66
7–10	43	49	60
>10	86	98	100

[a] Assuming a linear increase.

(i) risk of death and life-threatening events and
(ii) risk of syncopal recurrence.

Risk of death and life-threatening events. Based on the risk score shown in Table 16.1, the risk assessment for this patient indicates the following:

- *San Francisco Rule (SFR)*.[1] Low short-term risk at 7 days of life-threatening conditions and death.
- *Rose rule*.[2] Low short-term risk at 1 month of life-threatening conditions and death.
- *Martin*.[3] 16% risk of life-threatening arrhythmias or arrhythmic death at 1 year.
- *OESIL*.[4] 14–29% total mortality at 1 year.
- *EGSYS*.[5] 2% total mortality at 2 years and 2% probability of cardiac syncope.

In summary, the risk stratification of the patient indicates a low short-term risk of ominous events but contrasting results regarding long-term outcome; low probability of cardiac syncope.

Risk of syncopal recurrence. Table 16.7 provides recurrence rates in the pooled population of 590 patients >40 years, at low risk according ESC classification, who participated in the ISSUE 1 and ISSUE 2 studies. These individuals had unexplained syncope or suspected neurally mediated reflex syncope. Applying those data to this patient, our patient has an approximate 50% probability of a syncope recurrence within the next 2 years.[16]

Answer to question 1. Owing to the absence of an immediate risk, hospitalization is not necessary. On the other hand, there is uncertainty regarding long-term risk of death or life-threatening events. The high probability of syncope recurrence warrants further evaluation to determine the precise cause of syncope in order to find a specific therapy.

16.2.2.2 *Question 2 – Is an Arrhythmia Likely? (Pretest Probability)*

As discussed above, either reflex or primary arrhythmia may be responsible for syncope in this patient, and in fact several findings suggest that an arrhythmia is the likely cause of syncope. The absence or brevity of prodromes (Tables 16.5 and 16.6) and the presence of RBBB (Chapter 5, Table 5.6) support a cardiac arrhythmic cause. On the other hand, the low EGSYS score and several other features are more consistent with an atypical form of reflex syncope as was observed in patients enrolled in the ISSUE study, i.e., long-lasting recurrent syncope, without prodromes, starting in middle or old age (Fig. 8.2). The ISSUE study showed that among patients in whom syncope was recorded during follow-up, 54% these patients had a long pause documented by the implanted loop recorder.[16]

Answer to question 2. The pretest probability of an arrhythmic cause, either intrinsic cardiac or extrinsic reflex, is high enough to suggest pursuing additional investigations aimed to address this concern.

16.2.2.3   *Question 3* – Which Test Should Be Performed Next? (Identifying the Mechanism of Syncope)

Owing to the presence of BBB, both AHA/ACCF and ESC committees recommend further cardiac testing as initial step. According to the algorithm for cardiac syncope being "likely" (Fig. 16.2), ischemia evaluation and electrophysiological study (EPS) come first. In the present case, the absence of structural heart disease and the negative stress test tend to exclude clinically significant cardiac disease. EPS is justified by the presence of RBBB, though its diagnostic value would be higher in the case of bifascicular block or left bundle branch block, neither of which apply to this patient. On the other hand, implantable loop recorders (ILRs) are particularly useful in patients such as this with recurrent syncope (≥ 3 in the last 2 years) and in patients with BBB; randomized trials have shown a higher diagnostic yield of ILRs over conventional investigations including EPS (see Chapter 8).

Answer to question 3. Owing to the low risk status of the patient, a strategy of early ILR utilization instead of pursuing conventional laboratory investigation is the most cost-effective strategy. The risk of harm by waiting for another syncope event is very low, whereas the chance of establishing a solid diagnosis is important.

Acknowledgment   This chapter was prepared with the help of Ali Abdul Jabbar, MD, University of Nevada School of Medicine, Internal Medicine Department, Las Vegas, USA.

References

1. Quinn J, et al. Prospective validation of the San Francisco Syncope Rule to predict patients with serious outcomes. *Ann Emerg Med*. 2006;47:448–454.
2. Reed M, et al. Risk stratification of syncope in the emergency department: the ROSE study. *J Am Coll Cardiol*. 2010;55:713–721.
3. Martin TP, et al. Risk stratification of patients with syncope. *Ann Emerg Med*. 1997;29: 459–466.
4. Colivicchi F, et al. Development and prospective validation of a risk stratification system for patients with syncope in the emergency department: the OESIL risk score. *Eur Heart J*. 2003;24:811–819.

5. Del Rosso A, et al. Clinical predictors of cardiac syncope at initial evaluation in patients referred urgently to general hospital: the EGSYS score. *Heart*. 2008;94:1620–1626.
6. Huff JS, et al. Clinical policy: critical issues in the evaluation and management of adult patients presenting to the emergency department with syncope. *Ann Emerg Med*. 2007;49:431–444.
7. Moya A, et al. Guidelines for the Diagnosis and Management of Syncope (Version 2009). *Eur Heart J*. 2009;30:2631–2671.
8. Strickberger SA, et al. Scientific statement on the evaluation of syncope. *J Am Coll Cardiol*. 2006;47:473–484.
9. Ropper AH, Gorson KC. Concussion. *N Engl J Med*. 2007;356:166–172.
10. National Institute for Health and Clinical Excellence (2009) NICE clinical guideline 56. Head injury: triage, assessment, investigation and early management of head injury in infants, children and adults. September 2007. www.nice.org.uk
11. Haydel MJ, et al. Indications for computed tomography in patients with minor head injury. *N Engl J Med*. 2000;343:100–105.
12. Smits M, et al. External validation of the Canadian CT head rule and the New Orleans criteria for CT scanning in patients with minor head injury. *J Am Med Assoc*. 2005;294:1519–1525.
13. Stiell IG, et al. The Canadian CT head rule for patients with minor head injury. *Lancet*. 2001;357:1391–1396.
14. Calkins H, et al. The value of the clinical history in the differentiation of syncope due to ventricular tachycardia, atrioventricular block, and neurocardiogenic syncope. *Am J Med*. 1995;98:365–373.
15. Sud S, et al. Predicting the cause of syncope from clinical history in patients undergoing prolonged monitoring. *Heart Rhythm*. 2009;6:238–243.
16. Brignole M, et al. Indications for the use of diagnostic implantable and external ECG loop recorders. *Europace*. 2009;11:671–687.

Chapter 17
How to: Carotid Sinus Massage

Contents

Carotid sinus massage (CSM) is a clinical procedure used to identify patients with hypersensitive carotid sinus physiology and potentially disclose carotid sinus syndrome in patients with syncope. For the clinical value, indications, and interpretation of CSM responses, please also see Chapters 7 and 11.

17.1 Anatomy

The carotid sinus reflex arc is composed of an afferent limb arising from the mechanoreceptors of the carotid artery (principally located at the bifurcation of the common carotid artery) and terminating in midbrain centers, mainly the vagus nucleus and the vasomotor center. The efferent limb is via the vagus nerve and the parasympathetic ganglia to the sinus and atrioventricular nodes (and possibly more distally in the conduction system) as well as via the sympathetic nervous system to the heart and the blood vessels (Fig. 17.1). Usually, right-sided CSM tends to cause more of an effect on the sinus node, while left-sided CSM tends to have more impact on the atrioventricular node. However, this "rule" is often broken.

Whether the site of carotid sinus dysfunction resulting in a hypersensitive response to the massage is central at the level of brain stem nuclei or peripheral at the level of carotid baroreceptors is still a matter of debate.[1] There is evidence that both may play a role possibly in different patients. There is also evidence that abnormal afferent inputs from the proprioceptive nerves of the neck to the brain stem may contribute to inappropriate interpretation of neck movements and resulting changes induced locally on carotid arterial wall tension.

M. Brignole, D.G. Benditt, *Syncope*, DOI 10.1007/978-0-85729-201-8_17,
© Springer-Verlag London Limited 2011

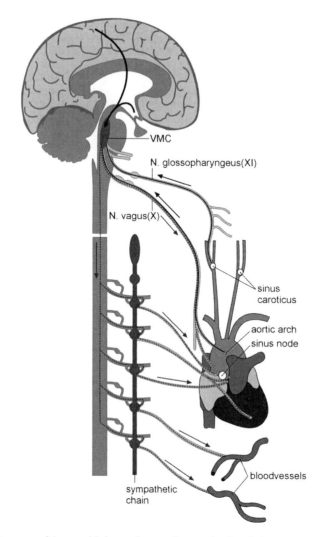

Fig. 17.1 Anatomy of the carotid sinus reflex arc. See text for description

17.2 Methodology and Response to Carotid Sinus Massage – The "Method of Symptoms"

There is general consensus that CSM should be performed with the patient in both supine and upright positions (usually on a tilt table). Continuous electrocardiographic (ECG) monitoring is required. Continuous blood pressure (BP) monitoring is also essential, preferably using a non-invasive beat-to-beat measurement device (e.g., Finometer®, Nexfin®); the latter is important as the vasodepressor response is rapid and cannot be adequately detected with devices which do not provide continuous beat-to-beat blood pressure.

Fig. 17.2 Carotid sinus massage. The carotid sinus located at the anterior margin of the sternocleidomastoid muscle at the level of the cricoid cartilage

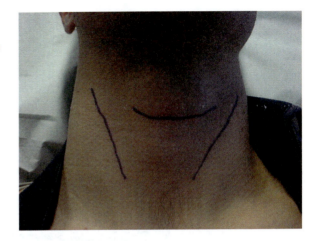

After baseline ECG and BP measurements, one carotid artery (usually the right as that is the side most physicians initiate the physical examination of patients) is firmly (but not so aggressively as to obstruct the vessel) massaged for 10 s (or less in case of induction of syncope) at the anterior margin of the sternocleidomastoid muscle at the level of the cricoid cartilage (Fig. 17.2). The massage is performed with the second, third, and fourth fingers of the preferred hand over the site of maximum pulsatility of the carotid artery (Fig. 17.3). After recovery of baseline conditions, a second massage is performed on the opposite side if the massage of the first side failed to yield a "positive" result. Then, the maneuver is repeated with the patient in an upright posture (usually on a tilt table) (Fig. 17.4). In order to assess the contribution of the vasodepressor component, which may otherwise be hidden if an asystolic response is evoked, CSM is repeated after intravenous administration of atropine

Fig. 17.3 Carotid sinus massage, supine position. The carotid sinus artery is firmly massaged for 10 s (or less in case of induction of syncope) at the anterior margin of the sternocleidomastoid muscle at the level of the cricoid cartilage. The massage is performed with the second, third, and fourth fingers of the preferred hand over the site of maximum pulsatility of the carotid artery

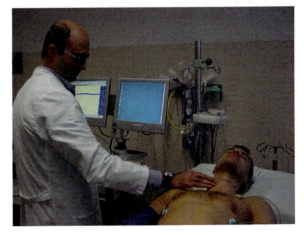

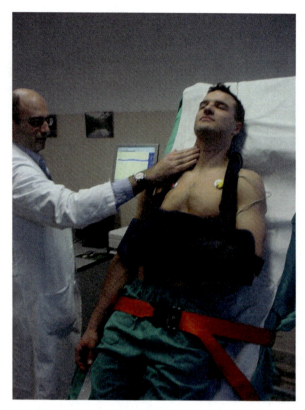

Fig. 17.4 Carotid sinus massage, upright position. The massage is repeated in upright position using a tilt table

(1 mg or 0.02 mg/kg body weight) (Figs. 17.5 and 17.6). Atropine administration is preferred to temporary dual-chamber pacing as it is simple, non-invasive, and easily reproducible. However, side effects such as dry eyes, dry mouth, constipation, and possible urinary retention are important to keep in mind and discuss with the patient in advance.

The response to CSM is generally classified as cardioinhibitory (i.e., marked bradycardia and/or asystole ≥3 s), vasodepressive (fall in systolic blood pressure ≥50 mmHg), or mixed. The mixed response is diagnosed by the association of an asystole of ≥3 s and a decline in systolic blood pressure of >50 mmHg from the baseline value on rhythm resumption. The test is positive (i.e., "*carotid sinus syndrome*") if syncope is reproduced in conjunction with asystole or hypotension and the finding is consistent with the patient's medical history. For this reason this methodology is also termed the "*method of symptoms*"[2] (Table 17.1). In experienced hands the reproducibility of response to CSM is >90%. However, the response does fatigue, and it cannot be induced repetitively if tests are repeated within a short time period.

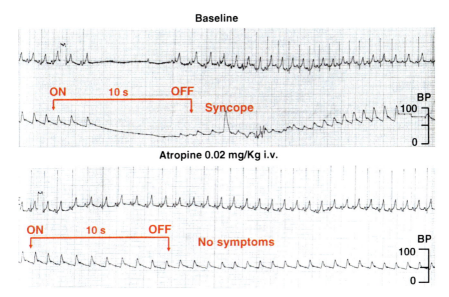

Fig. 17.5 Predominant cardioinhibitory form of carotid sinus syndrome diagnosed by carotid sinus massage performed according to the "method of symptoms." *Panel a*: The massage was performed during beat-to-beat, electrocardiographic (*top trace*), and systemic blood pressure monitoring (*bottom trace*) with the patient on a tilt table in upright 60° position. The *arrows* indicate the time of beginning and end of the massage. The massage was continued for 10 s. A 6.5-s asystole was induced soon after the beginning of the massage. The systolic blood pressure fell below 50 mmHg; the vasodepressor reflex persisted longer than the cardioinhibitory reflex. Syncope occurred after the end of the massage when the heart rhythm had already recovered. *Panel b*: In order to determine the relative contribution of the two components of the reflex, the cardioinhibitory component was suppressed by means of i.v. infusion of 0.02 mg/kg atropine and the massage repeated. Despite blood pressure fall to 75 mmHg, syncope could not be reproduced, thus showing that the cardioinhibitory component of the reflex was the major determinant of syncope in this patient

Since CSM carries potential hazards, the test should be performed by physicians who are aware that complications, especially of neurological origin, may occur. Even if these complications are rare, carotid massage should be avoided in patients with previous transient ischemic attacks and/or strokes within the past 3 months (with the possible exception that carotid Doppler studies have excluded significant stenosis) or in patients with carotid bruits. Rarely, CSM may elicit self-limited atrial fibrillation of little clinical significance.

There are several reasons to prefer the "method of symptoms":

- Although CSM is frequently performed with the patient in the supine position in clinical practice and in many studies, the importance of also undertaking massage with the patient in the upright position has become more widely recognized.[2–4] First, the syndrome may be missed in half of the cases if the massage

Baseline

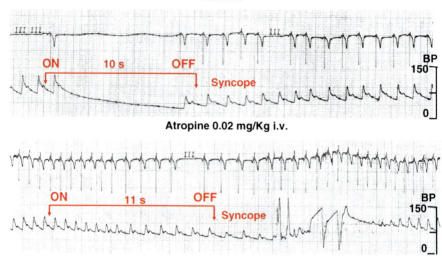

Fig. 17.6 Mixed form of carotid sinus syndrome diagnosed by carotid sinus massage performed according to the "method of symptoms." *Panel a*: The massage was performed during beat-to-beat, electrocardiographic (*top trace*), and systemic blood pressure monitoring (*bottom trace*) with the patient on a tilt table in upright 60° position. The *arrows* indicate the time of beginning and end of the massage. The massage was continued for 10 s. A 8.5-s asystole was induced soon after the beginning of the massage. The systolic blood pressure fell below 70 mmHg; the vasodepressor reflex persisted longer than the cardioinhibitory reflex. Syncope occurred after the end of the massage when the heart rhythm had already recovered. *Panel b*: In order to determine the relative contribution of the two components of the reflex, the cardioinhibitory component was suppressed by means of i.v. infusion of 0.02 mg/kg atropine and the massage repeated for 11 s. Despite persistence of normal heart rate, blood pressure fell of a similar magnitude and the patient had again syncope. Thus, the vasodepressor component of the reflex was the major determinant of syncope in this patient

is not performed in the upright position as the vasodepressor response may be underappreciated (Fig. 17.7). The evaluation of the magnitude of the vasodepressor component and the reproduction of symptoms frequently require the upright position (Fig. 17.8).

- Atropine administration is necessary in order to assess the vasodepressor response when an asystolic reflex is induced with CSM. Understanding the possible contribution of the vasodepressor component of the reflex is of practical importance for the choice of therapy. Pacemaker therapy has been shown to be less effective in mixed forms of CSS in which there is an important vasodepressor component, compared to those cases with dominant cardioinhibitory forms.[2,4]

- Six to nine seconds of asystole is usually necessary to cause syncope (there is position dependence to be factored in as well). This duration is consistent with that observed during spontaneous CSS episodes (median of 9 s, interquartile range 8–18) whereas episodes of asystole <6 s duration cause syncope in less than

Table 17.1 Carotid sinus massage: classification of positive responses

Predominant cardioinhibitory form
- Carotid sinus massage, baseline: asystole ≥ 3 s causes hypotension with reproduction of spontaneous symptoms
- Carotid sinus massage after atropine (1 mg or 0.02 mg/kg body weight): no inducibility of clinically significant hypotension by CSM and no further symptoms[a]

Mixed form
- Carotid sinus massage, baseline: asystole ≥ 3 s and fall in systolic blood pressure ≥ 50 mmHg with reproduction of spontaneous symptoms
- Carotid sinus massage after atropine (1 mg or 0.02 mg/kg body weight): milder symptoms due to systolic blood pressure fall ≥ 50 mmHg

Predominant vasodepressor form
- Carotid sinus massage, baseline: reproduction of the spontaneous symptoms due to systolic blood pressure fall ≥ 50 mmHg without asystole
- Carotid sinus massage after atropine (1 mg or 0.02 mg/kg body weight): inducibility of hypotension by CSM is unchanged

[a]In this case vasodepressor reflex is absent or, if present, asymptomatic

half of the cases. Therefore, shorter duration of the massage may underestimate positive responses.[5,6]

- Reproduction of symptoms by CSM is important for definitive diagnosis of CSS (although if the medical history is supportive, this level of evidence may not be essential in everyday clinical practice). The diagnostic value of asymptomatic abnormal responses ("*carotid sinus hypersensitivity*") is uncertain owing to its low specificity. Indeed, abnormal responses are frequently observed in subjects (especially older subjects) without syncope.[7–9] For example, an abnormal

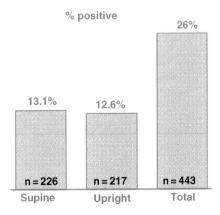

Fig. 17.7 Role of upright massage (from Puggioni et al.[2]). In this large population of 1,719 patients, syncope was induced in supine position in 13.1% of patients. In other 12.6%, syncope could be induced only in standing position. Thus, carotid sinus syndrome would have been missed in half of the cases if the massage were not performed also in the upright position

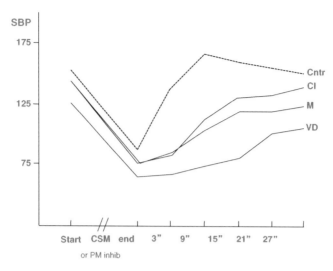

Fig. 17.8 The importance of the vasodepressor reflex in carotid sinus syndrome (from Gaggioli et al.[10]). Systolic blood pressure (SBP) curve during and up to 27 s after the end of the carotid sinus massage was calculated in patients with cardioinhibitory (CI, 47 pts), mixed (M, 10 pts), and vasodepressor (VD, 11 pts) forms of carotid sinus syndrome. The control group (Cntr) consisted of nine patients affected by third-degree atrioventricular block who had received the implant of a permanent pacemaker and were pacemaker dependent. By means of temporary inhibition of the pulse generator, a ventricular asystole was caused that was similar in length to that caused by carotid sinus massage in patients with carotid sinus syndrome. In other words, the control group indicates what happens to the blood pressure when a sudden prolonged pause occurs in the absence of abnormal carotid sinus reflexivity. The control group showed a marked decrease in systolic blood pressure immediately after pacemaker inhibition caused by the reduction in arterial capacity due to prolonged absence of flow during ventricular asystole and the time needed to refill the vascular bed, but blood pressure rapidly recovered with a compensatory overshoot. Compared to controls, all the patients with carotid sinus syndrome had a marked and prolonged decrease in blood pressure. The magnitude of the decrease in systolic blood pressure was greatest at the end of the massage itself and was similar in extent in all forms of carotid sinus syndrome. In patients with the CI form, the blood pressure progressively increased after massage and returned to the baseline value after a mean of 27 s. In patients with the VD form, blood pressure values were significantly lower than those in the other groups, starting from the third second after the end of the massage, and the remaining decreased for >27 s. Patients with the mixed form showed an intermediate pattern. The results point out the importance of the vasodepressor reflex in patients with carotid sinus syndrome. Indeed, the main result of this study is that an important vasodepressor effect is elicited by carotid sinus massage in all patients affected by carotid sinus syndrome, including those who are usually categorized as affected by the CI form. Abbreviations: Inhib, inhibition; PM, pacemaker

response was observed in 17–20% of patients affected by various types of cardiovascular diseases[7] and in 38% of patients with severe narrowing of the carotid arteries.[8] On the other hand, the reproduction of symptoms has shown better specificity, being positive in <10% of asymptomatic subjects. In one study,[9] while carotid sinus hypersensitivity was present in 35% of older asymptomatic subjects, syncope was induced in only 4% of these.

17.3 Case Study #3: Predominant Cardioinhibitory Carotid Sinus Syndrome

History taking

- *Present illness.* This 74-year-old male reports that he had an episode of sudden onset of loss of consciousness while driving a car. The event was not triggered by any known circumstance, but was preceded by a short prodrome ("feeling about to faint"). He could just stop the car before fainting. The loss of consciousness was very short, and the recovery was rapid and complete. The patient had two previous brief episodes of loss of consciousness during the previous year, without prodrome, while standing.
- *Past illnesses.* He has a history of coronary artery disease (chronic mild stable angina) for 10 years. He had a positive stress test years ago and is currently asymptomatic on medical management. He is also treated for hypertension and hyperlipidemia. He recently had an echocardiogram which was consistent with hypertensive heart disease with preserved left ventricular systolic function and a sclerotic aortic valve. He has chronic mild renal insufficiency (creatinine of 1.4 mg/dL). A Doppler arterial scan of the legs showed diffuse non-obstructive atherosclerosis.
- Medications: aspirin 100 mg, atenolol 100 mg, ramipril 5 mg, hydrochlorothiazide 25 mg, simvastatin 40 mg.

Physical Exam

- No apparent distress; alert; and oriented to time, place, and person.
- Vitals: Afebrile, BP 150/95 HR 52 supine and 140/100, 56 standing, respectively, RR 16 with oxygen saturation 98% on room air.
- Cardiovascular: regular rhythm, 2/6 systolic murmur heard in the aortic area and in the apex.
- Neurological: normal for age.
- Remainder of exam is unremarkable.

Standard 12-lead ECG

- Sinus rhythm at 52 bpm, left ventricular hypertrophy with ST segment depression and flat T waves.

Results from the initial evaluation: syncopal spell likely, but uncertain etiology; cardiac cause is likely.

Interpretation of the findings of the initial evaluation. Although non-diagnostic, some features of the initial evaluation suggest a possible cardiac arrhythmic cause of syncope. Factors supporting this possibility that are among those listed in Tables 5.3 and 5.6 are absent or are very short prodrome and stable coronary artery disease.

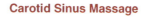

Right carotid sinus massage

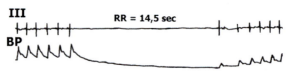

Fig. 17.9 A case of carotid sinus syncope diagnosed by carotid sinus massage in supine position (see text for explanation)

On the other hand, the EGSYS score, which is 3 in this patient, indicates a low probability of 13% of cardiac syncope.

The patient had already been evaluated by stress test and echocardiogram. Next step might reasonably be coronary angiography and electrophysiological study. However, all the syncopal episodes occurred at rest in the absence of chest pain, which makes an acute ischemic event as cause of syncope unlikely. Electrophysiological study is not indicated as it is usually of little value in this scenario in the absence of one or more of the following: previous myocardial infarction, a depressed EF, or bundle brunch block. Thus, the most useful evaluation should be prolonged ambulatory ECG monitoring by means of implantable loop recorder (see Chapter 8). However, before embarking on this diagnostic procedure, it is advisable to investigate other competitive causes of syncope, in particular atypical reflex syncope. It is known that in older males with atherosclerotic cardiovascular disease, carotid sinus massage is frequently positive. The clinical features are consistent with carotid sinus syndrome (high pretest probability).

Thus, carotid sinus massage (CSM) was performed. CSM with the patient supine induced syncope with an asystole of 14.5 s and systolic blood pressure (SBP) drop from 135 to 40 mmHg. The symptoms were recognized by the patient as similar to the spontaneous clinical syncope (Fig. 17.9). CSM standing (not shown in the figure) also induced syncope with an asystole of 12 s and a SBP drop from 120 to 40 mmHg; after atropine (0.02 mg/kg i.v.) there was no asystole or syncope.

Conclusion: Predominant cardioinhibitory carotid sinus syndrome. In this case, permanent cardiac pacing has a high probability of preventing syncope recurrences on long-term follow-up (see Chapter 11).

References

1. Thomas JE. Hyperactive carotid sinus reflex and carotid sinus syncope. *Mayo Clin Proc.* 1969;44:127–139.
2. Puggioni E, et al. Results and complications of the carotid sinus massage performed according to the "Methods of Symptoms". *Am J Cardiol.* 2002;89:599–601.
3. Parry SW, et al. Diagnosis of carotid sinus hypersensitivity in older adults: carotid sinus massage in the upright position is essential. *Heart.* 2000;83:22–23.

4. Almquist A, et al. Carotid sinus hypersensitivity: Evaluation of the vasodepressor component. *Circulation.* 1985;71:927–937.
5. Menozzi C, et al. Follow-up of asystolic episodes in patients with cardioinhibitory, neurally mediated syncope and VVI pacemaker. *Am J Cardiol.* 1993;72:1152–1155.
6. Maggi R, et al. Cardioinhibitory carotid sinus hypersensitivity predicts an asystolic mechanism of spontaneous neurally mediated syncope. *Europace.* 2007;9:563–567.
7. Brignole M, et al. The cardioinhibitory reflex evoked by carotid sinus stimulation in normal and in patients with cardiovascular disorders. *G Ital Cardiol.* 1985;15:514–519.
8. Brown KA, et al. Carotid sinus reflex in patients undergoing coronary angiography: relationship of degree and location of coronary artery disease to response to carotid sinus massage. *Circulation.* 1980;62:697–703.
9. Kerr SR, et al. Carotid sinus hypersensitivity in asymptomatic older persons: implications for diagnosis of syncope and falls. *Arch Intern Med.* 2006;166:515–520.
10. Gaggioli G, et al. Reappraisal of the vasodepressor reflex in carotid sinus syndrome. *Am J Cardiol.* 1995;75:518–521.

Chapter 18
How to: Tilt-Table Testing

Contents

18.1 Background

On moving from supine to erect posture there is a large gravitational shift of blood away from the chest to the distensible venous capacitance system below the diaphragm. This shift is estimated to total $\frac{1}{2}$–1 L of thoracic blood with most of the volume shift occurring in the first 10 s of upright posture. In addition, with prolonged standing, the high capillary transmural pressure in dependent parts of the body causes filtration of protein-free fluid into the interstitial spaces. It is estimated that this results in about a 15–20% (700 ml) decrease in plasma volume in 10 min in healthy humans. As a consequence of this gravitationally induced blood pooling and the superimposed decline in plasma volume, the return of venous blood to the heart is reduced; the result is rapid diminution of cardiac filling pressure and a consequent decrease in stroke volume. However, normally, despite decreased cardiac output, hypotension is prevented by compensatory vasoconstriction of the resistance and the capacitance vessels in the splanchnic, musculo-cutaneous, and renal vascular beds.

Vasoconstriction of systemic blood vessels is the key factor in the maintenance of arterial blood pressure in the upright posture. The main sensory receptors involved

M. Brignole, D.G. Benditt, *Syncope*, DOI 10.1007/978-0-85729-201-8_18,
© Springer-Verlag London Limited 2011

in the necessary orthostatic neural reflex adjustments are the arterial mechanoreceptors (baroreceptors) located in the aortic arch and carotid sinuses. Failure of these
compensatory adjustments either due to disease or as a result of inappropriate neural
reflexes is thought to play a crucial role in patients in whom syncope is triggered by
upright posture. Identifying this susceptibility to systemic hypotension with upright
posture forms the basis for the use of tilt-table testing in the evaluation of patients
with syncope.[1]

18.2 Tilt Test Protocols

Tilt-table testing was introduced for the evaluation of patients with syncope in
1986.[2] Since then, the test has been used extensively in many studies, and a variety of authors have proposed different protocols for diagnostic, investigational, and
therapeutic purposes. Tilt-table testing protocols have varied with respect to various
factors including the angle of the tilt table when upright, time duration of each phase
of the test (i.e., (1) supine rest, (2) upright tilt without drugs, (3) second supine rest
period, and (4) upright tilt with drug provocation), and the use of different provocative drugs. The following presents an overview of the most used and best validated
protocols (Table 18.1).

Table 18.1 Comparative synopsis of some tilt protocols

	Westminster	Low-dose isoproterenol	Italian protocol	Clomipramine
Sensitivity	+	+++	+++	+++
Specificity	+++	++	++	++
Adverse effects	+	+++	+	++
Duration	++	++	++	+++
Worldwide utilization	++	++	+++	+

18.2.1 Passive Only (the Westminster Protocol)

This protocol was first proposed by Kenny and Sutton[2] in 1986 and more fully
described by Fitzpatrick et al.[3] in 1991. The protocol calls for a drug-free tilt duration of 45–60 min at 60–70°. Assessment of the Westminster protocol revealed it to
exhibit a lower sensitivity with tilt angles = or <70°. The mean time to a positive
response in those cases in whom the test was positive was 24 ± 10 min.

> *Advantages*: physiologic; low false-positive rate (<5%); no complications
> *Disadvantages*: low positivity rate (25%); time consuming
>
> The best diagnostic accuracy is probably obtained with the following:
>
> *Protocol*: supine pre-tilt phase of at least 5 min without venous cannulation; tilt
> angle is 60–70°; passive phase of 45 min.

18.2.2 Low-Dose Isoproterenol Challenge

The isoproterenol provocation tilt-table test was proposed by Almquist et al.[4] and Waxman et al.[5] in 1989. The original protocol consists in isoproterenol infusion in progressive doses from 1 to 5 μg/min. The drug is administered with the patient in the supine position. When the heart rate stabilizes the patient is then tilted at 70° for 10 min. This maneuver is repeated at increasing doses up to 5 μg/min, with 5-min intervals between one step and the following step. Owing to the high rate of false-positive responses in subjects without syncope, a simplified protocol was proposed by Morillo et al.[6] and Natale et al.[7] in 1995. This consists of low-dose isoproterenol tilt testing, in which, after 15–20 min of baseline tilt at 60–70°, incremental doses of isoproterenol designed to increase average heart rate by about 20–25% over baseline (usually ≤3 μg/min) are administered with or without returning the patient to the supine position. Cardioinhibitory (asystolic) responses are only rarely induced because of the positive chronotropic action of isoproterenol.

> *Advantages*: high positivity rate (60%); short duration.
> *Disadvantages*: acceptable false positivity rate with low dose (<10%), higher with an infusion of 3 μg/min (25%); non-physiologic; drug-related adverse effects; relative contraindication in patients with structural heart disease due to risk of tachyarrhythmias and myocardial ischemia; need for cannulation.

The best diagnostic accuracy is probably obtained with the following:

> *Protocol*: supine pre-tilt phase of at least 10–15 min (venous cannulation); tilt angle of 60–70°, passive phase of 15–20 min; if negative the patient receives incremental infusion rate of isoproterenol from 1 up to 3 μg/min in order to increase average heart rate by about 20–25% over baseline, with or without returning the patient to the supine position, then tilt continued for 10 min.

18.2.3 Nitroglycerin Challenge (the Italian Protocol)

This protocol was proposed by Raviele et al. in 1994 with intravenous nitroglycerin infusion, then substituted by sublingual nitroglycerin 300 μg in 1995.[8,9] Several studies that have compared this test with isoproterenol showed essentially similar diagnostic accuracy, but nitroglycerin had no adverse effect. Moreover, unlike with isoproterenol, nitroglycerin protocol resulted in cardioinhibitory (asystolic) responses in up to 25% of positive responses. Finally, a simplified shortened protocol using 400 μg was proposed in 2000 by an Italian task force.[10]

> *Advantages*: high positivity rate (60%); short duration; no adverse effects, cardioinhibitory responses. Probably the protocol most widely used in clinical practice outside North America and the one that has been most thoroughly evaluated in clinical trials.

Disadvantages: acceptable false positivity rate (<10%) and may induce exaggerated responses (now called delayed orthostatic hypotension), especially in the older individuals (approximately 15%) that should be differentiated from the vasovagal responses.

The best diagnostic accuracy is probably obtained with the following:

Protocol: supine pre-tilt phase of at least 5 min without venous cannulation; tilt angle is 60–70°, passive phase of 15–20 min; if negative the patient receives a fixed dose of 400 μg nitroglycerin spray sublingually administered in the upright position, then tilt is continued for 15 min.

18.2.4 *Clomipramine Challenge*

The clomipramine test was proposed by Theodorakis et al.[11] in 2000 and in one study compared favorably with nitroglycerin.[12] Clomipramine, a central serotoninergic agent, is given intravenously during the first 5 min of tilting at a dose of 5 mg (1 mg/min). There is no passive phase. Following this, the patient remains in the upright position for the remaining 15 min.

There is only limited experience with this approach. However, it seems that clomipramine test could be complementary to nitroglycerin. While nitroglycerin acts mainly through peripheral vasodilatation, clomipramine seems to act through a central serotoninergic mechanism. These different mechanisms of action of the two drugs suggest that they could be able to differentiate two clinical forms of vasovagal syncope: those triggered by central mechanism (fear, pain, emotional distress, instrumentation, etc.) should be more sensitive to clomipramine, while those triggered by peripheral mechanisms (e.g., prolong standing or situational events) should be more sensitive to nitroglycerin.

Advantages: high positivity rate (70%) especially for those forms with central triggers, to be confirmed by other studies; short duration

Disadvantages: limited single center experience; acceptable false positivity rate (<10%); mild adverse effects of clomipramine (gastrointestinal); need of cannulation

Protocol: supine pre-tilt phase of at least 20 min (venous cannulation); tilt angle is 60–70°; no passive phase; 20 min of tilt at 60° with intravenous administration of 5 mg clomipramine during the first 5 min of tilting.

18.3 Procedures

Regardless of the protocol used, some general procedures may be suggested.[1] The room where the test is performed should be quiet and only dimly lit. The patients should fast for at least 2 h before the test. When venous cannulation is used, the patients should be in a supine position 20 min before tilting in order to decrease the likelihood of a vasovagal reaction in response to venous cannulation. With the protocols that do not use venous cannulation, time in supine position before tilting can be reduced to 5 min. The tilt table should be able to achieve the upright position smoothly and rapidly and be able to reset to the supine position quickly (<10 s) when the test is completed in order to avoid the consequences of prolonged loss of consciousness. Only tilt tables with foot-board support are appropriate for syncope evaluation. An experienced nurse or medical technician should be in attendance during the entire procedure. The need for a physician to be present throughout the tilt-test procedure is less well established because the risk to patients of such testing is very low. Therefore, it is sufficient that a physician is in proximity and immediately available should a problem arise.

Minimum monitoring should include continuous surface ECG leads and continuous beat-to-beat non-invasive arterial blood pressure. The most desirable devices for beat-to-beat non-invasive blood pressure are those that use the method of Penaz to record the arterial waveform indirectly from a finger (Fig. 18.1). Studies on the accuracy of this measurement system have suggested little systematic bias versus intra-arterial pressure but substantial variability. Intermittent measurement of pressure using a sphygmomanometer or automatic arm-cuff devices is discouraged because they are unable to detect blood pressure pattern and excessively interfere with autonomic state (due to the repetitive cuff inflations). Additional useful features are the continuous display of calculated hemodynamic parameters (cardiac output,

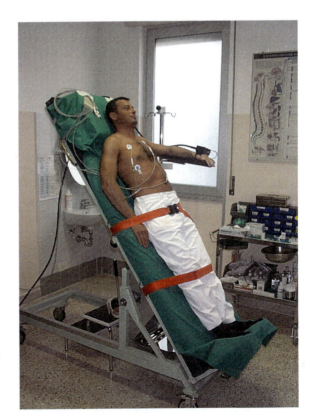

Fig. 18.1 Tilt-table testing. During the test the patient is monitored continuously with surface ECG leads and non-invasive beat-to-beat finger blood pressure. Note that the left arm is kept at the level of the heart in order to obtain finger blood pressure measures consistent with those at the level of the heart

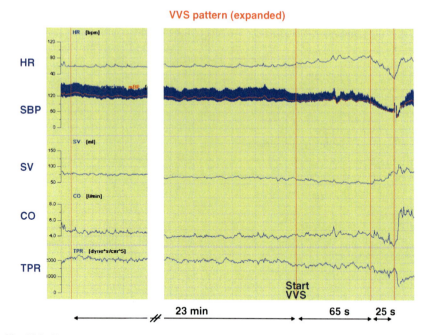

Fig. 18.2 Hemodynamic pattern of a patient with a mixed vasovagal syncope. The reflex reaction starts 23 min after standing. During the initial 65 s there is a compensatory phase which is characterized by mild drop in peripheral resistance and stroke volume, but only a slight blood pressure drop because of the activation of a compensatory tachycardia that preserves cardiac output. The start of the vagal reflex is evidenced by the progressive bradycardia. Cardiac output falls together with peripheral resistance and causes a decline of blood pressure to critical values insufficient to maintain sufficient cerebral blood flow and syncope occurs. Recorded by Task Force monitor (CNSystem, Austria)

stroke volume, peripheral resistances, and related parameters): even if not necessary for diagnosis of syncope, hemodynamic measurements are useful for a more precise understanding of the pathophysiological mechanism (Figs. 18.2 and 18.3). On the other hand, while the tilt-test findings identify susceptibility to reflex syncope, they cannot predict the basis of a spontaneous faint in the patient (although, induced prolonged asystole may have predictive value according to the ISSUE trial observations).

18.4 Case Study #4: Cardioinhibitory Vasovagal Syncope

18.4.1 Results from the Initial Evaluation

History taking

- *Present illness*. This 60-year-old female reports that she has been suffering syncopal episodes since her youth. In recent years the episodes

POH pattern

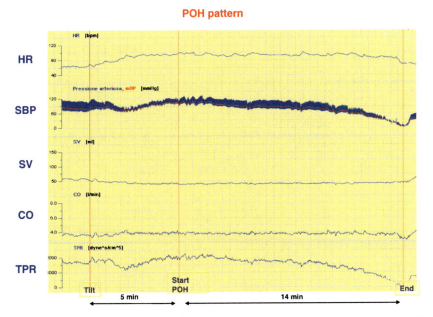

Fig. 18.3 Hemodynamic pattern of a patient with delayed orthostatic hypotension syndrome. The reflex reaction starts a few minutes after standing and the subsequent hypotensive phase is prolonged. After 5 min of standing (start), total vascular resistances decrease progressively together with systolic blood pressure (SBP), up to a critical value which causes presyncope (end). Stroke volume and cardiac output show minor variation. Recorded by Task Force monitor (CNSystem, Austria)

have become more frequent; they usually occurred in clusters of four to five episodes within a few hours. The events were not triggered by any known circumstance, but were frequently preceded by nausea and vomiting and long prodromes ("feeling to be about to faint"). The patient could not prevent the episodes even by assuming the supine position. Some of these occurred while already supine. The loss of consciousness was of brief duration, but it was followed by weakness and fatigue for 24 h during which she was incapacitated from her normal daily activity. She never had trauma as a consequence of faints, but she was very distressed.

– *Past illnesses.* No known cardiac or other diseases. Because of the recurrent syncopal episodes, she had already undergone several electrocardiograms, an echocardiogram, a 24-h Holter, a stress test, an electroencephalogram, a CT scan, and carotid echo-Doppler imaging; all of these were non-diagnostic. She is not taking any medication.

Physical Exam

– No apparent distress; alert; and oriented to time, place, and person.
– Vitals: BP 140/80, HR 62 supine and 140/90, 64 standing, respectively.
– Cardiovascular: regular rhythm, no murmur.

    – Neurological: nonfocal, no gait disturbance.
    – Remainder of exam is unremarkable.

Standard 12-lead ECG

    – Sinus rhythm at 74 bpm, normal.

Results from the initial evaluation: syncopal loss of consciousness, cardiac unlikely, recurrent and severe symptoms.

   Interpretation of the findings of the initial evaluation. Although non-diagnostic, some features of the initial evaluation suggest a possible reflex cause of syncope. Among those listed in Table 5.3 are the absence of structural heart disease, the long history of syncope, and the accompanying symptoms of autonomic activation (nausea and vomiting). Moreover, the EGSYS score value is –1 which suggests a reflex cause. However, the diagnostic criteria of the ESC guidelines for reflex syncope are not completely met because they require the evidence of a trigger, which in this case is unknown. Furthermore, the finding of syncope occurring in supine position is unusual for reflex syncope, being more frequent in cardiac syncope. Finally, the

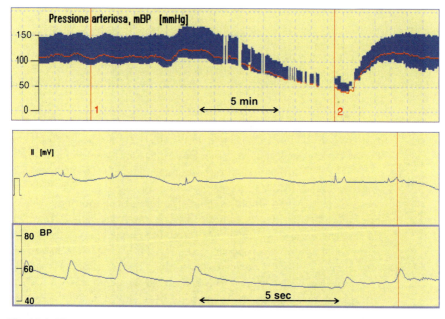

Fig. 18.4 *Upper panel*: The *top trace* shows systolic, diastolic, and mean blood pressure curves. Only drug challenge phase is shown (*vertical line 1*). Seven minutes after oral 400 μg spray nitroglycerin administration (*vertical line 2*), the patient showed a typical symptomatic hypotension reflex with drop in arterial blood pressure until 65 mmHg and syncope. At the time of syncope (expanded in the *lower panel*), the ECG showed progressive severe bradycardia with a maximum pause of 5 s. She recovered spontaneously and completely a few minutes after rhythm resumption, but she had vomiting and experienced severe weakness which persisted for a few hours. Recorded by Task Force monitor (CNSystem, Austria)

very long recovery period is uncommon in reflex syncopal patients (although prolonged periods of fatigue are relatively common). In any case, the likely diagnosis
is reflex syncope of an atypical form and further diagnostic evaluation by carotid
sinus massage and tilt-table testing is warranted (see also Table 11.5). Finally, apart
from its diagnostic value, tilt-table testing is also indicated in order to train the
patient to recognize reflex susceptibility and to permit the patient to start physical
maneuvers designed to prevent syncopal recurrences (see also biofeedback training,
Chapter 11).

Thus, carotid sinus massage and tilt testing were performed. Carotid sinus
massage was negative. Tilt-table testing induced, 3 min after administration of
nitroglycerin challenge, a cardioinhibitory response with an asystolic pause of 5 s
duration (Fig. 18.4). Syncope was preceded and followed by symptoms that the
patient recognized as very similar to the spontaneous ones.

Conclusion: Cardioinhibitory vasovagal syncope. The patient was trained in
counterpressure maneuvers and was scheduled for follow-up visit.

Follow-Up: The patient came for follow-up visit after 6 months. She reported
having had recently experienced three syncope episodes at rest, while supine, from
8 to 12 pm. She immediately started counterpressure maneuvers, but she felt so

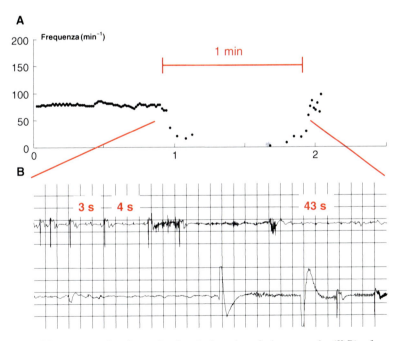

Fig. 18.5 ECG documentation, 3 months after the insertion of a loop recorder (ILR), of a spontaneous syncopal episode. The *upper panel* shows heart rate trend. At the time of syncope there is a
short and rapid decrease in heart rate followed by asystole. The expanded ECG at that time (*lower
panel*) shows sinus bradycardia plus AV block with multiple pauses, the longest of which was 43 s.
This pattern has been defined as form 1B of the ISSUE classification (see Chapter 8)

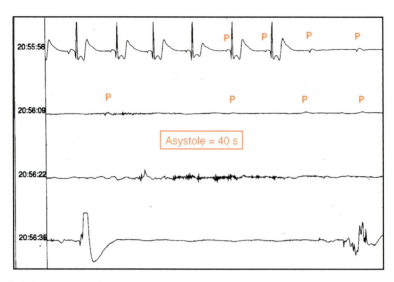

Fig. 18.6 Same patient of Fig. 18.5. The patient exhibits marked bradycardia in association with syncope. Subsequently, a few hours later, she had a second syncopal episode similar to this one. During the pause, initially there are three blocked P waves followed by prolonged sinus arrest

weak that she was unable to contract the muscles with sufficient strength. At this point, cardiac pacing can be considered due to the documentation of an asystolic pause during tilt testing. However, this is a weak indication for pacing, being ranked class IIB only in the ESC guidelines owing to contradictory results of randomized

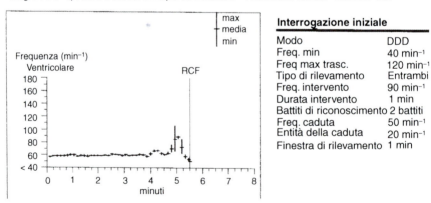

Fig. 18.7 Same patient of Figs. 18.5 and 18.6 after DDD pacemaker implantation provided with rate drop response feature. The pacemaker interrogation during a follow-up visit shows a likely vasovagal episode aborted by intervention of the pacemaker (RCF). After an initial increase of heart rate up to 90 bpm, there was a fall in heart rate up to the programmed value of intervention of rate hysteresis of the pacemaker. The patient was at rest and reported symptoms of impending syncope coincident with the recorded episode

trials and different opinions among clinicians. On the other hand, a recent ISSUE 2 sub-study[13] has shown that an asystolic pause during tilt-table testing is 80% predictive that spontaneous syncope is also due to asystole/severe bradycardia, thus potentially benefitting from cardiac pacing. However, this result comes from a small number of observations of a single study and cannot be regarded as definitive. The guidelines recommend attempting to document a spontaneous syncopal event before embarking in cardiac pacing (see Chapter 8).

An implantable loop recorder (ILR) was inserted which, 3 months later, documented two episodes of syncope: both were characterized by long pauses due to AV block plus sinus bradycardia (type 1B of the ISSUE classification) (Figs. 18.5 and 18.6). A DDD pacemaker with rate-drop features was finally implanted. During the subsequent 2 years the patient has had no more syncopes despite frequently a feeling of an impending faint. Interrogation of the pacemaker after one such occasion documented episodes of activation of the pacing function preceded by a typical phase of progressive increase and then decrease of heart rate (Fig. 18.7).

References

1. Benditt DG, et al. Tilt table testing for assessing syncope. ACC expert consensus document. *J Am Coll Cardiol.* 1996;28:263–275.
2. Kenny RA, et al. Head-up tilt: a useful test for investigating unexplained syncope. *Lancet.* 1986;14(1):1352–1355.
3. Fitzpatrick AP, et al. Methodology of head-up tilt testing in patients with unexplained syncope. *J Am Coll Cardiol.* 1991;17:125–130.
4. Almquist A, et al. Provocation of bradycardia and hypotension by isoproterenol and upright posture in patients with unexplained syncope. *N Engl J Med.* 1989;320:346–351.
5. Waxman MB, et al. Isoproterenol induction of vasodepressor-type reaction in vasodepressor-prone persons. *Am J Cardiol.* 1989;63:58–65.
6. Morillo CA, et al. Diagnostic accuracy of a low-dose isoproterenol head-up tilt protocol. *Am Heart J.* 1995;129:901–906.
7. Natale A, et al. Provocation of hypotension during head-up tilt testing in subjects with no history of syncope or presyncope. *Circulation.* 1995;92:54–58.
8. Raviele A, et al. Nitroglycerin infusion during upright tilt: a new test for the diagnosis of vasovagal syncope. *Am Heart J.* 1994;127:103–111.
9. Raviele A, et al. Value of head-up tilt testing potentiated with sublingual nitroglycerin to assess the origin of unexplained syncope. *Am J Cardiol.* 1995;76:267–272.
10. Bartoletti A, et al. 'The Italian Protocol': a simplified head-up tilt testing potentiated with oral nitroglycerin to assess patients with unexplained syncope. *Europace.* 2000;2:339–342.
11. Theodorakis GN, et al. Central serotonergic responsiveness in neurocardiogenic syncope: a clomipramine test challenge. *Circulation.* 1998;98:2724–2730.
12. Flevari P, et al. Recurrent vasovagal syncope: comparison between clomipramine and nitroglycerin as drug challenges during head-up tilt testing. *Eur Heart J.* 2009;30:2249–2253.
13. Moya A, et al. Reproducibility of electrocardiographic findings in patients with neurally-mediated syncope. *Am J Cardiol.* 2009;102:1518–1523.

Chapter 19
How to: Prolonged Ambulatory ECG Monitoring

Contents

19.1 External and Implantable Loop Recorders

Prolonged electrocardiographic (ECG) monitoring is among the most valuable tools for determining if T-LOC is due to syncope, and thereafter substantiating the cause of syncope. Currently, the available prolonged ECG monitoring techniques include in-hospital telemetry, 1- to 7-day ambulatory Holter monitoring, external loop recorders (ELRs), remote (at home) telemetry, and implantable loop recorders (ILRs).[1,2] Certain of the most common ILRs are shown in Fig. 19.1 and their characteristics are listed in Table 19.1. All have in common the possibility of manual and automatic recording and the possibility of remote transmission to medical center. However, the modalities of recording and transmission vary from model to model and at present, only one offers automatic remote telemetry (although this latter device is not currently being distributed commercially). Some of the most common ELRs and remote telemetric monitors are shown in Figs. 19.2 and 19.3 and their characteristics are listed in Table 19.2. As was the case with IRs, all have in common the possibility of manual and automatic recording and the possibility of remote transmission to the medical center. Since the diagnostic criteria are the same

M. Brignole, D.G. Benditt, *Syncope*, DOI 10.1007/978-0-85729-201-8_19,
© Springer-Verlag London Limited 2011

for all ECG monitoring systems, the choice of device is a function of the risk of life-threatening events and of the frequency of symptoms (i.e., effectiveness is limited by the relation between recording duration and expected likelihood of an episode occurring during that time period) (Table 19.3).

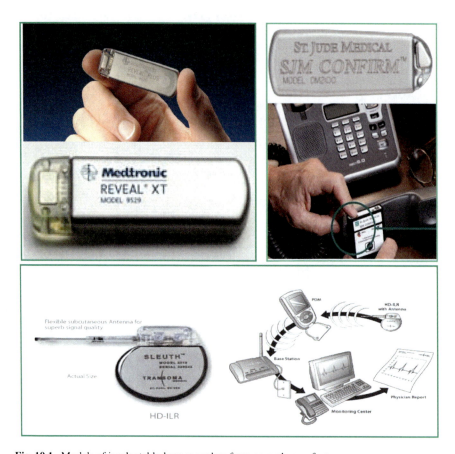

Fig. 19.1 Models of implantable loop recorders from several manufacturers

Table 19.1 Most common implantable loop recorders

Device/company	Expected monitoring duration	Total memory	Loop memory (patient activated)	Brady algorithms (auto-activated)	Tachy algorithms (auto-activated)	AF detection algorithms	Remote data transmission	Additional features
Reveal DX, Medtronic	3 years	49.5 min	6.5′ pre+1′ post each (× 3 episodes)	Asystole and bradycardia (physician defined)	SVT and VT discrimination: 16 consecutive intervals and probabilistic fast tachycardia (12/16 intervals), programmable rate boundary	No	Data stored in the device are sent on demand through a telephone transmission to a web server. Physician accesses data via internet with a secure log-in. Full access to all actual and historical diagnostic data and episodes	Sensing and detection algorithm; MRI conditional (1.5 and 3 T)

Table 19.1 (continued)

Device/company	Expected monitoring duration	Total memory	Loop memory (patient activated)	Brady algorithms (auto-activated)	Tachy algorithms (auto-activated)	AF detection algorithms	Remote data transmission	Additional features
Reveal XT, Medtronic	3 years	49.5 min	6.5' pre+1' post each (× 3 episodes)	Asystole and bradycardia (physician defined)	SVT and VT discrimination: 16 consecutive intervals and probabilistic fast tachycardia (12/16 intervals), programmable rate boundary	Yes	Data stored in the device are sent on demand through a telephone transmission to a web server. Physician accesses data via Internet with a secure log-in. Full access to all actual and historical diagnostic data and episodes	As reveal DX + AF burden (incl. trend), HR variability, HR day/night, patient activity, V-rate histograms

Table 19.1 (continued)

Device/company	Expected monitoring duration	Total memory	Loop memory (patient activated)	Brady algorithms (auto-activated)	Tachy algorithms (auto-activated)	AF detection algorithms	Remote data transmission	Additional features
Sleuth, Transoma[a]	28 months	630 min	3+2 min	When one R–R interval is less than the low heart rate setting	When six of eight consecutive R–R intervals are greater than the high heart rate setting	No	Wireless (real-time) to personal data manager and then trans-telephonic to service center. Daily + urgent reports from service center to physician	HR trending data every 4 h
Confirm DM2100 St Jude	3 years	48 min (147 episodes)	1'–6' pre + 0.5'–1' post	Asystole and bradycardia (physician defined)	Tachycardia (physician defined)	No	Data stored in the device are sent on demand through an analogic telephone transmission to physician. Local software for analysis	HR trending data

Table 19.1 (continued)

Device/company	Expected monitoring duration	Total memory	Loop memory (patient activated)	Brady algorithms (auto-activated)	Tachy algorithms (auto-activated)	AF detection algorithms	Remote data transmission	Additional features
Confirm DM 2102 St Jude	3 years	48 min (147 episodes)	1′–6′ pre + 0.5′–1′ post	Asystole and bradycardia (physician defined)	SVT and VT discrimination algorithm programmable rate boundary	Yes	Data stored in the device are sent on demand through an analogic telephone transmission to physician. Local software for analysis	AF burden

ᵃNot in commerce currently.

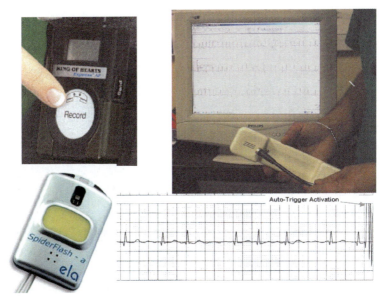

Fig. 19.2 Examples of models of external loop recorders that use dial-in trans-telephonic transmission systems

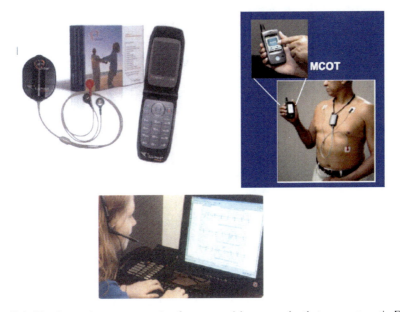

Fig. 19.3 The figure shows an example of an external loop recorder that uses automatic ECG transmission of predefined events via Bluetooth wireless link to service center. Then, daily as well as urgent recordings (those meeting pre-determined physician-selected criteria) are reported to an experienced ECG reared at a service center and then if appropriate sent from the service center to the patient's physician

Table 19.2 Most common external loop recorders and mobile (remote) telemetric monitors

Device/company	Expected monitoring duration[a]	Total memory	Loop memory (patient activated)	Brady algorithms (auto-activated)	Tachy algorithms (auto-activated)	AF detection algorithms	Remote data transmission	Additional features
Nuvant, Corventis	Few weeks	1 week	15″ pre + 30″ post	Asystole and bradycardia, 15″ pre + 30″ post	A and V tachycardia, AV block, rhythm during fall	Yes	*Continuous* or 24-h loop memory, wireless (real-time) to personal data manager and then trans-telephonic to service center. Physician accesses data via Internet with a secure log-in. Full access to all actual and historical diagnostic data and episodes	HR trending data
MCOT[a], Cardionet	Few weeks	21 days continuous monitoring	Patient's notes	Asystole and bradycardia, programmable duration	Rhythm changes and morphology	Yes (if applicable)	*Continuous* or 24-h loop memory, wireless (real-time) to personal data manager and then trans-telephonic to service center. Daily + urgent reports from service center to physician	HR trending data

Table 19.2 (continued)

Device/company	Expected monitoring duration[a]	Total memory	Loop memory (patient activated)	Brady algorithms (auto-activated)	Tachy algorithms (auto-activated)	AF detection algorithms	Remote data transmission	Additional features
LifeStar ACT, LifeWatch	Few weeks	21 days retrievable monitoring	1' pre + 0.5' post (total 20')	Asystole and bradycardia, programmable duration	No	Yes	Automatic ECG transmission of predefined events via Bluetooth wireless link to service center. Daily + urgent reports from service center to physician	Remotely programmable. Daily summary reports
LifeStar, LifeWatch	Few weeks	10 min	1' pre + 0.5' post (total 9')	Asystole and bradycardia, programmable duration	No	Yes (when enabled)	Dial-in trans-telephonic (delayed on demand) or via service center (fax, e-mail) or when the device is returned. Local software for analysis	

Table 19.2 (continued)

Device/company	Expected monitoring duration[a]	Total memory	Loop memory (patient activated)	Brady algorithms (auto-activated)	Tachy algorithms (auto-activated)	AF detection algorithms	Remote data transmission	Additional features
eVolution, eCardio	Few weeks	30 min	Six events (total 9')	Asystole and bradycardia, programmable duration	No	Yes	Automatic ECG transmission of predefined events via Bluetooth wireless link or over telephone line. Physician accesses data via Internet with a secure log-in	
3300 BT, Vitaphone	Few weeks	20 min	5 pre-/post-time settings, max 15 events	Asystole and bradycardia	Tachycardia	Yes	Automatic ECG transmission of predefined events via Bluetooth wireless link. Physician accesses data via Internet with a secure log-in	Display and acoustic feedback

Table 19.2 (continued)

Device/company	Expected monitoring duration[a]	Total memory	Loop memory (patient activated)	Brady algorithms (auto-activated)	Tachy algorithms (auto-activated)	AF detection algorithms	Remote data transmission	Additional features
V-PATCH, Medical System	Few weeks	30 h	30 s pre-/30 s post	Asystole and bradycardia	Tachycardia	No	Automatic ECG transmission of predefined events via Bluetooth wireless link. Physician accesses data via Internet with a secure log-in	
King of the Heart, Instromedics	Few weeks	6 min	1–60 events	Bradycardia (physician defined)	Tachycardia (physician defined)	Yes	Dial-in trans-telephonic (delayed on demand) or via service center (fax, e-mail) or when the device is returned. Local software for analysis	
SpiderFlash, Sorin	Few weeks	Several hours[c]	7.5′–15′ pre + 7.5′–15′ post (× 1–2 episodes)	No	No	No	Dial-in trans-telephonic (delayed on demand) or when the device is returned. Local software for analysis	Daily auto-trigger ECG (max 15 min)

Table 19.2 (continued)

Device/company	Expected monitoring duration[a]	Total memory	Loop memory (patient activated)	Brady algorithms (auto-activated)	Tachy algorithms (auto-activated)	AF detection algorithms	Remote data transmission	Additional features
Cardiocall, Reynolds Esaote	Few weeks	18 min	3'–16 pre + 1'–2' post	No	No	No	Dial-in trans-telephonic (delayed on demand) or when the device is returned	
Super, I-Cardia	Depends on patient compliance	Two recordings	40 s + 40 s each (× 2 episodes)	No	No	No	Trans-telephonic (delayed on demand) or via service center (fax, e-mail)	Disposable
Cardio PAL, Medicomp	Depends on patient compliance	NA	No	No	No	Yes	Via service center (fax, e-mail)	AF burden detection (real-time analysis)

[a] Monitoring duration is determined by average maximum patients' compliance for external devices.
[b] Mobile cardiac outpatient telemetry.
[c] Depends on memory card capacity.

Table 19.3 Table depicting recommendations for the best choice of ECG monitoring devices

Risk or symptoms frequency	In-hospital telemetry	1- to 7-day Holter	ELR	Remote (home) telemetry	ILR
High-risk criteria (see Chapter 6)	X				
≥ 1 event/week		X			
≥ 1 event/month			X	X	
≥ 1 event/year					X

19.2 Case Study # 4: Spontaneous Cardioinhibitory Vasovagal Syncope

Case study # 4, described in Chapter 18, provides an example of the use of ILR in order to confirm a suspected cardioinhibitory vasovagal syncope; the ILR was used before considering permanent cardiac pacing in a patient with recurrent severe syncope and an asystolic response during tilt testing (Fig. 18.4). The ILR (Figs. 18.5 and Fig. 18.6) documented long pauses due to AV block plus sinus bradycardia (type 1B of the ISSUE classification [3]). This case represents an example of class II indication for ILR according to the recent European guidelines and a class IIA indication for cardiac pacing. In the ISSUE 2 study, the patients with type 1 collapse pattern who received a pacemaker implant had a 90% risk reduction of recurrences compared to those who were not paced: syncope recurred in 9% versus 31%, respectively, during a follow-up of 2 years.[3] See also Chapter 8.

19.3 Case Study # 5: Spontaneous Syncope Without Heart Rate Variations

Case study # 5 provides an example of the use of an ILR to determine the mechanism of syncope in a 56-year-old patient with recurrent severe apparent syncope episodes. An ILR was implanted which documented no variations of heart rate at the time of "syncope" recurrence (Fig. 19.4). This is an example of type 3 pattern of the ISSUE classification.[4] Contrary to case #4, this patient had a mixed response during tilt testing. The ISSUE 2 study showed that the mixed pattern observed during tilting was poorly correlated with that observed during spontaneous syncope and, therefore, a documentation of spontaneous syncope was still necessary for diagnosis.[5] In the ISSUE 2 study, the probability of an asystolic spontaneous syncope in patients with mixed response to tilt testing was 31%. Therefore, an empirical pacemaker implantation is unlikely to prevent recurrences. Indeed, pacemaker implantation is ranked as class III in the European guidelines. This case represents an example of class IIA indication for ILR according to the recent European guidelines. See also Chapter 8.

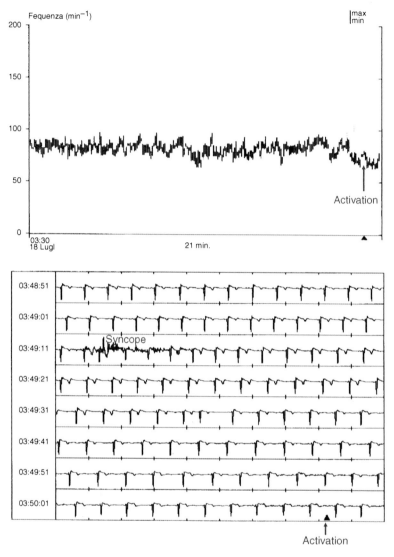

Fig. 19.4 Type 3 pattern of the ISSUE classification (see Chapter 8). *Upper panel*: Heart rate trend which shows no apparent variations before manual activation of the ILR immediately after the syncopal event. ECG findings are confirmed by the expanded tracing at the time of syncope (*lower panel*)

19.4   Case Study # 6: Differentiating Intrinsic Versus Extrinsic Intermittent Sinoatrial Block

Differentiating intrinsic versus extrinsic intermittent sinoatrial block is often challenging. However, the ECG documentation of spontaneous episodes is helpful for differentiating intrinsic disease of the sinoatrial node which causes impairment of its automatic properties (Fig. 19.5) from an extrinsic abnormal reflex vagal output which temporarily inhibits the function of an otherwise normal sinoatrial node (Fig. 19.6). This differentiation is not only of pathophysiological interest but also of practical importance for therapy. Indeed, while cardiac pacing is usually always useful when an intrinsic disorder is present, its use should be individually and carefully

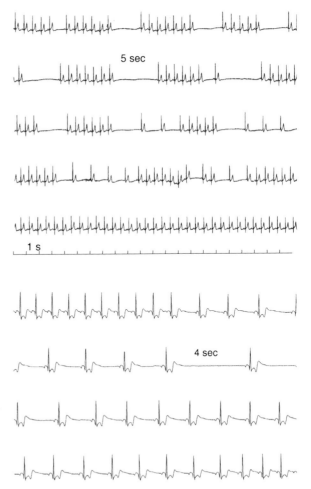

Fig. 19.5 ECG traces from a patient who had normal sinus rhythm interrupted by repetitive episodes of sinoatrial block. The episodes of sinoatrial block occur suddenly and the pauses are multiple of the sinus cycle length. This feature suggests an intrinsic disease of the sinoatrial node (sick sinus syndrome)

Fig. 19.6 ECG traces from a patient who had a progressive sinus bradycardia, then a longer pause of 4 s and finally a progressive resumption of the baseline rhythm. This pattern has been described as "type 1A" in the ISSUE classification (see Chapter 8). This feature suggests an extrinsic (reflex) mechanism

considered for treatment of reflex forms based on the frequency and severity of symptoms and age of the patient (i.e., avoiding unneeded implatation of pacemakers in the young).

19.5 Case Study # 7: Swallowing Syncope

19.5.1 Initial Evaluation

This 43-year-old female reports that she has experienced several episodes of T-LOC during the past 2 weeks. The episodes occurred suddenly during painful swallowing and have occurred both in supine and in upright position; they were not preceded by prodromes, but were followed by jerking movements and rapid recovery of consciousness. Minor trauma had occurred in some cases. The patient indicated that she was suffering, at the same period, of throat pain localized in the right side of the neck with exacerbation during swallowing and to have taken antibiotic therapy in the previous days for fever. She was unable to drink or to eat because every attempt at swallowing caused symptoms.

Results from the initial evaluation: The history of the present illness is sufficient to diagnose "swallow (reflex) syncope" (see Chapter 5). Investigation, however, is useful in order to determine the exact mechanism of syncope, its etiology, and the proper therapy.

Management: The patient was admitted to the cardiology department. During continuous ECG and blood pressure monitoring, the patient was asked to swallow some food. Again she had pain during swallowing immediately followed by loss of consciousness; at that time the ECG showed bradycardia with some pauses, the longest of which was of 12.5 s and a fall of systolic blood pressure to 50 mmHg (Fig. 19.7). The test was repeated after intravenous atropine administration (0.02 mg/kg); the drug was able to prevent bradycardia, hypotension, and syncope.

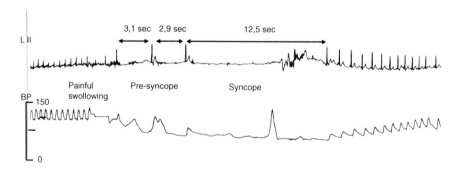

Fig. 19.7 Swallow syncope. For explanation, see text

The patient was initially treated with atropine 1 mg i.v. every 4 h for 24 h which prevented further episodes. Moreover, a back-up temporary pacemaker was positioned via right jugular vein which intervened properly any time that the patients had bradycardia thus avoiding symptom relapse.

Otorhinolaryngological and neurological evaluation showed the presence of hyperesthesia of the right glossopharyngeal nerve that, during the visit, triggered the cardioinhibitory syncope. A diagnosis of glossopharyngeal neuralgia was made and treatment with gabapentin 900 mg/day (300 mg t.i.d.) was started. Five days from the onset of that treatment the painful pharyngeal spasm completely disappeared; the patient has had no further episodes of asystole and/or syncope, and temporary pacemaker could be removed. She was discharged on the seventh day and continued therapy for 1 month. During the following 2 years she had no syncope recurrences.

Conclusion: reflex syncope, situational (swallowing), and glossopharyngeal neuralgia

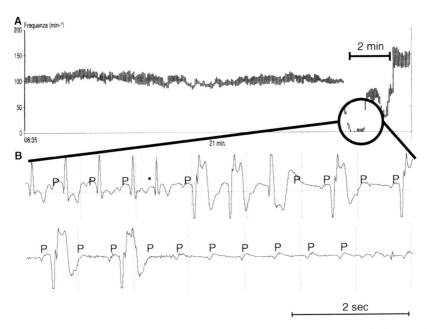

Fig. 19.8 Recordings from a patient who had sudden-onset AV block (and ventricular pause) triggered by an atrial premature beats. This pattern has been described as "type 1C" in the ISSUE classification (see Chapter 8). This feature suggests an intrinsic His–Purkinje disease. *Panel a*: Heart rate trend during the whole 21-min loop recording. Initially, the heart rate is stable at 100 bpm and suddenly falls at the time of the syncope. *Panel b*: Expanded ECG shows a premature atrial beat (∗) that seems to trigger the AV block. Initially during the block, there are seven idioventricular beats, then prolonged asystole occurs

19.6 Case Study # 8: Spontaneous Stokes–Adams Syncopal Attack

Patients with syncope and bundle branch block (BBB) are at high risk of developing atrioventricular block, but syncope can also be due to other etiologies such as ventricular and supraventricular tachycardia, carotid sinus syndrome, and neurally mediated or orthostatic hypotension. If syncope remains unexplained after complete workup, including an electrophysiological study, then it is prudent to try and document the cause of syncope by means of an ILR. This is a class I indication for an ILR according to the recent European guidelines as syncope may not recur in 1/2 of patients for more than 2 years [6], and without an ILR, making an accurate diagnosis would be almost impossible.

Figure 19.8 shows the case of a 67-year-old male with unexplained syncope and BBB who, after 77 days from ILR implantation, had a syncopal recurrence that was documented to be due to paroxysmal AV block. Cardiac pacing was indicated based on this definitive observation.

References

1. Moya A, et al. Guidelines for the Diagnosis and Management of Syncope (Version 2009). *Eur Heart J*. 2009;30:2631–2671.
2. Brignole M, et al. Indications for the use of diagnostic implantable and external ECG loop recorders. *Europace*. 2009;11:671–687.
3. Brignole M, et al. Early application of an implantable loop recorder allows effective specific therapy in patients with recurrent suspected neutrally-mediated syncope. *Eur Heart J*. 2006;27:1085–1092.
4. Brignole M, et al. Proposed electrocardiographic classification of spontaneous syncope documented by an Implantable Loop Recorder. *Europace*. 2005;7:14–18.
5. Brignole M, et al. Lack of correlation between the responses to tilt testing and adenosine triphosphate test and the mechanism of spontaneous neurally-mediated syncope. *Eur Heart J*. 2006;27:2232–2239.
6. Brignole M, et al. The mechanism of syncope in patients with bundle branch block and negative electrophysiologic test. *Circulation*. 2001;104:2045–2050.

Chapter 20
When and How: Electrophysiological Study (EPS)

Contents

20.1 Introduction

The gold standard for diagnosis of arrhythmia-induced syncope is correlation of abnormal ECG findings of spontaneous cardiac arrhythmias with symptoms (i.e., syncope). Obtaining such documentation is usually best achieved by ambulatory electrocardiographic (ECG) recording (e.g., "Holter" monitors, "event" recorders, mobile cardiac outpatient telemetry (MCOT), or insertable loop recorders (ILRs)). However, in many patients it may not be possible to obtain such documentation due to the infrequency of symptomatic events, or concerns regarding patient safety should a spontaneous recurrence be associated with a life-threatening circumstance or potential for physical injury. In such cases, electrophysiological study (EPS) may be warranted in an attempt to obtain at least a plausible cause for the symptoms. This is particularly the case in those individuals with an abnormal ECG and/or evidence underlying structural heart disease.

The role of EPS in the laboratory evaluation of syncope patients was introduced in Chapter 7. Here we provide a more comprehensive treatment of EPS indications and methodology.

M. Brignole, D.G. Benditt, *Syncope*, DOI 10.1007/978-0-85729-201-8_20,
© Springer-Verlag London Limited 2011

The diagnostic utility of EPS is highly dependent on the degree of suspicion of a conduction disturbance or arrhythmic cause of symptoms (pretest probability), the stimulation protocol, and the criteria used for diagnosis of clinically significant abnormalities. In the management of syncope, EPS may play a role in determining whether the fainter is susceptible to certain cardiac arrhythmias or conduction disturbances that may have been responsible for the symptoms. As a consequence, EPS observations may provide valuable, albeit usually inferential, evidence of the cause of syncope and thereby allow initiation of an effective treatment strategy.

Arrhythmic syncope, potentially amenable to EPS assessment, may be caused by either bradycardias or tachycardias; careful application of EPS techniques by experienced practitioners may help to elucidate the precise cause(s). The most important categories of arrhythmias subject to EPS evaluation are

- sinus node dysfunction (including bradycardia–tachycardia syndrome),
- atrioventricular (AV) conduction system disease,
- paroxysmal supraventricular tachycardia (including preexcitation),
- ventricular tachycardia, including certain inherited syndromes (e.g., long QT syndrome, Brugada syndrome), and
- implanted device (pacemaker, defibrillator) malfunction.

20.2 EPS Indications in Syncope

As has been emphasized throughout this volume, the optimal evaluation of syncope patients begins with a careful medical history taking a thorough physical examination and if necessary certain non-invasive tests such as a 12-lead ECG, an echocardiogram, and possibly ambulatory ECG (AECG) monitoring. These initial steps are discussed in detail in other chapters.

EPS should be reserved for those cases in which initial evaluation is non-diagnostic (i.e., the medical history does not provide a solid diagnosis, ambulatory ECG recordings are unable to obtain a spontaneous symptom-ECG correlation, etc.) (Table 20.1).[1] In this regard, EPS is typically of greatest value in patients with known structural heart disease.[1,2] However, EPS testing may also be very effective in a number of other selected scenarios in which structural disease may not be present or at least not immediately apparent (e.g., patients with paroxysmal supraventricular tachycardia (PSVT) and patients with idiopathic ventricular tachycardia). Additionally, although more controversial, EPS may be helpful in assessing patients with suspected Brugada syndrome or with arrhythmogenic right ventricular dysplasia/cardiomyopathy (ARVD/C).

In syncope patients with an abnormal ECG (apart from the preexcitation syndromes and channelopathies) and/or evidence of structural heart disease, cardiac conduction system disease and/or ventricular tachyarrhythmias (VTs) are a major clinical concern (Table 20.2). In such cases (absent direct ambulatory ECG recordings during spontaneous events), demonstration of a "fragile" conduction system, or

Table 20.1 Indications for electrophysiological testing for syncope[1]

Class I

• EPS is indicated when the initial evaluation suggests an arrhythmic cause of syncope. Risk factor include
  – abnormal electrocardiography
  – structural heart disease
  – syncope associated with palpitations or chest pain
  – syncope during exertion or in the supine position
  – family history of sudden death

Class II

• To evaluate the nature of an arrhythmia that has already been identified as the cause of the syncope
• In patients with high-risk occupations, in whom every effort to exclude a cardiac cause of syncope is warranted

Class III

• In patients with normal ECG, no structural heart disease or palpitations

Table 20.2 ECG abnormalities suggesting an arrhythmic syncope

• Bifascicular block (defined as either left bundle branch block or right bundle branch block combined with left anterior or left posterior fascicular block)
• Intraventricular conduction abnormalities resulting in wide QRS duration ≥ 0.12 s
• Mobitz I second-degree atrioventricular block
• Asymptomatic sinus bradycardia (<50 bpm), sinoatrial block, or sinus pause ≥ 3 s in the absence of negatively chronotropic medications
• Preexcited QRS complexes
• Prolonged QT interval
• Right bundle branch block pattern with ST elevation in leads V_1–V_3 (Brugada syndrome)
• Negative T waves in right precordial leads, epsilon waves, and ventricular late potentials suggestive of arrhythmogenic right ventricular dysplasia (ARVD/C)
• Q waves suggesting myocardial infarction

alternatively induction of a reproducible tachycardia by cardiac stimulation during EPS, may be interpreted to be a plausible basis for symptoms. In this context though, eliciting AV block at rapid pacing rates (>130/min) and initiating polymorphous VT or ventricular fibrillation (VF) are usually not considered relevant observations. In patients with syncope and preexcitation syndrome (e.g., Wolff–Parkinson–White syndrome), EPS also offers the possibility of assessing hemodynamic risk of very rapid heart rates by evaluating accessory connection conduction properties and susceptibility to tachyarrhythmias. In the channelopathies (i.e., long/short QT syndrome, Brugada syndrome) the role of EPS is less certain and more needs to be learned; however, it may have prognostic value.

In syncope patients without either evident structural heart disease or an abnormal baseline ECG, EPS is best used for assessing susceptibility to paroxysmal supraventricular tachycardias (PSVT) as the probable cause or, more rarely, susceptibility to certain idiopathic VTs (e.g., fascicular VTs). In the latter situation (i.e., idiopathic VT), however, ambulatory ECG (AECG) monitoring may be the preferred approach since the suspected arrhythmias are not typically life-threatening, and sustained VT is often difficult to induce. This is also true in the presence of left ventricular hypertrophy as well as in some other more minor forms of structural heart disease in which there is no evidence of clinically significant ventricular dysfunction.

20.3 EPS Techniques

20.3.1 Essential Diagnostic Measurements

As a rule, a conventional EPS procedure requires placement of one or more multi-polar electrode catheters into the heart for recording and stimulation using conventional vascular access techniques (via the great veins and more rarely via arterial access) (Fig. 20.1). These catheters are usually placed at the high right atrium (HRA) near the sinus node region, in the vicinity of the tricuspid valve annulus at the His bundle area (HBE), at the right ventricular apex (RVA), and occasionally within the coronary sinus (CS) vein for left atrial recording and stimulation. Most studies require only venous access (usually the femoral vein). However, arterial access with recording from and stimulation of the left ventricle (LV) may be needed in some circumstances (particularly for evaluation of susceptibility to certain VTs and some PSVTs). Further, arterial access allows for the ready monitoring of systemic pressure. The latter can be a distinct advantage when trying to ascertain the hemodynamic importance of an induced arrhythmia (bearing in mind that the study is carried out with the patient supine, whereas most instances of syncope occur in upright individuals). Finally, use of trans-septal puncture in order to access the left atrium directly has become increasingly important for certain procedures (e.g., mapping and ablation of left-sided accessory AV connections or left atrial tachycardias, isolation of pulmonary veins for treatment of paroxysmal atrial fibrillation). The latter is facilitated by availability of intra-cardiac ultrasound imaging (ICE) to identify the foramen ovale and to confirm positioning of catheters safely in the left atrial chamber.

Baseline EPS measurements usually include (Table 20.3) the following:

- RR interval – the cardiac "rate" measured in terms of cycle length
- PA interval – the interval from onset of atrial electrical activity to the inscription of the low septal right atrial electrogram
- AH interval – the interval from the low right atrial electrogram to the onset of the His bundle potential which provides a measure of conduction time through the AV node
- HV interval – the interval from onset of the His bundle electrogram to the earliest onset of ventricular activation on intra-cardiac or surface ECG provides an estimate of conduction time through the His–Purkinje system
- QRS duration and QT interval

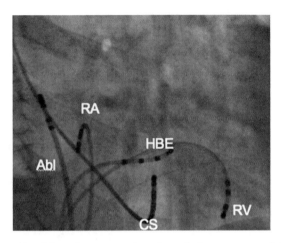

Fig. 20.1 Right anterior oblique fluoroscopy view of a typical arrangement of electrode catheters during EPS. Depending on the circumstances, catheter positions will differ; sometimes including left atrial and left ventricular sites are needed. The catheters in this case are as follows: Abl, an ablation catheter currently resting in the right atrium near the sinus node region; CS, catheter within the coronary sinus; HBE, catheter recording His bundle potentials; RA, catheter at the lateral right atrial wall; RV, catheter at right ventricular apex

Table 20.3 Minimal electrophysiological testing protocol for syncope evaluation

- Measurement of sinus node recovery time (SNRT) and corrected sinus node recovery time (CSRT) by repeated sequences of atrial pacing for 30–60 s with at least one low and two high pacing rates. Suggested "low" pacing rate is started at 10–20 beats above sinus rate. The "higher" rates are then an additional 20–30 bpm above the "low" value. Autonomic blockade may be applied if needed[a]
- Assessment of the His–Purkinje system includes measurement of the HV interval during initial baseline rhythm and again during "stress" of His–Purkinje conduction by incremental atrial pacing (i.e., pacing at increasingly rapid rates until AV block occurs). If HV interval is moderately prolonged, pharmacological provocation is recommended unless contraindicated. Suggested drugs include ajmaline 1 mg/kg or procainamide 10 mg/kg
- Assessment of ventricular arrhythmia inducibility performed by programmed electrical stimulation using up to two extrastimuli (usually with coupling interval not below 180–200 ms) from two right ventricular sites (apex and outflow tract) at two to three drive cycle lengths (typically 600 ms and 500 ms and 400 ms). A third extrastimuli may be added to enhance sensitivity at the cost of reduced specificity
- Assessment of supraventricular arrhythmia inducibility by atrial pacing and premature stimulation protocol. Generally this entails "burst" pacing at cycle lengths as short as 300 ms and use of up to two extrastimuli at two to three drive cycle lengths (typically 600 ms and 500 ms and 400 ms)
- Isoproterenol at doses ranging from 1 to 5 μg/min may be used to facilitate ventricular and supraventricular initiation. Atropine 0.5–1 mg may be used to facilitate induction of supraventricular tachyarrhythmias. However, when these provocative agents are used, care must be taken in the interpretation of the induced arrhythmias to be sure that the observations are consistent with the clinical presentation

[a]Pharmacological autonomic blockade as discussed in the text.

20.3.2 Assessment of Sinus Node Dysfunction (SND)

A transient bradycardia due to SND (also termed sick sinus syndrome or sinus node disease) should be suspected in evaluating a patient with syncope when there is a consistent sinus bradycardia (<50 bpm, excluding sleep or very physically fit individuals) or sinus pause >3 s. or a prolonged asystole after spontaneous termination or cardioversion of atrial fibrillation (Fig. 20.2).[3–6] Conversely, intermittent rapid rhythms (usually atrial fibrillation) may be the problem in SND patients. In either case, however, while these findings may be suspicious, they can only be considered as inferential for the cause of syncope in the absence of occurrence of symptoms at the time of the documented arrhythmia. Usually, symptom–rhythm correlation requires long-term AECG recordings. A MCOT (mobile cardiac outpatient telemetry) or ILR (insertable loop recorder) are the most effective means of obtaining such correlation.[7]

Apart from AECG recordings, assessment of sinus node function should include assessment of sinus node automaticity at baseline (including intrinsic heart rate measured by pharmacologic blockade using combined atropine and beta-blocker pre-treatment) and during symptom-limited exercise (to assess chronotropic competence).[3] Thereafter, in the absence of a convincing diagnosis, EPS evaluation of sinus node function may help to clarify if suspected SND is present. However, all tests designed to search for SND are only indirect measures of sinus node function with relatively poor positive predictive value.

Although there have been many techniques proposed to assess sinus node function, only sinus node recovery time (SNRT) and sinoatrial conduction time (SACT) are commonly used. The sensitivity and specificity of combined SNRT and SACT testing to detect SND are in the range of 70% and 90%, respectively. However, identifying the presence of SND does not necessarily provide conclusive evidence that SND was responsible for syncope (i.e., poor positive predictive value). Further, even if SND is responsible, since SND-related symptoms may be due to brady- or tachyarrhythmias, or both, the precise arrhythmic mechanism for syncope usually cannot be addressed convincingly by EPS. On the other hand, in difficult to diagnose situations, evidence of the presence of SND may help focus subsequent evaluation.

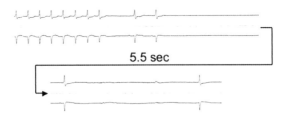

Fig. 20.2 ECG recording obtained during spontaneous termination of atrial tachyarrhythmia. The overall duration of the asystolic pause was approximately 8 s. Approximately 5.5 s of asystole was deleted between the two otherwise sequential traces

The most widely used EPS test of sinus node function takes advantage of a physiologic characteristic of native pacemakers, namely "overdrive suppression." This property, by which cardiac pacemaker cells can be suppressed by pacing at rapid rates, has been used since the early 1970s as a technique to assess the health of sinus node pacemaker function. Specifically, the time taken for sinus node activity to return following termination of a period of rapid atrial stimulation (i.e., the sinus node recovery time or SNRT) is used to identify underlying sinus node dysfunction. SNRT is usually measured after 30–60 s of pacing at various pacing cycle lengths starting with a pacing cycle length about 20 ms shorter than the baseline sinus rate. The longest recovery time ($SNRT_{max}$) is documented along with pacing cycle length at which it occurred (Fig. 20.3).

The SNRT measurement is dependent on multiple factors such as autonomic tone, sinoatrial conduction properties, the patient's sinus cycle length at time of study, and the magnitude of sinus arrhythmia present. To account for some of these variables, SNRT is usually corrected for baseline sinus cycle length (i.e., corrected SNRT or CSNRT). Most commonly, this correction is obtained by subtracting the baseline (pre-pacing) sinus cycle length from the SNRT:

$$CSNRT = SNRT - \text{sinus cycle length}.$$

In normal subjects, SNRT increases as pacing rate increases up to a maximum value after which it declines due to presumed entrance block of very rapid paced impulses into the node. Usually SNRT reaches a maximum value ($SNRT_{max}$) at pacing cycle lengths in the range of 500–400 ms (i.e., 120–150 beats/min). $SNRT_{max}$ >1,500–1,720 ms or corrected $SNRT_{max}$ ($CSNRT_{max}$) >525 is considered abnormal, with sensitivity of 50–80% and specificity of >95%, respectively, for detecting SND. Further, an $SNRT_{max}$ occurring at cycle lengths ≥600 ms

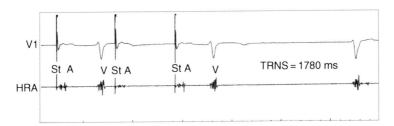

Fig. 20.3 Abnormal sinus node recovery time (SNRT). At the cessation of rapid right atrial pacing (St) at a rate of 100 bpm, a pause of 1,780 ms occurs which is followed by an escape junctional beat which obscures recovery of normal sinus rhythm. Therefore, the SNRT is ≥1,780 ms. Such a pause indicates an impairment of the automatic properties of a diseased sinus node and consequent inability to resume a stable rhythm promptly; the mechanism is the pause after the spontaneous termination of atrial tachyarrhythmia shown in Fig. 20.2. Note that there is also an abnormality of AV conduction as evidenced by the induction of a second-degree Wenckebach AV block during atrial pacing. Thus, findings in this record indicate bi-nodal disease. St, stimulus; HRA, high right atriogram; A, atrial wave; V, ventricular wave

Table 20.4 Diagnostic value of electrophysiologic study (EPS) findings[1]

Class I

- EPS is diagnostic, and usually no additional tests are required, in the following cases
- Sinus bradycardia and a very prolonged CSNRT
- Bifascicular block and

  o A baseline HV interval of ≥ 100 ms or
  o Second- or third-degree His–Purkinje block is during incremental atrial pacing or
  o High-degree His–Purkinje block is provoked by intravenous administration of ajmaline or procainamide

- Induction of sustained monomorphic ventricular tachycardia
- Induction of supraventricular arrhythmia which reproduces spontaneous symptoms (this rare unless the patient is upright) or that causes hypotension of sufficient severity in the supine patient to be consistent with a basis for syncope

Class II

- EPS diagnostic value is less well established if

  o HV interval of >70 ms but <100 ms
  o Induction of polymorphic ventricular tachycardia or ventricular fibrillation in patients with Brugada syndrome, arrhythmogenic right ventricular dysplasia, and patients resuscitated from cardiac arrest

Class III

- EPS is non-diagnostic if polymorphic ventricular tachycardia or ventricular fibrillation is induced in patients with ischemic or dilated cardiomyopathy

Note: Normal EPS findings cannot exclude an arrhythmic cause of syncope; if the presentation suggests that an arrhythmia is likely, further evaluations (for example, loop recording) are recommended.

(≤ 100 bpm) suggests compromise of the conduction into the sinus node and provides indirect additional evidence of SND (Table 20.4).

Sinoatrial conduction time (SACT) is estimated by calculating the time it takes for an impulse to enter and leave the sinus node. This is most commonly estimated by inserting single premature atrial extrastimuli during sinus rhythm as part of the EPS procedure. If inserted early enough in the cardiac cycle (usually between 50% and 75% of the cycle) the premature beat will enter the sinus node and reset it. When the next sinus beat emerges, the pause between the premature beat and the emerging sinus beat will be (approximately) the sinus cycle length plus the sum of the conduction time into and out of the sinus node. If multiple such measures are consistent, one can calculate an estimate of SACT. There are other methods to make the same measure, but a complete discussion lies outside the realm of this chapter (see Benditt et al.[3]).

Assessment of sinus node function is more reliable and reproducible after pharmacologic autonomic blockade as it permits clearer assessment of intrinsic sinus node activity.[8–12] In this regard, autonomic blockade is usually achieved by combined administration of intravenous propranolol (0.2 mg/kg) and atropine (0.04 mg/kg). However, lower doses should be used in the elderly patient to diminish risk of adverse drug effects (particularly that of atropine). Intrinsic heart rate (i.e., heart rate after complete autonomic blockade) has an approximately linear relationship to age, which equals 118.1 (0.57 × age). Testing of sinus node function is often positive in patients with abnormal intrinsic heart rate after pharmacologic autonomic blockade when it might otherwise have been non-diagnostic.

Other less frequently utilized measures of sinus node function include

- unexpected prolongation of subsequent post-pacing cycles ("secondary pauses"),
- assessment of the paced cycle length at which entrance block first occurs,
- direct recording of sinus node electrograms, and thereby obtaining direct estimate of SACT (feasible but infrequently used as the recordings are difficult to obtain),
- sinus node effective refractory period (SNERP),
- measurement of the duration of the sinus node electrogram.

As noted earlier, whereas EPS findings may suggest that SND is present, they cannot as yet cannot delineate the precise basis of syncope in these patients. In one study, however, a prolonged CSNRT was associated with patients benefiting from cardiac pacing.[12] The predictive value of SNRT as a marker of syncope and potential benefit of pacing increases with longer SNRT. Patients with a CSNRT of >800 ms have an eight times higher risk of syncope than patients with a CSNRT below this value.[13] The following diagnostic criteria are widely used for defining sinus node dysfunction: 1.6 or 2 s for SNRT or 525 ms for CSNRT. Marked $SNRT_{max}$ prolongation (longer than 3 s) has been suggested to substantially increase the possibility that SND may be responsible for syncope. It is the opinion of the ESC Syncope Task Force panel that, in the presence of an SNRT > 2.0 s or CSNRT > 1.0 s, SND may be reasonably surmised to be the cause of syncope if no other diagnostic candidates remain.[1]

20.3.3 EPS and Conduction System Disease

Intermittent AV block is an important cause of syncope in patients with underlying disease of the cardiac conduction system. However, confirming the relation between symptoms and AV block may be difficult. Long-term ambulatory ECG recording with an ILR or MCOT system may be the most desirable method of establishing a diagnosis. The ISSUE study,[14–16] in which ILRs were used in an attempt to obtain ECG-symptom correlation, revealed that intermittent AV block was a frequent cause of syncope in patients with intra-ventricular conduction system disease. However, if documentation of a spontaneous event is either not possible or is impracticable, then EPS may be a reasonable alternative.

In patients with syncope and suspected conduction system disease, EPS is used mainly to evaluate intra- and infra-His conduction. A prolonged HV interval is associated with a higher risk of developing AV block. The progression rate to AV block is 2–4% in patients with a normal (<55 ms) or slightly prolonged (55–60 ms) HV interval and increases to 21% and 24%, when HV interval ≥70 and ≥100 ms, respectively. Incremental atrial pacing and pharmacological provocation with sodium-channel blocking drugs are often used to increase the diagnostic yield of EPS when HV interval is only marginally prolonged.

Development of intra- or infra-His block during incremental atrial pacing (i.e., pacing the atria at progressively more rapid rates to stress the adequacy of the

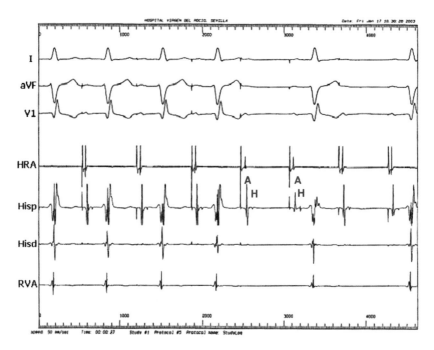

Fig. 20.4 Infra-Hisian AV block induced by atrial pacing. The fifth and the seventh paced atrial beats are blocked. A and H waves are not followed by V wave; thus meaning that the site of block is distal to His deflection and is located in the His–Purkinje system

AV conduction system) is rare (perhaps about 5% of cases) but highly predictive of impending AV block[15–21] (Fig. 20.4). For example, in the study by Gronda et al.,[20] HV prolongation of >10 ms was observed in 6% and second-degree AV block in 5% of cases. Complete AV block developed in 40% of these patients during a mean follow-up of 42 months. In the study by Dini et al,[21] pacing-induced AV block occurred in 7% with progression to complete AV block in 30% within 2 years.

In patients with moderate prolongation of HV interval, acute pharmacological stress testing of the His–Purkinje system may be used to assess His–Purkinje system "reserve." Such stress testing of the His–Purkinje system has been performed with several class IA antiarrhythmic substances: ajmaline, procainamide, and disopyramide.[1,20–23] A substantial increase of HV interval duration (i.e., HV >100 ms or the precipitation of second- or third-degree infra-His block) following pharmacological challenge with or without incremental atrial pacing was predictive of subsequent spontaneous AV block (Fig. 20.5). On average from multiple reports, pharmacological stress was able to elicit susceptibility to high-degree AV block in 15% of patients studied. Spontaneous AV block developed in approximately 68% of these patients during follow-up for a period of 2–5 years.

Apart from susceptibility to intermittent AV block, patients with bundle branch block also exhibit increased mortality risk, especially in the presence of structural heart disease. Age, congestive heart failure, and coronary artery disease are

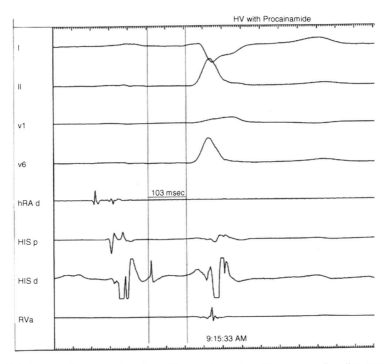

Fig. 20.5 Intra-cardiac recordings in a 68-year-old male with syncope. Baseline recording revealed an HV interval of 85 ms. However, further prolongation to >100 ms after procainamide infusion as illustrated in the His bundle electrogram (HIS d) tended to support a diagnosis of conduction system disease as a basis for syncope

associated with higher risk of death. It appears that neither syncope nor a prolonged HV interval is substantially associated with high risk of death; it is the underlying disease process. Thus, pacemaker therapy reduces syncope recurrence but does not decrease the mortality risk. The mechanism of sudden cardiac death is believed to be due to ventricular tachyarrhythmia or electromechanical dissociation rather than a bradycardia. A sustained ventricular tachyarrhythmia is frequently induced in patients with bundle branch block (32%).

In summary, in patients with syncope and bifascicular block, EPS is highly sensitive in identifying patients with intermittent or impending high-degree AV block (Table 20.4).[1] This block is likely the cause of syncope in most cases, but does not account for the increased mortality. The latter seems to be mainly related to underlying structural heart disease and ventricular tachyarrhythmias. Unfortunately, EPS does not seem to be able to correctly identify the high-risk patients.

20.3.4 Supraventricular Tachycardias

Reentrant paroxysmal supraventricular tachycardias (PSVT) are not a frequent cause of syncope, but should be considered as a possibility in syncope patients

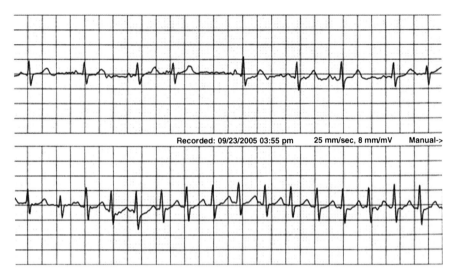

Recorded: 09/23/2005 03:55 pm   25 mm/sec, 8 mm/mV   Manual->

Fig. 20.6 Abrupt onset of PSVT associated with "light-headedness" detected by AECG monitoring in a patient with recurrent syncope

with palpitations (Fig. 20.6), especially if there is no evidence of structural heart disease.[24] In such cases, syncope can occur at the onset of an attack (Fig. 20.6) or just after its termination when a pause may ensue before normal sinus function is restored. Pharmacologic challenge (usually intravenous isoproterenol and/or atropine) may be very effective in helping to elicit susceptibility to PSVT and for evaluating the hemodynamic effects of tachycardia.

The EPS procedure requires transvenous placement of multiple electrode catheters to specific intra-cardiac sites usually including the coronary sinus. Burst pacing and extrastimulus pacing are used to initiate the arrhythmia. Thereafter various techniques are used to prove that the mechanism is reentry, and in most cases to define the optimal site for ablation of the reentry circuit.

Recognition of PSVT as a cause of syncope is important, as most of these arrhythmia are curable by radiofrequency ablation. In terms of assessing hemodynamic impact of a tachycardia (i.e., to provide evidence that it may have caused cerebral hypoperfusion), it is important to position the patient in an upright posture (e.g., using a tilt table). This latter aspect of the procedure is not often done, but may be of value if the cause of syncope remains in doubt.

In addition to PSVT, other supraventricular tachyarrhythmias can be responsible for triggering syncope. In the case of atrial fibrillation, syncope may be due to insufficient ventricular filling, inadequate reflex vascular compensation at the onset of an episode, or delayed return of normal rhythm at the termination of an episode. In certain cases, and particularly in patients with preexcitation syndrome, syncope may occur due to atrial fibrillation resulting in excessively rapid ventricular rates.

In selected atrial fibrillation patients, EPS may be useful to determine whether the arrhythmia is occurring as a consequence of another treatable rhythm (e.g., PSVT degenerating to atrial fibrillation) or is the primary problem itself. This is particularly the case in younger individuals with the so-called lone atrial fibrillation (i.e., without apparent cause for the arrhythmia). Furthermore, atrial fibrillation can be treated by transcatheter ablation in some patients, while in others (almost exclusively older individuals) ablation of the His bundle and placement of a cardiac pacemaker can be very effective in preventing excessively rapid heart rates during atrial fibrillation from inducing hypotension and syncope. Finally, EPS may help to identify the very infrequent patient in whom an atrial antitachycardia pacemaker can be helpful.

20.3.5 Ventricular Tachycardias (VT)

Ventricular tachyarrhythmias (VT) tend to be more closely associated with syncope than are SVTs probably due to the fact that most VTs occur in the setting of more severe heart disease. However, polymorphous VT causing syncope also occurs in some individuals with structurally relatively normal hearts, particularly in the setting of so-called channelopathies (e.g., long QT syndrome, Brugada syndrome, short-QT syndrome, and idiopathic ventricular fibrillation, and possibly including those with recently described infero-lateral ST segment "early repolarization") (Fig. 20.7).[25–27]

Ventricular tachycardia may present as syncope with or without palpitations or other accompanying symptoms such as chest pain and dyspnea. Table 20.5 summarizes important clinical factors that, if present, should increase suspicion that VT is a possible cause of syncope. Indications for undertaking EPS in syncope patients are summarized in Tables 20.1 and 20.6.

A major limitation of EPS for assessing the possible contribution of ventricular arrhythmia in the evaluation of syncope patients is the uncertain sensitivity and specificity in various clinical settings. Inasmuch as published reports have often used a variety of different cardiac stimulation protocols, it is difficult to derive solid conclusions. Generally speaking, EPS is thought to be a sensitive tool in patients with chronic ischemic heart disease (particularly a prior myocardial infarction) and spontaneous monomorphic VT, but has a lower predictive value in patients with non-ischemic dilated cardiomyopathy. In any event, with regard to the syncope evaluation, EPS can reasonably be considered to be diagnostic if monomorphic VT is initiated (Fig. 20.8); induction of polymorphous VT is not of solid diagnostic value (Fig. 20.9). Lacroix et al.[28] showed that, while EPS reproduced the spontaneous

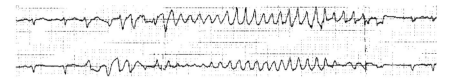

Fig. 20.7 Brief episode of torsades-de pointes polymorphous VT associated with syncope, detected by AECG

Table 20.5 Clinical findings, the presence of which, increase the likelihood that VT caused syncope

1. Prior history of sustained monomorphic VT
2. Medical history positive for coronary artery disease (particularly previous myocardial infarction) or cardiomyopathy (including HCM or ARVD/C)
3. Diminished left ventricular ejection fraction of any cause
4. Evidence of left ventricular hypertrophy
5. Previous cardiac surgery for congenital anomalies, revascularization, valve replacement/repair, or tumor removal
6. ECG evidence of long QT syndrome, short QT syndrome, or Brugada syndrome
7. Positive signal-averaged electrocardiogram (SAECG) or T-wave alternans study
8. Advanced age

Table 20.6 Syncope due to cardiac arrhythmias: indications for EPS[1]

- Class I
  - o Abnormal ECG suggesting conduction system cause
  - o Syncope during exertion or in supine position or with important structural heart disease
  - o Syncope with palpitations or angina-like chest pain
  - o Family history of sudden death
- Class II
  - o Define/ablate an arrhythmia that has already been identified
  - o In patients with high-risk occupations
- Class III
  Absence of risk factors above, unless suspected paroxysmal supraventricular tachycardia

arrhythmia in 13 of 17 cases, a non-specific atrial or ventricular arrhythmia was also induced in 31 of 44 cases.

ICDs offer a valuable tool for the follow-up and better understanding of the role of EPS in assessing high-risk populations. In this setting, a number of studies[29-35] have evaluated the utility of ICD in high selected patients with syncope (Table 20.7). Findings suggest that among those syncope patients in whom VT was inducible and ICDs were implanted, appropriate shock frequency was high in the first 1–2 years of follow-up (20–50% of patients). Together, these findings provide indirect evidence that EPS may be helpful in predicting the basis of syncope in the setting of suspected ventricular tachyarrhythmias. However, syncope may still recur in some patients due to the time delay in detection of tachycardia and a long battery charge time. In this regard, an examination of data gleaned from the Sudden Cardiac Death in Heart Failure Trial (SCD-HeFT) demonstrated that[36]

- rates of syncope did not differ between the three treatment arms (ICD versus amiodarone versus placebo),
- patients with syncope (either before or after randomization) were more likely to have appropriate ICD shocks, and
- syncope after randomization was associated with an increased risk of death, independent of treatment arm.

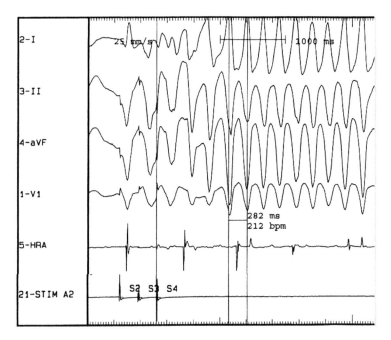

Fig. 20.8 Induction of ventricular tachycardia by means of premature ventricular stimulation in a patient with previous myocardial infarction. A short coupling sequence of three premature ventricular beats (S2, S3 and S4) induces ventricular tachycardia. Atrial rhythm is dissociated (HRA lead)

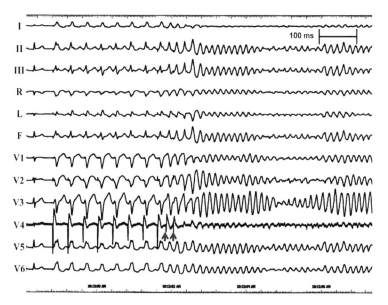

Fig. 20.9 Induction of ventricular fibrillation by means of premature ventricular stimulation. After an overdrive ventricular pacing sequence of eight beats, a short coupling sequence of two premature ventricular beats induces ventricular fibrillation

Table 20.7 ICD therapy in syncope patients with syncope and suspected ventricular tachyarrhythmias

Study	Population	ICD therapies in follow-up
Link et al.[30]	50 ICM	22% at 1 year, 50% at 3 years
Militianu et al.[31]	33 (ICM, NICM)	36% at 17 months
Mittal et al.[32]	67 ICM	41% of EPS inducible at 1 year
Andrews et al.[33]	54 ICM	
	– 22 inducible VT	57% at 1 year
	– 32 syncopal VT	50% at 1 year
Pires et al.[34]	178 ICM inducible VT	55% at 2 years
Knight et al.[29]	NICM	
	– 14 sync inducible VT	50% at 2 years
	– 19 VF arrest	42% at 2 years

In brief, EPS is an effective adjunctive diagnostic tool in patients with coronary artery disease, markedly depressed cardiac function, and unexplained syncope. Its utility is more questionable in patients with non-ischemic dilated cardiomyopathy. Patients who undergo implantation of an automatic defibrillator have a high incidence of spontaneous ventricular arrhythmia requiring device therapy and suppression of syncope recurrences. However, these results applied to a highly selected, high-risk referral population that might be not representative of typical patients encountered in the clinical practice.

20.4 Ablation of Arrhythmias

The potential to identify and cure certain arrhythmias is a major benefit of invasive EPS in syncope patients. In this regard, transcatheter ablation using radiofrequency energy (or other energy delivery systems, such as cryothermia) is now an integral part of most EPS laboratory capabilities. Transcatheter ablation can be used to cure a number of arrhythmias that may be responsible for syncope, including

- preexcitation syndromes (e.g., Wolff–Parkinson–White syndrome – WPW syndrome and its variants),
- PSVT due to AV nodal reentry or accessory connections,
- ectopic atrial tachycardias,
- atrial flutter,
- idiopathic VT arising from the right or left ventricles (including idiopathic fascicular VT and bundle-branch reentry VT),
- paroxysmal and persistent atrial fibrillation (a developing technique not nearly so advanced as the others).

20.5 Clinical Perspective

EPS is indicated when initial evaluation points to an arrhythmic cause of syncope particularly in patients with an abnormal ECG and/or structural heart disease or syncope associated with palpitations. Such testing may also be appropriate in the absence of structural heart disease or an abnormal ECG when PSVT is suspected or when non-invasive diagnostic evaluation has been unproductive. Finally, EPS may also be recommended:

- For diagnostic reasons to evaluate the exact nature of an arrhythmia which has been already identified as the cause of the syncope especially when ablation is a consideration.
- For prognostic reasons in patients with cardiac disorders, in which arrhythmia induction has a bearing on the selection of therapy, and in patients with high-risk occupations (e.g., pilots) in whom every effort to exclude a cardiac cause of syncope is warranted.

Although EPS accurately delineates abnormalities in patients with fixed cardiac conduction defects, its sensitivity for identifying transient rhythm disturbances is relatively low (PSVT is an important exception). Consequently, normal EPS findings cannot completely exclude an arrhythmic cause of syncope. When an arrhythmia seems likely, continued attempts to obtain symptom–rhythm correlation are essential. An ILR will likely be required. Conversely, depending on the clinical context, abnormal EPS findings may not be diagnostic of the cause of syncope; false positives are a concern. In all cases, the physician must carefully consider whether the EPS findings are consistent with the clinical history.

References

1. Moya A, et al. Guidelines for the diagnosis and management of syncope (version 2009). *Eur Heart J.* 2009;30:2631–2671.
2. Brignole M, et al. Standardized care pathway vs usual management of syncope patients presenting as emergencies at general hospitals. *Europace.* 2006;8:644–650.
3. Benditt DG, et al. Indications for electrophysiologic testing in the diagnosis and assessment of sinus node dysfunction. *Circulation.* 1987;75(III):93–102.
4. De Sisti A, et al. Electrophysiologic characteristics of the atrium in sinus node dysfunction: atrial refractoriness and conduction. *J Cardiovasc Electrophysiol.* 2000;11:30–33.
5. Yee R, Strauss HC. Electrophysiologic mechanisms: sinus node dysfunction. *Circulation.* 1987;75(III):12–18.
6. Bergfeldt L, et al. Sinus node recovery time assessment revisited: role of pharmacological blockade of the autonomic nervous system. *J Cardiovasc Electrophysiol.* 1996;7:95–101.
7. Rothman SA, et al. The diagnosis of cardiac arrhythmias: a prospective multi-center randomized study comparing mobile cardiac outpatient telemetry versus standard loop event monitoring. *J Cardiovasc Electrophysiol.* 2007;18:241–247.
8. Narula OS, et al. Significance of the sinus-node recovery time. *Circulation.* 1972;45:140–148.
9. de Marneffe M, et al. Variations of normal sinus node function in relation to age: role of autonomic influence. *Eur Heart J.* 1986;7:662–666.
10. de Marneffe M, et al. The sinus node function: normal and pathological. *Eur Heart J.* 1993;14:649–654.
11. Brignole M. Sick sinus syndrome. *Clin Geriatr Med.* 2002;18:211–227.
12. Gann D, et al. Electrophysiologic evaluation of elderly patients with sinus bradycardia: a long-term follow-up study. *Ann Intern Med.* 1979;90:24–29.

13. Menozzi C, et al. The natural course of untreated sick sinus syndrome and identification of the variables predictive of unfavourable outcome. *Am J Cardiol.* 1998;82:1205–1209.

14. Brignole M, et al. Mechanism of syncope in patients with bundle branch block and negative electrophysiologic test. *Circulation.* 2001;104:2045–2050.

15. Menozzi C, et al. Mechanism of syncope in patients with heart disease and negative electrophysiologic test. *Circulation.* 2002;105:2741–2745.

16. Moya A, et al. Mechanism of syncope in patients with isolated syncope and in patients with tilt-positive syncope. *Circulation.* 2001;104:1261–1267.

17. Dhingra RC, et al. Significance of block distal to the His bundle induced by atrial pacing in patients with chronic bifascicular block. *Circulation.* 1979;60:1455–1464.

18. Petrac D, et al. Prospective evaluation of infrahisal second-degree AV block induced by atrial pacing in the presence of chronic bundle branch block and syncope. *Pacing Clin Electrophysiol.* 1996;19:679–687.

19. Click R, et al. Role of invasive electrophysiologic testing in patients with symptomatic bundle branch block. *Am J Cardiol.* 1987;59:817–823.

20. Gronda M, et al. Electrophysiologic study of atrio-ventricular block and ventricular conduction defects. *G Ital Cardiol.* 1984;14:768–773.

21. Dini P, et al. Prognostic value of His-ventricular conduction after ajmaline administration. In: Masoni A, Alboni P, eds. *Cardiac Electrophysiology Today.* London: Academic Press; 1982:pp 515–522.

22. Englund A, et al. Pharmacological stress testing of the His-Purkinje system in patients with bifascicular block. *Pacing Cardiac Electrophysiol.* 1998;21:1979–1987.

23. Fei L, Trohman RG. Advances in cardiac electrophysiology and pacing. *Crit Care Clin.* 2001;17:337–364.

24. Camm AJ, Lau C-P. Syncope of undetermined origin: diagnosis and management. *Prog Cardiol.* 1988;1:139–156.

25. Moss AJ, et al. ECG T-wave patterns in genetically distinct forms of the hereditary long QT syndrome. *Circulation.* 1995;92:2929–2934.

26. Zipes DP, et al. ACC/AHA/ESC 2006 guidelines for management of patients with ventricular arrhythmias and the prevention of sudden cardiac death. *Circulation.* 2006;114: e385–e484.

27. Priori S. Long QT and Brugada syndromes. From genetics to clinical management. *J Cardiovasc Electrophysiol.* 2000;11:1174–1180.

28. Lacroix D, et al. Evaluation of arrhythmic causes of syncope: correlation between Holter monitoring, electrophysiologic testing, and body surface potential mapping. *Am Heart J.* 1991;122:1346–1354.

29. Knight B, et al. Outcome of patients with nonischemic dilated cardiomyopathy and unexplained syncope treated with an implantable defibrillator. *J Am Coll Cardiol.* 1999;33: 1964–1970.

30. Link MS, et al. High incidence of appropriate implantable cardioverter-defibrillator therapy in patients with syncope of unknown etiology and inducible ventricular tachycardia. *J Am Coll Cardiol.* 1997;29:370–375.

31. Militianu A, et al. Implantable cardioverter defibrillator utilization among device recipients presenting exclusively with syncope or near-syncope. *J Cardiovasc Electrophysiol.* 1997;8:1087–1097.

32. Mittal S, et al. Long-term outcome of patients with unexplained syncope treated with an electrophysiologic-guided approach in the implantable cardioverter-defibrillator era. *J Am Coll Cardiol.* 1999;34:1082–1089.

33. Andrews N, et al. Implantable defibrillator event rates in patients with unexplained syncope and inducible sustained ventricular tachyarrhythmias. *J Am Coll Cardiol.* 1999;34: 2023–2030.

34. Pires L, et al. Comparison of event rates and survival in patients with unexplained syncope without documented ventricular tachyarrhythmias versus patients with documented sustained

ventricular tachyarrhythmias both treated with implantable cardioverter-defibrillator. *Am J Cardiol.* 2000;85:725–728.

35. Fonarow G, et al. Improved survival in patients with nonischemic advanced heart failure and syncope treated with an implantable cardioverter-defibrillator. *Am J Cardiol.* 2000;85: 981–985.

36. Olshansky B, et al. Syncope predicts the outcome of cardiomyopathy patients: Analysis of the SCD-HeFT study. *J Am Coll Cardiol.* 2008;51:1277–1282.

Chapter 21
How to: Physical Maneuvers for Reflex and Orthostatic Syncope

Contents

Non-pharmacological "physical" treatments (physical maneuvers) are emerging as a new front-line treatment of orthostatic intolerance syndromes (reflex syncope and orthostatic hypotension), instead of or in addition to other therapies.

21.1 Counterpressure Maneuvers

Counterpressure maneuvers are the only therapy ranked as class I (level of evidence B) indication for reflex syncope; consequently in many cases (when warning symptoms are present) they are the therapy of first choice. These same maneuvers are class IIB (level of evidence C) in patients with orthostatic hypotension. The most used maneuvers are arm tensing, handgrip, and leg crossing[1,2] (Fig. 21.1). Whichever of these maneuvers is employed, they are able to increase blood pressure rapidly thus aborting syncope for a sufficient period of time to permit the affected individual to achieve a safe position (e.g., if driving then pull the car to the side of the road or if standing then sit down or lie down) (Fig. 21.2).

M. Brignole, D.G. Benditt, *Syncope*, DOI 10.1007/978-0-85729-201-8_21,
© Springer-Verlag London Limited 2011

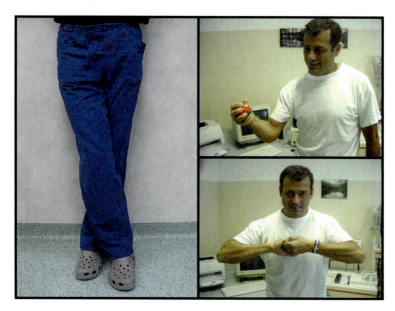

Fig. 21.1 Most common counterpressure maneuvers. Patients with known susceptibility to reflex or orthostatic faints should be instructed to use them as preventive measures when they experience any symptoms of impending fainting. *Handgrip* consists of the maximal voluntary contraction of a rubber ball (approximately of 5–6 cm diameter) taken in the dominant hand for the maximum tolerated time or until to complete disappearance of symptoms. *Arm tensing* consists of the maximum tolerated isometric contraction of the two arms achieved by gripping one hand with the other and contemporarily abducting (pushing away) the arms for the maximum tolerated time or until to complete disappearance of symptoms. *Leg crossing* consists of leg crossing combined with tensing of leg, abdominal, and buttock muscles for the maximum tolerated time or until to complete disappearance of symptoms

21.1.1 Instruction for Use (for Physicians)

Physical maneuvers for interrupting reflex or orthostatic faints[1,2] (Fig. 21.1):

- *Handgrip.* Consists of the maximal voluntary contraction of a rubber ball (approximately of 5–6 cm diameter) or comparable soft object taken in the dominant hand for the maximum tolerated time or until complete disappearance of symptoms.
- *Arm tensing.* Consists of the maximum tolerated isometric contraction of the two arms achieved by gripping one hand with the other and at the same time abducting (pulling away) the arms for the maximum tolerated time or until complete disappearance of symptoms.
- *Leg crossing.* Consists of leg crossing combined with maximum tensing of leg, abdominal, and buttock muscles for the maximum tolerated time or until complete disappearance of symptoms. This procedure is sometimes described in the literature as leg crossing with muscle tensing. Leg crossing alone has also been shown to be useful but is less powerful in terms of preventing hypotension.

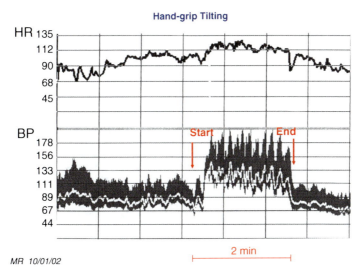

Fig. 21.2 *Handgrip*: The start of the maneuver causes a rapid rise in blood pressure, which persists as long as the contraction was maintained; initially, heart rate slightly increases and then slightly decreases

21.1.2 Counseling Information for Patients (for Reflex or Orthostatic Faints)

21.1.2.1 Purpose

Patients should be trained in the various physical maneuvers. They should be advised to use leg crossing, handgrip, and/or arm tensing in case they experience symptoms of impending syncope. Patients will be instructed to maintain the maneuver they choose as long as possible and eventually move on to a second/third maneuver if useful (while at the same time seeking a safe posture, e.g., sitting down). Patients are allowed to choose the maneuver and the sequence of their administration, but they should take note of them in a logbook so that the effectiveness can be later reviewed by their physician.

21.1.2.2 Typical Biofeedback Training Session Protocol

Duration maximum 1 h:

- Explanation of purpose and session program
- Simple explanation of physiology and vasovagal reflexes
- Demonstration and explanation of the three maneuvers
- *Instrumentation*. Non-invasive beat-to-beat blood pressure and ECG monitoring attached to not-dominant hand
- Practising of all three maneuvers using blood pressure recordings as biofeedback signal (Fig. 21.3)
- Offer the patient instruction sheet with photographs

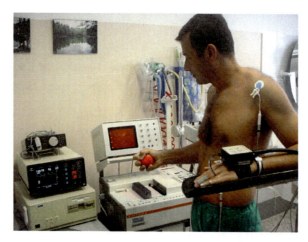

Fig. 21.3 Biofeedback training. The patient is trained in the maneuver while watching his continuous blood pressure and ECG monitors. Biofeedback training allows him to perceive immediately the effect on his blood pressure and heart rate of the maneuver that he is performing and what is the most muscle strength that he has to exert

21.2 Instruction Sheet for the Patient

21.2.1 What Happens During Syncope Triggered by Upright Posture Including the "Common Faint"?

With standing up from a supine position blood pressure drops as the volume of blood usually delivered to the chest and heart is diverted under the influence of gravity to the abdomen and legs. As a result, the heart cannot fill with as much blood as is necessary and the amount of blood the heart can pump diminishes. Without countermeasures blood pressure will drop. Usually the body reacts with narrowing of the blood vessels in the abdomen and legs and by making the heartbeat faster. Under normal conditions more blood will stay in the upper part of the body and blood pressure will rise again. These measures are taken by the autonomic (involuntary) part of the nervous system. Some people display insufficient countermeasures in specific situations and as a consequence the fainting reaction occurs. Blood vessels dilate (i.e., become wider) instead of constricting (narrower), and somewhat later the heart rate slows down (or at least fails to speed up adequately). As a result of this faulty response the heart cannot pump enough blood to the brain and the retina of the eye; the result is dimming or "blackout" of the vision, and if severe enough loss of consciousness. By sitting or lying down, gravity can be used to help fill the heart again with blood and consciousness will be restored. Why this reaction happens more often to some people than to other is unknown.

21.2.2 When Does a Fainting Response Occur?

Most people know under which circumstances they might expect to experience a reflex faint (e.g., common or vasovagal faint) or an orthostatic (upright posture induced) faint. Specifically, susceptible individuals often display symptoms in the following situations:

- During emotional circumstances (seeing blood or being in pain, during religious services)
- After a long period of standing (such as standing in a line or at a reception)
- In a warm surrounding (in a sauna, warm weather, under a hot shower)
- Directly after exercise
- Soon after dinner
- For women, during the menstrual period
- When you have not had enough rest
- During illness
- After getting out of a warm bed or bath
- After standing-up quickly (may occur immediately or a few moments later)

21.2.3 Symptoms

The prodromal symptoms most often reported by people with neural reflex or orthostatic fainting reactions are light-headedness, seeing spots, nausea, and/or a sense of abdominal discomfort, and then loss of consciousness. Before, during, and after the episode the affected individual looks pale, may sweat profusely, and may be nauseous. After the patient has regained consciousness he/she often stays tired for a long period of time (especially with vasovagal faints). Not all reflex or orthostatic fainting reactions are accompanied by these typical responses.

21.2.4 Advice

Being susceptible to fainting reactions is not a serious disease, but can be very annoying, may lead to injury or accidents, and can have restrictive lifestyle consequences to the patient and their family. The treatment of patients with fainting reactions consists of advice that is designed to diminish susceptibility and may cause the fainting reactions to diminish or even stop. Such advice to the affected individual includes the following:

- It is important to understand as completely as possible what is going on with you. Ask your physician for a more detailed explanation if you do not fully understand what fainting is, or if you have other questions.
- Try to find out during which circumstances you are susceptible to fainting. Try to avoid these circumstances.

- If you recognize any symptoms of the fainting reaction, sit down or lie down if possible.
- Follow your physician's advice regarding increase of your salt and volume intake. This is an important step for most reflex and orthostatic fainters, but may be limited in some by concomitant presence of high blood pressure (hypertension).
- Avoid excessive use of alcohol.
- Make sure your body is in good shape, but do not exercise excessively as this may cause dehydration and increase the risk of fainting.

21.2.5 Tilt Training (Standing Training)

In highly motivated young patients with recurrent vasovagal symptoms triggered by orthostatic stress, the prescription of progressively prolonged periods of enforced upright posture (so-called tilt training or standing training) may reduce syncope recurrence over the long term. The goal is to improve the body's autonomic reaction to upright posture. However, this treatment is hampered by low compliance of patients in persisting with the training over a long period; some randomized controlled trials failed to confirm short-term effectiveness of tilt training in reducing the positive response rate of tilt testing.[3] For this reason tilt training is ranked class IIB indication for therapy of reflex syncope.

Patients are instructed to perform tilt training at home by standing with their back gently against a wall (with the ankles placed together about 20 cm from the wall). The training is undertaken from twice a day to three times per week for a planned duration starting as short as 5 min per session and increasing up to 30 min per session, depending on the subject's orthostatic tolerance (Fig. 21.4). Patients are instructed to maintain the standing position (without moving leg or thigh muscles) until pre-syncopal symptoms appear or otherwise to the planned termination of their session. Patients are asked to perform tilt-training sessions in a comfortable and safe environment in order to avoid the risk of trauma; if possible the supervision of a family member may be helpful to enhance safety. Sometimes it is useful to test the effect of tilt training by tilt-table testing at the end of the 1–2 months of at-home tilt-training program. Generally, tilt training must be maintained consistently into the future, albeit at a reduced number of sessions per week. Little is yet known about the optimal frequency or duration.

21.2.6 Compression Stockings and Abdominal Binders

Gravitational venous pooling in older patients can be treated with abdominal binders or compression stockings. Abdominal binders and/or support stockings to reduce venous pooling may be indicated are class IIB therapies in the ESC guidelines on syncope. Since support stockings are often difficult for patients (especially older patients) to apply, "biker's pants" may be a useful alternative.

Fig. 21.4 Tilt-training
(standing training) session

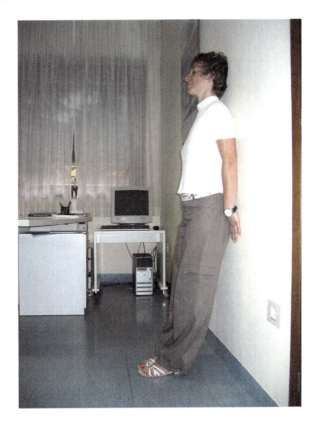

21.3 Symptom Questionnaire

The syndromes of orthostatic intolerance are characterized by frequent non-syncopal posture-related symptoms (dizziness, fatigue, weakness, palpitations, hearing disturbances, etc.); syncope occurs infrequently. These syndromes can be evaluated by the self-administered Specific Symptom Scale questionnaire for Orthostatic Intolerance (SSS-OI) shown in Table 21.1.[4]

The most common posturally related symptoms (Table 21.1) are included in a self-administered Specific Symptom Scale questionnaire for Orthostatic Intolerance (SSS-OI).[4] The questionnaire evaluates the following symptoms grouped in seven items: dizziness and presyncope; visual disturbances (including blurring, color changes, white-out, graying-out, enhanced brightness, darkening or blackening, and tunnel vision); syncope; hearing disturbances (including impaired hearing, crackles, and tinnitus); pain in the neck (occipital/paracervical and shoulder region), low back pain, or precordial pain; weakness, fatigue, lethargy; palpitations and hyperhidrosis. The patients are asked to assess the severity of each of the above symptoms on a visual scale from 0 to 10 (10 maximum entity of the symptom). The sum of scores

Table 21.1 Specific symptom score for orthostatic intolerance at 1-month visit

Symptom	Score of the symptom on a 1–10 scale
1. Dizziness and presyncope	
2. Visual disturbances	
3. Syncope	
4. Hearing disturbances	
5. Pain in the neck, low back pain, or precordial region	
6. Weakness, fatigue, and lethargy	
7. Palpitations and hyperhidrosis	
Total (0–70)	

of the seven items was the total symptom score (70 maximum score). The questionnaire is administered at baseline before therapy and can be repeated after a period (1 to several months) of treatment. In one study,[4] the mean baseline SSS-OI score in patients was 35.2 ± 12.1 with dizziness, weakness, and palpitations accounting for 64% of the total score; the SSS score decreased to 22.5 ± 11.3 after 1 month of therapy with elastic stockings ($p = 0.01$), which means a relative reduction of 34% (95% confidence interval 28–38). By comparison, the mean SSS-OI score in control subjects was 10.4 ± 5.6.

21.4 Acute Tilt-Table Study

The acute tilt-table study can be used in order to evaluate the ability of compression stockings or abdominal binders to prevent orthostatic hypotension and to reduce the symptoms of orthostatic intolerance before prescribing long-term treatment. The patient undergoes two tilt tests during the same day, at least 1 h apart. During active compression treatment, elastic bandage is applied over the legs (with a pressure of 40–60 mmHg at the ankles and 30–40 mmHg at the hip) for 10 min, and then abdominal binder is added for further 10 min (with a pressure of 20–30 mmHg). During sham treatment, the same elastic bandages are applied with a pressure of 5 mmHg overall (Figs. 21.5 and 21.6). A cuff manometer is used to calibrate the appropriate pressure of the bandage. The type of treatment is blind to the patient.

21.5 Follow-Up

If elastic compression is effective and well tolerated during the acute test, patients are trained to apply daily elastic leg compression stockings and/or abdominal binders (Fig. 21.7). Both elastic compression stockings and abdominal binders are available commercially. In the case of leg compression they have a nominal degree of compression of 40–60 mmHg at the level of the ankles and of 30–40 mmHg at the level of the hip. One should avoid compression stockings that only come

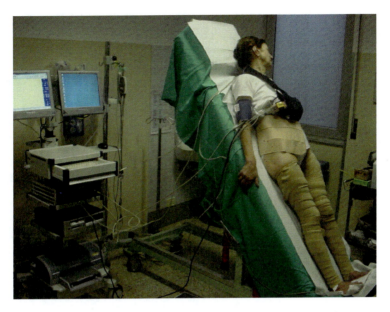

Fig. 21.5 Elastic compression stockings (bandage) during an acute tilt-table study

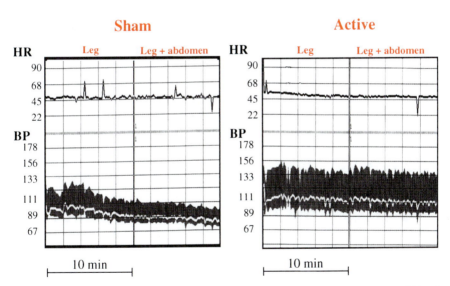

Fig. 21.6 Same patient case of Fig. 21.5. From *top to bottom* are shown heart rate and blood pressure (systolic, diastolic, and mean) traces. *Left panel: Sham treatment*. There is absence of appropriate adaptation of blood pressure to the *upright* position. Blood pressure declines slightly and progressively throughout the test. Systolic blood pressure declines below 80 mmHg. Heart rate remains stable at about 50 beats/min (chronotropic incompetence pattern). *Right panel: Active treatment*. Treatment increases blood pressure during the test. Heart rate remains stable at about 50 beats/min (chronotropic incompetence pattern). Abbreviations: HR, heart rate; BP, blood pressure

Fig. 21.7 Elastic stocking
therapy during the follow-up

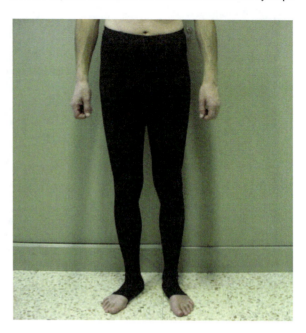

as high as the knee or thigh. These are inadequate and may compromise venous
return.

For many older frail patients it is difficult to put on conventional support stockings. Furthermore, younger patients often do not want to use them. In such cases,
"bikers shorts" may be an option. They provide support, are easier to get into, and
can be more comfortably worn under conventional clothing.

References

1. van Dijk N, et al. Effectiveness of physical counterpressure maneuvers in preventing vasovagal syncope: the Physical Counterpressure Manoeuvres Trial (PC-Trial). *J Am Coll Cardiol.*
   2006;48:1652–1657.
2. Brignole M, et al. Isometric arm counter-pressure maneuvers to abort impending vasovagal
   syncope. *J Am Coll Cardiol.* 2002;40:2054–2060.
3. Foglia-Manzillo G, et al. Efficacy of tilt training in the treatment of neurally mediated syncope.
   A randomized study. *Europace.* 2004;6:199–204.
4. Podoleanu C, et al. Lower limb and abdominal compression bandages prevent progressive
   orthostatic hypotension in the elderly. A randomized placebo-controlled study. *J Am Coll
   Cardiol.* 2006;48:1425–1432.

Index

M. Brignole, D.G. Benditt, *Syncope*, DOI 10.1007/978-0-85729-201-8,
© Springer-Verlag London Limited 2011